Medical Translator pocket

Patient interviews in 14 foreign languages

MW00488365

Editor: Andrea Rauneker
Production: Natascha Choffat, Anne Herhold
Cover Illustration: Janin Schroth
Publisher: Börm Bruckmeier Publishing LLC, www.media4u.com

IMPORTANT NOTICE - PLEASE READ!
This book is based on information from sources believed to be reliable, and every effort has
been made to make the book as complete and accurate as possible and to describe generally
accepted practices based on information available as of the printing date, but its accuracy
and completeness cannot be guaranteed. Despite the best efforts of author and publisher,
the book may contain errors, and the reader should use the book only as a general guide
and not as the ultimate source of information about the subject matter.
This book is not intended to reprint all of the information available to the author or
publisher on the subject, but rather to simplify, complement and supplement other available
sources. The reader is encouraged to read all available material and to consult the package
insert and other references to learn as much as possible about the subject.
This book is sold without warranties of any kind, expressed or implied, and the publisher and
author disclaim any liability, loss or damage caused by the content of this book.
IF YOU DO NOT WISH TO BE BOUND BY THE FOREGOING CAUTIONS AND CONDITIONS , YOU
MAY RETURN THIS BOOK TO THE PUBLISHER FOR A FULL REFUND.

Printed in China
ISBN 978-1-59103-235-9

Preface

Language barriers constantly interfere with doctor-patient communication. Every physician has a legal obligation to ensure that non-English-speaking patients understand all the essential information covered in a consultation. And competent interpreters are not always readily available.

Medical Translator pocket has the cure. It takes doctors and patients systematically through the medical history, examination, diagnosis, and treatment recommendations in 14 languages.

Whether it's an emergency situation, infection, headache, or chronic illness, a total of 581 useful questions, sentences, and phrases from everyday medical practise will provide for better understanding in various clinical communication situations. All of these expressions are grouped thematically into 25 chapters for quick navigation.

Phonetic guides help with the pronounciation of possibly unfamiliar sounds. Transliterations are also provided for all non-Latin scripts.

We hope that our Medical Translator pocket will make communication with non-English-speaking patients easier for all physicians, medical students, and auxiliary medical staff.

As always, we are happy to receive your suggestions at info@media4u.com.

The Editorial Team   Grünwald, April 2007

Additional titles in this series:

Börm Bruckmeier Publishing LLC on the Internet:
www.media4u.com

6 Inhalt

1 Reception

Hello, I am Dr. ...

ES Hola, soy el Dr. ...

ZH 嗨, 我是 ... 医生
wǒ shì ... yī shēng

FR Bonjour, Je suis le Dr. ...

DE Hallo, ich bin Dr. ...

VI Xin chào, tôi là bác sĩ. ...

IT Buongiorno, sono il Dr. ...

KO 안녕하세요, 저는 의사 ... 입니다
an-nyeong-ha-se-yo, jeo-neun ui-sa ... im-ni-da

RU Здравствуйте, я доктор ...
Zdravstvuyte, ya doctor ...

PL Dzień dobry, jestem dr. ...

AR مرحباً, انا الدكتور ...
Marhaban, ana ad-doktor ...

PT Como está? Sou o Dr. ...

FK Alo, mwen se Doktè ...

EL Γεια σας. Ειμαι ο / η γιατρός ...
geeA sas. EEme o / ee geeatrOs ...

HI नमस्ते, मैं डॉक्टर हूं ...
Namaste, main Doctor hun ...

Do you understand me?

ES	¿Me comprende?
ZH	你明白我说的话吗？ nǐ míng bái wǒ shuō de huà ma?
FR	Est-ce que vous me comprenez?
DE	Verstehen Sie mich?
VI	Quý vị có hiểu tôi nói không?
IT	Mi capisce?
KO	이해하십니까? i-hae-ha-sim-ni-kka?
RU	Вы меня понимаете? Vy menya ponimaete?
PL	Czy pan(i) mnie rozumie?
AR	هل تفهمني \ تفهميني؟ Hal tifhamni / tifhameeni?
PT	Percebe o que digo?
FK	Eske ou konprenn mwen?
EL	Με καταλαβαίνετε; me katalabEnete?
HI	क्या आप मुझे समझ रहे हैं? Kya aap mujhe samajh rahe hain?

Please arrange a translator to be with you.

ES Por favor, hágase acompañar de un traductor.

ZH 请找一个帮你翻译的人.
qǐng zhǎo yī gè bāng nǐ fān yì de rén.

FR S'il vous plaît, arrangez-vous pour venir avec un traducteur.

DE Bitte bringen Sie einen Übersetzer mit.

VI Vui lòng thu xếp đi cùng để thông dịch giúp cho quý vị.

IT Per favore, chieda l'aiuto di un traduttore.

KO 통역을 준비하십시오.
tong-yeo-geul jun-bi-ha-sip-si-o

RU Пожалуйста, приведите с собой переводчика.
Pozhaluysta, privedite s soboy perevodchika.

PL Proszę zapewnić sobie obecność tłumacza.

AR لطفاً رتب \ رتبي حضور مترجم معك.
Lutfan rattib / rattibi hudhoor mutarjim ma'ak.

PT Terá que trazer consigo uma pessoa para traduzir.

FK Tanpri fè aranjman pou gen yon tradiktè avèk ou.

EL Παρακαλώ να κανονίσετε να είναι μαζί σας ένας διερμηνέας.
ParakalO na kanonEEsete na EEne mazEE sas Enas dee-ermeenEas.

HI कृपया अपने साथ एक अनुवादक का प्रबंध करें।
kripya apne saath ek anuvadak ka prabandh karein?

How are you?

ES	¿Cómo está usted?
ZH	你好吗？ nǐ hǎo ma?
FR	Comment allez-vous?
DE	Wie geht es Ihnen?
VI	Quý vị có khỏe không?
IT	Come sta?
KO	안녕하세요? an-nyeong-ha-se-yo?
RU	Как ваше здоровье? Kak vashe zdorov'ye?
PL	Jak się pan(i) miewa?
AR	كيف حالك؟ Kayf haalak?
PT	Como está?
FK	Ki jan ou ye?
EL	Πώς είστε; Pos EEste?
HI	आप कैसे हैं? ... Aap kaise hain?

(very) well / sick / weak / tired / depressed / exhausted / confused

ES (muy) bien / mal / débil / cansado / deprimido / agotado / confundido

ZH （很）好 / 有病 / 虚弱 / 疲乏 / 抑郁 / 精疲力竭 / 脑子乱
(hén) hǎo / yǒu bìng / xū ruò / pí fá / yì yù / jīng pí lì jié / nǎo zī luàn

FR (Très)bien / malade / faible / fatigué(e) / déprimé(e) / exténué(e) / troublé(e)

DE (sehr) gut / krank / schwach / müde / depremiert / erschöpft / verwirrt

VI (rất) khỏe / ốm / yếu / mệt / suy nhược / kiệt sức / hay nhầm lẫn

IT (molto) bene / male / debole / stanco / depresso / esausto / confuso

KO (아주)좋다 / 아프다 / 힘이 없다 / 피곤하다 / 우울하다 / 기지맥진하다 /
혼란스럽다
(a-ju)jo-ta / a-peu-da / hi-mi eop-da / pi-gon-ha-da / u-ul-ha-da / gi-jin-maek-
jin-ha-da / hol-lan-seu-reop-da

RU (очень) хорошо / я болен / слаб / устал / подавлен / истощён /
дезориентирован
(ochen') khorosho / ya bolen / slab / ustal / podavlen / istoshchyon / dezorientirovan

PL (Bardzo) dobrze / jestem chory(a) słaby(a) / przygnębiony(a) /
zdezorientowany(a)

AR بخير \ مريض، مريضة \ ضعيف، ضعيفة \ تعبان \ تعبانة \ مكتئب، مكتئبة \ مرهق، مرهقة \ متحير،
متحيرة (جدا)
Bakhayr / mareedh [male], mareedhah [female] / dha"eef [male], dha"eefah [female] /
ta"baan [male], ta"baanah [female] / mukta'ib [male], mukta'ibah [female] / murhaq
[male], murhaqah [female] / mutahayyir [male], mutahayyirah [female] (jiddan)

PT (muito) bem / doente / fraco(a) / cansado(a) / deprimido(a) / exausto(a) / confuso(a)

FK (tre) byen / malad / fèb / fatige / deprime / ekstreman fatige / konfuzyon

EL (πολύ) καλά / άρρωστοι / αδύναμοι / κουρασμένοι / κατεθλιμμένοι /
εξασθενισμένοι / συγκεχυμένοι
(polEE) kalA / Arostee / adEEnamee / kurasmEnee / katethleemEnee / exastheneesmEnee /
seegeheemEnee

HI (बहुत) अच्छा / बीमार / कमजोर / थका हुआ / तनावग्रस्त / निढाल / भ्रमित
(Bahut) achchha / beemaar / kamjor / thaka hua / tanavgrast / niDhaal / bhramit

How do you feel?

ES	¿Cómo se siente?

ZH 你感觉如何？
nǐ gǎn jué rú hé?

FR Comment vous sentez-vous?

DE Wie fühlen Sie sich?

VI Quý vị cảm thấy thế nào?

IT Come si sente?

KO 기분이 어떠세요?
gi-bu-ni eo-tteo-se-yo?

RU Как вы себя чувствуете?
Kak vy sebya chuvstvuete?

PL Jak się Pan(i) czuje?

AR كيف تشعر \ تشعرين؟
Kayf tish"ur [male] / tish"ureen [female]?

PT Como se sente?

FK Ki jan ou santi w?

EL Πώς νιώθετε;
Pos neeOthete?

HI आप कैसा महसूस कर रहे हैं? ...
Aap kaisa mahsoos kar rahe hain?

well / don't feel well / sick / so-so

ES bien / no me siento bien / enfermo / más o menos

ZH 好 / 不好 / 有病 / 一般般
hǎo / bù hǎo / yǒu bìng / yī bān bān

FR Bien / je ne me sens pas bien / malade / comme ci, comme ça

DE gut / schlecht / krank / so lala

VI khỏe / không cảm thấy khỏe / ốm / bình thường

IT mi sento bene / non mi sento bene / sto male / così-così

KO 좋다 / 안 좋다 / 아프다 / 그저 그렇다
jo-ta / an jo-ta / a-peu-da / geu-jeo geu-reo-ta

RU хорошо / нехорошо / больным / неважно
khorosho / nekhorosho / bol'nym / nevazhno

PL dobrze / nie czuję się zbyt dobrze / czuję się chory(a) / tak sobie

AR بخير \ لا اشعر بخير \ مريض، مريضة \ لا بأس، ماشي الحال
Bakhayr / la ash"ur bakhayr / mareedh [male], mareedhah [female] / laa ba's, maashi al-haal

PT Bem / não me sinto bem / doente / mais ou menos

FK byen / pa santi w byen / malad / konsi konsa.

EL καλά / δεν νιώθετε καλά / άρρωστοι / μέτρια
kalA / den neeOthete kalA / Arostee / mEtreea

HI अच्छा / अच्छा महसूस नहीं कर रहा / बीमार / ठीक-ठाक
Achchha / achchha mahsoos nahi kar raha / beemaar / theek-thak

2 Admission

Have you been here before? When?

ES	¿Ya había estado aquí antes? ¿Cuándo?
ZH	你以前来过这里吗？什么时候？ nǐ yǐ qián lái guò zhè lǐ ma? shén me shí hòu?
FR	Etes-vous déjà venu(e) auparavant? Quand?
DE	Waren Sie schon einmal hier? Wann?
VI	Quý vị đã bao giờ tới đây chưa? Khi nào?
IT	È già stato / a qui? Quando?
KO	여기에 오신 적이 있습니까? 언제? Yeo-gi-e o-sin jeo-gi it-seum-ni-kka? Eon-je?
RU	Вы здесь раньше были? Когда? Vy zdes' ran'she byli? Kogda?
PL	Czy był(a) Pan(i) już kiedyś w tym ośrodku? Kiedy?
AR	هل كنت هنا من قبل؟ متى؟ Hal kunta / kunti henaa min qabl? Mattaa?
PT	Já aqui esteve antes? Quando?
FK	Eske ou te janm isi a deja? Ki lè?
EL	Έχετε έρθει ξανά εδώ; Πότε; Ehete Erthee xanA edO? POte?
HI	क्या आप पहले यहाँ आ चुके है? कब? kya aap pehle yahan aa chuke hain? kab?

What is your name?

ES	¿Me dice su nombre?
ZH	你叫什么名字？ nǐ jiào shén me míng zi?
FR	Quel est votre nom?
DE	Wie heißen Sie?
VI	Quý vị tên là gì?
IT	Come si chiama?
KO	이름이 어떻게 되십니까? I-reu-mi eo-tteo-ke doe-sim-ni-kka?
RU	Как вас зовут? Kak vas zovut?
PL	Jak się Pan(i) nazywa?
AR	ما اسمك؟ Maa ismak?
PT	Como se chama?
FK	Kijan ou rele?
EL	Ποιο είναι το όνομά σας; peeO EEne to OnomA sas?
HI	आपका नाम क्या है? aapka naam kya hai?

What is your address / telephone number?

ES ¿Cuál es su dirección / número telefónico?

ZH 你的地址 / 电话号码是什么？
nǐ de dì zhǐ / diàn huà hào mǎ shì shén me?

FR Quelle est votre adresse / votre numéro de téléphone?

DE Wie ist Ihre Adresse / Telefonnummer?

VI Địa chỉ / số điện thoại của quý vị là gì?

IT Qual è il Suo indirizzo / numero telefonico?

KO 주소 / 전화번호가 어떻게 되십니까?
Ju-so / jeon-hwa-beon-ho-ga eo-tteo-ke doe-sim-ni-kka?

RU Какой ваш адрес / номер телефона?
Kakoy vash adres / nomer telefona?

PL Jaki jest Pana(i) adres / numer telefonu?

AR ما هو عنوان سكنك \ رقم تلفونك؟
Ma huwa "anwaan sakanak / raqam telefonak?

PT Qual é o seu endereço / número de telefone?

FK Ki adrès ou / nimewo telefòn ou ?

EL Ποια / Ποιος είναι η διεύθυνση / τηλεφωνικός αριθμός;
peea / peeos EEne ee deeEftheensee / teelefoneekOs areethOs?

HI आपका पता / टेलिफोन नंबर क्या है?
aapka pataa / telephone number kya hai?

Where did you come from?

ES	¿De dónde viene usted?
ZH	你从什么地方来？ nǐ cóng shén me dì fāng lái?
FR	D'où venez-vous?
DE	Wo kommen Sie her?
VI	Quý vị từ đâu tới?
IT	Da dove è arrivato?
KO	어디서 오셨습니까? Eo-di-seo o-syeot-seum-ni-kka?
RU	Откуда вы приехали? Otkuda vy priekhali?
PL	Skąd Pan(Pani) pochodzi?
AR	من أين جئت ؟ Min ayna ji't?
PT	De onde é?
FK	Ki bò ou fèt?
EL	Από πού έρχεστε; apO pu Erheste?
HI	आप कहां से आए हैं? aap kahan se aaye hain?

Please show it to me

ES	Por favor muéstremelo
ZH	让我看看 ràng wǒ kàn kàn
FR	S'il vous plaît, montrez-le moi
DE	Bitte zeigen Sie es mir
VI	Xin cho tôi xem chỗ đó
IT	Mi faccia vedere, per favore
KO	제게 보여 주세요 Je-ge bo-yeo ju-se-yo
RU	Пожалуйста, покажите мне это Pozhaluysta, pokazhite mne eto
PL	Proszę mi to pokazać
AR	ارني \ اريني إياه رجاءاً Arini / areeni iyyaahu rajaa'an
PT	Mostre-me isso
FK	Tanpri montre m
EL	Παρακαλώ δείξτε το μου parakalO dEExte to mu
HI	कृपया यह मुझे दिखायें kripyaa yeh mujhe dikhayen

Please write it down

ES Por favor anótelo

ZH 请写下来
qǐng xiě xià lái

FR S'il vous plaît, veuillez l'écrire

DE Bitte schreiben Sie es auf

VI Xin ghi ra giấy

IT Lo scriva, per favore

KO 써 주세요
Sseo ju-se-yo

RU Пожалуйста, запишите это
Pozhaluysta, zapishite eto

PL Proszę to zapisać

AR اكتبه \ اكتبيه رجاءاً
Uktubuh / iktubeehe rajaa'an

PT Escreva sobre isso

FK Tanpri ekri l

EL Παρακαλώ γράψτε το
parakalO grApse to

HI कृपया इसे लिख लें
kripyaa ise likh lein

Please bring it with you

ES	Por favor tráigalo a la consulta
ZH	请带在身上 qǐng dài zài shēn shàng
FR	S'il vous plaît, apportez-le avec vous
DE	Bitte bringen Sie es mit
VI	Xin mang theo cùng với quý vị
IT	Lo / la porti con sé, per favore
KO	가지고 오세요 Ga-ji-go o-se-yo
RU	Пожалуйста, принесите это с собой Pozhaluysta, prinesite eto s soboi
PL	Proszę to przynieść ze sobą
AR	احضره / احضريه معك رجاءاً Ahdhiruh / adhdhireehi ma"ak rajaa'an
PT	Traga isso consigo por favor
FK	Tanpri pote l ave w
EL	Παρακαλώ φέρτε το μαζί σας parakalO fErte to mazEE sas
HI	कृपया इसे अपने साथ लाएं kripyaa ise apne saath laayen

Yes / no / I don't know

ES Sì / no / no sé

ZH 是的 / 不是 / 我不知道
shì de / bú shì / wǒ bù zhī dào

FR Oui / non / Je ne sais pas

DE Ja / nein / Ich weiß es nicht

VI Có / không / tôi không biết

IT Sì / no / non lo so

KO 네 / 아니오 / 몰라요
Ne / A-ni-o / Mol-la-yo

RU Да / нет / я не знаю
Da / net / ya ne znayu

PL Tak / nie / nie wiem

AR نعم \ لا \ انا لا ادري
Na"m / laa / ana laa adri

PT Sim / não / não sei

FK Wi / non / mwen pa konin

EL Ναι / Όχι / Δεν γνωρίζω
ne / Ochee / den gnorEEzo

HI हां /ना /मुझे पता नही
haan / naa / mujhe pataa nahi

last name / first name / date of birth (place of birth) / telephone number / country

ES apellidos / nombre / fecha de nacimiento (lugar de nacimiento) / número telefónico / país

ZH 姓 / 名字 / 出生日期 / （出生地） / 电话号码 / 国家
xìng / míng zi / chū shēng rì qī / (chū shēng dì) / diàn huà hào mǎ / guó jiā

FR Nom / prénom / date de naissance (lieu de naissance), numéro de téléphone, pays

DE Nachname / Vorname / Geburtsdatum (-ort) / Adresse / Telefonnummer / Land

VI tên họ / tên gọi / ngày tháng năm sinh (nơi sinh) / số điện thoại / quốc gia

IT cognome / nome / data di nascita (luogo di nascita) numero telefonico / paese

KO 성 / 이름 / 생년월일(출생지) / 전화번호 / 국가
seong / i-reum / saeng-nyeon-wo-ril(chul-saeng-ji) / jeon-hwa-beon-ho / guk-ga

RU фамилия / имя / дата рождения (место рождения) / номер телефона / страна
familiya / imya / data rozhdeniya (mesto rozhdeniya) / nomer telefona / strana

PL nazwisko / imię / data urodzenia (miejsce urodzenia) / numer telefonu / kraj

AR اسم العائلة \ الاسم الأول (محلّ ولادتك) تأريخ ولادتك \ رقم التلفون \ البلد
Ism al-"aa'ilah \ al-ism al-'awwal taareekh wilaadtak (mahall wilaadtak) / raqam telefonak / al-balad

PT apelido / nome próprio / data de nascimento (local onde nasceu) / telefone / país

FK siyati / non w / dat nesans (kote ouf è) / nimewo telefòn / payi

EL επώνυμο / πρώτο όνομα / ημερομηνία γέννησης (τόπος γέννησης) / τηλεφωνικός αριθμός / χώρα
epOneemo / prOto Onoma / eemeromeenEEa gEneesees (tOpos gEEneesees) / teelefoneekOs areethmOs / hOra

HI अंतिम नाम / प्रथम नाम / जन्म तिथि (जन्म स्थान) / टेलिफोन नंबर / देश
antim naam / pratham naam / janam tithi (janam sthaan) / telephone number / desh

How old are you? How old is he / she?

ES   ¿Qué edad tiene usted? ¿Qué edad tiene él / ella?

ZH   你多大岁数了？他 / 她多大年纪？
nǐ duō dà sui shù le? tā / tā duō dà nián jì?

FR   Quel âge avez-vous? Quel âge a-t-il (elle)?

DE   Wie alt sind Sie? Wie alt ist er / sie?

VI   Quý vị bao nhiêu tuổi? Anh ấy / cô ấy bao nhiêu tuổi?

IT   Quanti anni ha? Quanti anni ha lui / lei?

KO   나이가 어떻게 되십니까? 그 분은 몇 살입니까?
Na-i-ga eo-tteo-ke doe-sim-ni-kka? geu bu-neun myeot sa-rim-ni-kka?

RU   Сколько вам лет? Сколько ему / ей лет?
Skol'ko vam let? Skol'ko emu / ey let?

PL   Ile Pan(i) ma lat? Ile on(a) ma lat?

AR   كم عمرك؟ كم عمره \ عمرها؟
Kam "umrak? Kam "umroh / "umrhaa?

PT   Que idade tem? Que idade tem ele / ela?

FK   Ki laj ou? Ki laj li?

EL   Πόσο χρονών είστε; Πόσο χρονών είναι αυτός / αυτή;
pOso hronOn EEste? pOso hronOn EEne aftOs / aftEE?

HI   आपकी आयु कितनी है? उसकी आयु क्या है?
Aapki aayu kitni hai? Uski aayu kya hai?

What is your marital status?

ES ¿Cuál es su estado civil?

ZH 你的婚姻情况怎样？
nǐ de hūn yīn qíng kuàng zěn yàng?

FR Quel est votre état civil?

DE Wie ist Ihr Familienstand?

VI Tình trạng hôn nhân của quý vị là gì?

IT Qual è il Suo stato civile?

KO 배우자 유무는(결혼하셨습니까)?
Bae-u-ja yu-mu-neun(gyeol-hon-ha-syeot-seum-ni-kka)?

RU Какое у вас семейное положение?
Kakoe u vas semeynoe polozhenie?

PL Jaki jest Pana(i) stan cywilny?

AR ما حالتك الزوجية؟
Maa haalatak az-zaujiyyah?

PT Qual é o seu estado civil?

FK Ki eta sivil ou?

EL Ποια είναι η οικογενειακή κατάστασή σας;
peeA EEne ee eekogeneeakE katAstasEE sas?

HI आपकी वैवाहिक स्थिति क्या है?
Aapki vaivahik sthiti kya hai?

married / single / divorced / widowed

ES	casado(a) / soltero(a) / divorciado(a) / viudo(a)
ZH	已婚 / 单身 / 离婚 / 寡居 yī hūn / dān shēn / lí hūn / guǎ jū
FR	marié(e), célibataire / divorcé(e), veuf (-euve)
DE	verheiratet / alleinstehend / geschieden / verwitwet
VI	đã lập gia đình / độc thân / đã ly dị / góa chồng (vợ)
IT	sposato / a / celibe / nubile / divorziato / a / vedovo / a
KO	결혼함 / 혼자 / 이혼 / 미망인(홀아비) gyeol-hon-ham / hon-ja / i-hon / mi-mang-in(ho-ra-bi)
RU	женат, замужем / холостой, незамужняя / разведен, разведена / вдовец, вдова zhenat, zamuzhem / kholostoy, nezamuzhnyaya / razveden, razvedena / vdovets, vdova
PL	Żonaty, zamężna / wolny(a) / rozwiedziony(a) / wdowiec, wdowa
AR	متزوّج \ متزوجة \ أعزب \ عزباء \ مطلّق \ مطلقة \ مترمّل \ أرملة Mutazawwij / mutazawwijah / a"azab / "azbaa' / mutallaq / mutallaqah / mutarammil / armalah
PT	casado(a) / solteiro(a) / divorciado(a) / viúvo(a)
FK	marye / selibatè / divose / vev[vef]
EL	παντρεμένος / η / άγαμος / η / διαζευγμένος / η / χήρος / α pandremEnos / ee / Agamos / ee / deeazevmEnos / ee / hEEros / a
HI	विवाहित / अविवाहित / तलाकशुदा / विदुर Vivahit / A-vivahit / talaakshuda / vidur

Whom may we call? Phone number?

ES	¿A quién podemos llamar? ¿Número de teléfono?
ZH	谁是联系人？电话是多少？ shéi shì lián xì rén? diàn huà shì duō shǎo?
FR	Qui pouvons-nous appeler? Numéro de téléphone?
DE	Wen können wir anrufen? Telefonnummer?
VI	Chúng tôi có thể gọi cho ai? Số điện thoại?
IT	A chi possiamo telefonare? Numero telefonico?
KO	누구한테 전화를 할까요? 전화번호는? Nu-gu-han-te jeon-hwa-reul hal-kka-yo? Jeon-hwa-beon-ho-neun?
RU	Кому мы можем позвонить? Номер телефона? Komu my mozhem pozvonit'? Nomer telefona?
PL	Do kogo możemy dzwonić? Numer telefonu?
AR	بمن يمكن أن نتّصل؟ ما هو رقم التلفون؟ Biman yimkin an nattasil? Maa huwa raqam at-telefon?
PT	A quem podemos telefonar? Número de telefone?
FK	Ki moun nou gendwa rele? Nimewo telefòn?
EL	Ποιον μπορούμε να καλέσουμε; Τηλεφωνικό αριθμό; peeOn borUme na kalEsume? TeelefoneekO areethmO?
HI	हम किसे कॉल कर सकते हैं? फोन नंबर? Hum kise call kar sakte hain? Phone number?

What is the name of your primary care physician?

ES ¿Cómo se llama su médico familiar?

ZH 你的主管医师叫什么名字？
nǐ de zhǔ guǎn yī shī jiào shén me míng zi?

FR Quel est le nom de votre médecin de famille?

DE Wie ist der Name Ihres Hausarztes?

VI Tên của bác sĩ chăm sóc chính của quý vị là gì?

IT Come si chiama il Suo medico?

KO 주치의 이름이 무엇입니까?
Ju-chi-ui i-reu-mi mu-eo-sim-ni-kka?

RU Как зовут вашего семейного врача?
Kak zovut vashego semeynogo vracha?

PL Jak się nazywa Pana(i) lekarz rodzinny?

AR ما اسم طبيب العناية الأولية لديك؟
Maa ism tabeeb al-"inaayah al-'awwaliyah ladayk?

PT Qual é o nome do seu médico principal?

FK Ki jan doktè regilye w rele?

EL Ποιο είναι το όνομα του οικογενειακού γιατρού σας;
peeO eene to Onoma tu eekogeneeakU geeatrU sas?

HI आपके प्राथमिक परिचर्या चिकित्सक का क्या नाम है?
Aapke prathmik paricharya chikitsak ka kya naam hai?

What is your profession? Are you (a) ...

ES ¿A qué se dedica usted? ¿Es usted ...

ZH 你的职业是什么？你是做 ...
nǐ de zhí yè shì shén me? nǐ shì zuò ...

FR Quelle est votre profession? Etes-vous un (e) ...

DE Was arbeiten Sie? Sind Sie ...

VI Quý vị làm nghề gì? Quý vị là ...

IT Qual è la Sua professione? Lei è (un / una) ...

KO 직업이 무엇입니까? ... 입니까?
Ji-geo-bi mu-eo-sim-ni-kka? ... sim-ni-kka?

RU Какая у вас профессия? Вы ...
Kakaya u vas professiya? Vy ...

PL Jaki jest Pana(i) zawód? Czy jest Pan(i) ... ?

AR ما مهنتك؟ هل انت ...
Maa mehnatak? Hal inta (male) / inti (female) ...

PT Qual é a sua profissão? Está ou é ...

FK Ki pwofesyon w? Eske ou se (yon) ...

EL Ποιο είναι το επάγγελμά σας; Είστε ...
peeO EEne to epAgelmA sas? EEste ...

HI आपका पेशा क्या है? क्या आप (ए)...हैं
Aapka pesha kya hai? Kya aap (a) ... hain

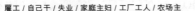

employed / self-employed / unemployed / housewife / factory worker / farmer

ES empleado / autoempleado / desempleado / ama de casa / obrero / agricultor

ZH 雇工 / 自己干 / 失业 / 家庭主妇 / 工厂工人 / 农场主
gù gōng / zì jǐ gàn / shī yè / jiā tíng zhǔ fù / gōng chǎng gōng rén / nóng chǎng zhǔ

FR employé(e) / indépendant(e) / sans emploi / femme au foyer / ouvrier d'usine / fermier

DE angestellt / selbstständig / arbeitslos / Hausfrau / Fabrikarbeiter / Landwirt

VI nhân viên làm thuê / tự kinh doanh / thất nghiệp / nội trợ / công nhân nhà máy / nông dân

IT impiegato / a lavoratore autonomo / disoccupato / a casalinga / operaio / agricoltore

KO 직업이 있는 / 자영업하는 / 무직장의 / 주부 / 공장 근로자 / 농부
ji-geo-bi in-neun / ja-yeong-eop-ha-neun / mu-jik-jang-ui / ju-bu / gong-jang
geul-lo-ja / nong-bu

RU работаете по найму / работаете на себя / безработный / домохозяйка /
работник предприятия / фермер
rabotaete po naymu / rabotaete na sebya / bezrabotnyi / domohozyaika /
rabotnik predpriyatiya / fermer

PL Zatrudniony(a) / prowadzi własne przedsiębiorstwo / bezrobotny(a) / gospodynią
domową / pracownikiem fabryki / rolnikiem?

AR متوظف \ متوظفة \ صاحب \ صاحبة مهنة حرة \ عاطل \ عاطلة عن العمل \ ربّة بيت \ عامل \
عاملة مصنع \ مزارع \ مزارعة
Mutawadhdhif / sahib / sahibat mehnah hurrah / "aatil" / "aatilah "anil-"amal /
rabbat bayt / "aamil / "aamilat masna" / muzaari" / muzaari"ah

PT empregado / trabalha por conta própria / desempregado / dona de casa / trabalhador(a)
de fábrica / lavrador

FK anplwaye / travay pou tèt ou / ou pap travay / fenm fwaye / anplwaye faktori / kiltivatè

EL εργαζόμενος / αυτοαπασχολούμενος / άνεργος / νοικοκυρά / εργάτης
εργοστασίου / αγρότης
ergazOmenos / aftoapasholUmenos / Anergos / neekokeerA / ergAtees ergostasEEu /
agrOtees

HI कार्यरत / स्व–नियोजित / बेरोजगार / गृहणी / फैक्ट्री कार्यकर्ता / किसान
Karyarat / swa-niyojitt / berojgar / grahNi / factory karyakarta / Kisaan

Do you have health insurance? Private?

ES	¿Tiene algún seguro médico? ¿Privado?
ZH	你有健康保险吗？私人的吗？ nǐ yǒu jiàn kāng bǎo xiǎn ma? sī rén de ma?
FR	Avez-vous une assurance soins de santé? Privée?
DE	Sind Sie krankenversichert? Privat?
VI	Quý vị có bảo hiểm sức khỏe không? Bảo hiểm tư?
IT	Ha un'assicurazione sanitaria? Privata?
KO	의료보험이 있으십니까? 사적 보험? Ui-ryo-bo-heo-mi i-seu-sim-ni-kka? Sa-jeok bo-heom?
RU	У вас есть медицинская страховка? От частной компании? U vas est' meditsinskaya strakhovka? Ot chastnoy kompanii?
PL	Czy posiada Pan(i) ubezpieczenie zdrowotne? Prywatne?
AR	هل لديك تأمين صحة؟ تأمين صحة خاص؟ Hal ladayk ta'meen sihhah? / ta'meen sihhah khaas?
PT	Tem seguro médico? Privado?
FK	Eske ou gen asirans lasante? Prive?
EL	Έχετε ασφάλεια υγείας; Ιδιωτική; Ehete asfAleea eegEEas? EedeeoteekEE?
HI	क्या आपका स्वास्थ्य बीमा है? निजी? Kya aapka swasthya beema hai? Niji?

Who is your insurance carrier?

ES	¿Cuál es su compañia o institución aseguradora?
ZH	哪一家保险公司？ nǎ yī jiā bǎo xiǎn gōng sī?
FR	Quelle est votre compagnie d'assurance de soins de santé?
DE	Bei welcher Versicherung?
VI	Hãng bảo hiểm sức khỏe của quý vị là hãng nào?
IT	Con quale compagnia assicurativa è assicurato / a?
KO	보험회사 이름이 무엇입니까? Bo-heom-hoe-sa i-reu-mi mu-eo-sim-ni-kka?
RU	В какой компании вы застрахованы? V kakoy kompanii vy zastrakhovany?
PL	W jakiej firmie jest Pan(i) ubezpieczony(a)?
AR	ما هي الجهة الحاملة لتأمين صحتك؟ Maa hiya al-jihhah al-haamilah li-ta'meen sihhtak?
PT	Qual é a sua companhia de seguros médicos?
FK	Kijan konpani asirans ou rele?
EL	Ποιος είναι ο ασφαλιστικός φορέας σας; peeOs EEne o asfaleesteekOs forEas sas?
HI	आपका बीमाकर्ता कौन है? Aapka beema kartaa kuan hai?

Do you have your insurance card with you?

ES ¿Trae consigo su credencial del seguro?

ZH 你有没有带保险卡？
 nǐ yǒu méi yǒu dài bǎo xiǎn kǎ?

FR Avez-vous votre carte d'assurance avec vous?

DE Haben Sie Ihre Versicherungskarte dabei?

VI Quý vị có mang theo thẻ bảo hiểm không?

IT Ha con sé la tesserina dell'assicurazione?

KO 보험 카드를 가지고 오셨습니까?
Bo-heom ka-deu-reul ga-ji-go o-syeot-seum-ni-kka?

RU У вас с собой есть страховая карта?
U vas s soboy est' strakhovaya karta?

PL Czy ma Pan(i) przy sobie legitymację ubezpieczeniową?

AR هل معك بطاقة تأمينك؟
Hal ma"ak bitaaqat ta'meenak?

PT Tem o seu cartão do seguro consigo?

FK Eske ou gen kat asirans ou an avèk ou?

EL Έχετε την κάρτα ασφάλισης σας μαζί σας;
Ehete teen kArta asfAlesees sas mazEE sas?

HI क्या आपके पास अपना बीमा कार्ड है?
Kya aapke paas apna beema card hai?

Please wait in the waiting room

ES Por favor, pase a la sala de espera

ZH 请在这个休息室等一下
qǐng zài zhè gè xiū xī shì děng yī xià

FR S'il vous plaît, veuillez attendre dans la salle d'attente;

DE Bitte warten Sie hier im Wartezimmer

VI Xin đợi ở phòng chờ

IT Per cortesia, attenda in sala d'aspetto

KO 대기실에서 기다려 주십시오
Dae-gi-si-re-seo gi-da-ryeo ju-sip-si-o

RU Пожалуйста, подождите в приёмной
Pozhaluysta, podozhdite v priyomnoy

PL Proszę poczekać w poczekalni

AR الرجاء الإنتظار فى غرفة الإنتظار
Ar-rajaa' al-intidhaar fi ghurfatil-intidhaar

PT Queira aguardar na sala de espera

FK Tanpri al tan nan sal atnat lan?

EL Παρακαλώ περιμένετε στην αίθουσα αναμονής
parakalO pereemEnete steen Ethusa anamonees

HI कृपया प्रतीक्षा कक्ष में इंतजार करें
Kripya pratikSha KakSh mein Intzaar karein

Please return at ... AM / PM

ES	Por favor regrese a las ... am / pm
ZH	请在上午 / 下午 ... 点钟返回来 qǐng zài shàng wǔ / xià wǔ ... diǎn zhōng fǎn huí lái
FR	S'il vous plaît, revenez à ... heures
DE	Bitte kommen Sie um ... Uhr wieder
VI	Xin quay trở lại lúc ... giờ sáng / giờ chiều
IT	Per cortesia, torni alle ore ...
KO	오전 / 오후 ... 에 돌아오십시오 O-jeon / o-hu ... e do-ra-o-sip-si-o
RU	Пожалуйста, вернитесь в ... часов утра / дня / вечера Pozhaluysta, vernites' v ... chasov utra / dnya / vechera
PL	Proszę przyjść z powrotem o ...
AR	الرجاء العودة في ... صباحاً / بعد الظهر Ar-rajaa' al-"audah fi ... sabaahan / ba"d adh-dhuhr
PT	Queira voltar às ... horas
FK	Tanpri tounin a ... Matin / Apremidi
EL	Παρακαλώ επιστρέψτε στις ... ΠΜ / ΜΜ parakalO epeestEpste stees ... pro meseemvrEEas / metA meseemvrEEas
HI	कृपया .... बजे सुबह / शाम लौट आएं Kripya ... baje subah / shaam laut aayein

3 Main Symptoms

What makes you come to me / us?

ES Dígame, ¿qué lo trae por aquí?

ZH 你哪里不舒服？
nǐ nǎ lǐ bù shū fú?

FR Qu'est-ce qui vous amène à me / nous consulter?

DE Was führt Sie zu mir / uns?

VI Vì sao quý vị tới gặp tôi / chúng tôi?

IT Che cosa La ha spinta a venire da me / noi?

KO 저한테 / 여기에 무슨 일로 오셨습니까?
Jeo-han-te / yeo-gi-e mu-seun il-lo o-syeot-seum-ni-kka?

RU Что привело вас ко мне / к нам?
Chto privelo vas ko mne / k nam?

PL Co Pana / Panią do mnie sprowadza?

AR ما هو سبب زيارتك إليَّ \ إلينا؟
Maa huwa sabab ziyaaratak ilayy? / Ilayna?

PT O que é que o(a) levou a consultar-me / nos?

FK Kisa ki fè ou vin jwenn mwen / nou?

EL Γιατί ήρθατε σε μένα / μας;
geeatEE EErthate se mEna / mas?

HI आप मेरे / हमारे पास किसलिए आए हैं?
aap mere / hamaare paas kisliye aaye hain?

Are you ill / injured?

ES	¿Ha estado enfermo / se lastimó?
ZH	你病了 / 受伤了吗？ nǐ bìng le / shòu shāng le ma?
FR	Etes-vous malade / blessé(e)?
DE	Sind Sie krank / verletzt?
VI	Quý vị có bị ốm / chấn thương không?
IT	Sta male / si è fatto / a male?
KO	아프십니까? / 다치셨습니까? A-peu-sim-ni-kka? / Da-chi-syeot-seum-ni-kka?
RU	Вы больны / травмированы? Vy bol'ny / travmirovany?
PL	Czy jest Pan(i) chory(a) / ranny(a)?
AR	هل انت مصاب / مصابة بمرض / بجرح؟ Hal inta / inti musaab / musaabah bi-maradh / bi-jarh?
PT	Está doente / ferido?
FK	Eskeou malad / blese?
EL	Είστε άρρωστοι / τραυματισμένοι; EEste Arostee / travmateesmEnee?
HI	क्या आप बीमार / घायल हैं? kya aap beemar / ghayal hain?

What happened?

ES	¿Qué ha sucedido?
ZH	怎么回事？ zěn me huí shì?
FR	Qu'est-ce qu'il se passe?
DE	Was ist passiert?
VI	Chuyện gì đã xảy ra?
IT	Cosa è successo?
KO	무슨 일이 있었습니까? Mu-seun i-ri i-seot-seum-nikka?
RU	Что случилось? Chto sluchilos'?
PL	Co się stało?
AR	ماذا حدث؟ Madhaa hadadh?
PT	O que é que aconteceu?
FK	Sak pase?
EL	Τι συνέβη; tee seenEvee?
HI	क्या हुआ? kya hua?

What caused the wound you have?

ES ¿Cómo se causó esa herida?

ZH 怎么受的伤？
    zěn me shòu de shāng?

FR Qu'est-ce qui a causé la blessure que vous avez?

DE Was hat die Wunde verursacht?

VI Vì sao quý vị lại bị thương như thế này?

IT Cosa ha provocato la Sua ferita?

KO 이 상처는 어떻게 생긴 겁니까?
    I sang-cheo-neun eo-tteo-ke saeng-gin- geom-ni-kka?

RU От чего ваша рана?
    Ot chego vasha rana?

PL Skąd się wzięła ta rana?

AR ما هو سبب الجرح الذي تعاني \ تعانين منه؟
    Maa huwa sabab al-jarh iladhi tu"aani / tu"aaneen minhu?

PT O que é que causou o ferimento que tem?

FK Kisa ki lakòz blesi ou genyen an?

EL Τι προκάλεσε το τραύμα που έχετε;
    tee prokAlese to trAvma pu Ehete?

HI आपको यह घाव कैसे हुआ?
    aapko yeh ghaav kaise hua?

Did you vomit?

ES ¿Vomitó?

ZH 有没有呕吐？
yǒu méi yǒu ǒu tù?

FR Avez-vous vomi?

DE Haben Sie erbrochen?

VI Quý vị có bị ói mửa không?

IT Ha vomitato?

KO 토하셨습니까?
To-ha-syeot-seum-ni-kka?

RU Была ли у вас рвота?
Byla li u vas rvota?

PL Czy Pan(i) wymiotował(a)?

AR هل تقيأت؟
Hal taqayya't?

PT Vomitou?

FK Eske ou vomi?

EL Κάνατε εμετό;
kAnate emetO?

HI क्या आपको उलटी हुई?
kya aapko ulti hui?

Did you have a (car) accident?

ES	¿Tuvo un accidente de coche?
ZH	你有过外伤（车祸）吗？ nǐ yǒu guò wài shāng (chē huò) ma?
FR	Avez-vous eu un accident (de voiture)?
DE	Hatten Sie einen (Auto)Unfall?
VI	Quý vị có bị tai nạn (xe hơi) không?
IT	Ha avuto un incidente (automobilistico?)
KO	(자동차) 사고가 있었습니까? (Ja-dong-cha) sa-go-ga i-seot-seum-ni-kka?
RU	Вы попали в (автомобильную) аварию? Vy popali v (avtomobil'nuyu) avariyu?
PL	Czy był(a) Pan(i) w wypadku samochodowym?
AR	هل كنت في حادث (سيارة)؟ Hal kunta (male) / kunti (female) fi haadith (sayyarah)?
PT	Teve um acidente (de viação)?
FK	Eske ou te fè yon aksidan (machinn)?
EL	Είχατε (αυτοκινητιστικό) ατύχημα; EEhate (aftokeeneeteesteekO) atEEheema?
HI	क्या आपकी (कार) दुर्घटनाग्रस्त हुई? kya aapki(car)durghatnagrast hui?

Did you sustain cuts / impact injuries / crush injuries?

ES ¿Sufrió cortaduras / contusiones / aplastamiento?

ZH 你是否被割伤 / 挤压 / 碾伤？
nǐ shì fǒu bèi gē shāng / jǐ yā / niǎn shāng?

FR Avez-vous subi des coupures / un choc / un écrasement?

DE Haben Sie sich geschnitten / gestoßen / gequetscht?

VI Quý vị có bị các vết cắt / chấn thương do va chạm / chấn thương do bị đè bẹp không?

IT Si è tagliato / a / ha subito lesioni da impatto / ferite da schiacciamento?

KO 베인 상처 / 충돌 상해 / 짓눌임 상해를 입으셨습니까?
Be-in sang-cheo / chung-dol sang-hae / jin-nu-rim sang-hae-reuli-beu-syeot-seum-ni-kka?

RU Вы получили порезы / травмы от удара / размозженные раны?
Vy poluchili porezy / travmy ot udara / razmozzhennye rany?

PL Czy odniósł (odniosła) Pan(i) rany cięte / obrażenia spowodowane uderzeniem / zmiażdżeniem?

AR هل اصبت بجروح قاطعة \ ضارية \ ساحقة؟
Hal usibt bi-jurooh qaati"ah / dhaaribah / saahiqah?

PT Sofreu cortes / lesões devido a impacto / lesões devido a esmagamento?

FK Eske ou vin blese pou sinyin / domaj inpakt / andomajman kraze?

EL Έχετε υποστεί κοψίματα / τραυματισμούς από σύγκρουση / τραυματισμούς από σύνθλιψη;
Ehete eepostEE kopsEEmata / travmateesmUs apO sEEgrusee / travmateesmUs apO sEEnthleepsee?

HI क्या आपको कट /आघात चोट /रगड़ से हुए घाव हैं?
kya aapko cut / aaghat chot / ragad se huae ghaav hain

Did you have a fall?

ES	¿Se cayó?
ZH	跌伤过吗？ diē shāng guò ma?
FR	Avez-vous fait une chute?
DE	Sind Sie (hin)gefallen?
VI	Quý vị có bị ngã không?
IT	È caduto / a?
KO	넘어지거나 떨어지셨습니까? Neo-meo-ji-geo-na tteol-o-ji-syeot-seum-ni-kka?
RU	Вы падали? Vy padali?
PL	Czy Pan(i) upadł(a)?
AR	هل سقطت؟ Hal saqat-ta / saqat-ti ?
PT	Sofreu uma queda?
FK	Eske ou tonbe?
EL	Πέσατε; pEsate?
HI	क्या आप गिरे थे? kya aap gire the?

Where you involved in a physical fight?

ES ¿Se peleó a golpes?

ZH 哪个地方被打了？
nǎ gè dì fāng bèi dá le?

FR Où avez-vous été impliqué(e) dans un combat physique?

DE Waren Sie in einen Kampf verwickelt?

VI Quý vị đã đánh lộn ở đâu?

IT Ha partecipato a una lotta fisica?

KO 싸움을 하셨습니까?
Ssa-um-eul ha-syeot-seum-ni-kka?

RU Вы участвовали в драке?
Vy uchastvovali v drake?

PL Czy brał(a) Pan(i) udział w bijatyce?

AR هل كنت في صراع جسماني؟
Hal kunta (male) / kunti (female) fi siraa" jismaani

PT Esteve envolvido(a) numa luta física?

FK Eske ou te nan yon batay?

EL Είχατε εμπλακεί σε σωματική διαμάχη;
EEhate eblakEE se somateekEE deeamAhee?

HI आप शारीरिक लड़ाई में कहां शामिल हुए थे?
aap sharirik ladai mein kahan shamil hue the?

Have you been beaten (stick / stone / fist)?

ES ¿Lo golpearon con algo (palo / piedra / el puño)?

ZH 有没有被打伤（刺伤 / 石头砸伤 / 拳头打）？
yǒu méi yǒu bèi dǎ shāng (cì shāng / shí tóu zá / quán tóu dǎ)?

FR Avez-vous été frappé(e) (bâton / pierre / poing)?

DE Wurden Sie geschlagen (Stock / Stein / Faust)?

VI Quý vị có bị đánh (bằng gậy / ném đá / đấm) không?

IT È stato / a picchiato / a (bastone / pietra / pugno)?

KO 맞으셨습니까 (몽둥이 / 돌 / 주먹)?
Ma-jeu-syeot-seum-ni-kka (mong-dung-i / dol / ju-meok)?

RU Вас били (палкой / камнем / кулаком)?
Vas bili (palkoi / kamnem / kulakom)?

PL Czy został(a) Pan(i) pobity(a) / ukłuty(a) / uderzony(a) kijem / kamieniem / pięścią?

AR هل اصيت بضربات (بالعصا \ بالحجارة \ بالحجارة \ بالقبضة)؟
Hal usibt bi-dharbaat (bil-asaa / bil-hijaarah / bil-hijaarah / bil-qabdhah)?

PT Foi agredido com (um pau / uma pedra / um punho)?

FK Eske yo te janm bat ou (baton / wòch / kout pwin)?

EL Σας χτύπησαν με (ράβδο / κοτρόνα / γροθιά);
sas htEEpeesan me (rAvdo / kotrOna / grothEEa)?

HI क्या आपको (छड़ी / पत्थर / मुक्का) मारा गया था?
kya aapko (chhadi / patthar / mukka)maara gaya tha?

Have you sustained knife injuries?

ES ¿Lo lesionaron con un cuchillo o navaja?

ZH 被刀刺了吗？
bèi dāo cì le ma?

FR Avez-vous subi une blessure par un instrument tranchant?

DE Wurden Sie mit einem Messer verletzt?

VI Quý vị có bị thương do dao cắt không?

IT Ha subito ferite da coltello?

KO 칼로 베이셨습니까?
Kal-lo be-i-syeot-seum-ni-kka?

RU Вы получили ножевые ранения?
Vy poluchili nozhevye raneniya?

PL Czy zadano Panu(Pani) rany nożem?

AR هل اصيب بجروح ناتجة عن سكينة؟
Hal usibt bi-jurooh naatijah "an sikkinah?

PT Sofreu lesões infligidas por uma faca?

FK Eske ou te jan resevwa yon kout kouto?

EL Έχετε υποστεί τραυματισμούς από μαχαίρι;
Ehete eepostEE travmateesmUs apO mahEree?

HI क्या आपको चाकू से घाव हुआ था?
kya aapko chaaku se ghaav hua tha?

Have you sustained a bone fracture?

ES	¿Se fracturó algún hueso?
ZH	有骨折吗？ yǒu gǔ zhé ma?
FR	Avez-vous subi une fracture?
DE	Haben Sie sich einen Knochen gebrochen?
VI	Có quý vị có bị gãy xương không?
IT	Si è rotto / a un osso?
KO	뼈가 골절되었습니까? Ppyeo-ga gol-jeol-doe-eot-seum-ni-kka?
RU	У вас были переломаны кости? U vas byli perelomany kósti?
PL	Czy doznał(a) Pan(i) złamania kości?
AR	هل اصبت بكسر في عظم من عظامك؟ Hal usibt bi-kasrin fi "adhm min "idhaamak?
PT	Sofreu uma fractura óssea?
FK	Eske ou gen yon zò w ki kase?
EL	Έχετε υποστεί κάταγμα οστού; Ehete eepostEE kAtagma ostU?
HI	क्या आपकी हड्डी टूटी है? kya aapki haddi tutee hai?

Have you been raped?

ES	¿Fue víctima de violación?
ZH	你有没有被强奸？ nǐ yǒu méi yǒu bèi qiáng jiān?
FR	Avez-vous été violée?
DE	Wurden Sie vergewaltigt?
VI	Có phải quý vị đã bị hãm hiếp không?
IT	È stato / a violentato / a?
KO	강간당하셨습니까? Gang-gan-dang-ha-syeot-seum-ni-kka?
RU	Вас изнасиловали? Vas iznasilovali?
PL	Czy została Pani zgwałcona?
AR	هل تعرضت للاغتصاب؟ Hal ta"arradhti lil-ightisaab?
PT	Foi violada(o)?
FK	Eske yo fè kadejak sou ou?
EL	Σας βίασαν; sas vEEasan?
HI	क्या आपका बलात्कार हुआ है? kya aapka balaatkaar hua hai?

Have you sustained firearm injuries?

ES ¿Le lesionaron con un arma de fuego?

ZH 你被枪打伤了吗？
nǐ bèi qiāng dǎ shāng le ma?

FR Avez-vous été blessé(e) par une arme à feu?

DE Wurden Sie angeschossen?

VI Có phải quý vị đã bị thương do hỏa hoạn không?

IT Ha subito ferite da arma da fuoco?

KO 화기로 상해를 입으셨습니까?
Hwa-gi-ro sang-hae-reul i-beu-syeot-seum-ni-kka?

RU Вы получили огнестрельные ранения?
Vy poluchili ognestrel'nye raneniya?

PL Czy został(a) Pan(i) postrzelony(a) z broni palnej?

AR هل اصبت بجروح ناتجة عن اسلحة نارية؟
Hal usibt bi-jurouh naatijah "an aslihah naariyah?

PT Sofreu lesões infligidas por uma arma de fogo?

FK Eske ou resevwa blesi de yon kout zam?

EL Έχετε υποστεί τραυματισμούς από πυροβόλο όπλο;
Ehete eepostEE travmateesmUs apO peerovOlo Oplo?

HI क्या आपको बंदूक की गोली से घाव हुए हैं?
kya aapko bandook ki goli se ghaav hue hain?

Have you been bitten by a dog / snake?

ES ¿Lo mordió un perro / víbora?

ZH 被狗 / 蛇咬过吗？
bèi gǒu / shé yǎo guò ma?

FR Avez-vous été mordu(e) par un chien / un serpent?

DE Wurden Sie von einem Hund / einer Schlange gebissen?

VI Quý vị có bị chó / rắn cắn không?

IT È stato / a morso / a da un cane / serpente?

KO 개 / 뱀에 물리셨습니까?
Gae / bae-me mul-li-syeot-seum-ni-kka?

RU Вас укусила собака / змея?
Vas ukusila sobaka / zmeya?

PL Czy został(a) Pan(i) ugryziony(a) przez psa / ukąszony(a) przez węża?

AR هل تعرضت لعض كلب \ ثعبان؟
Hal ta"arradht li-"adhdh kalb / tha"baan?

PT Foi mordido(a) por um cão / uma cobra?

FK Eske yon chyen / koulèv mode w?

EL Σας δάγκωσε σκύλος / φίδι;
sas dAgose skEElos / fEEdee?

HI क्या आपको कुत्ते/सांप ने काटा है?
kya aapko kutte / saanp ne kaata hai?

Did an insect sting you?

ES	¿Lo picó un insecto?
ZH	被昆虫叮了吗？ bèi kūn chóng dīng le ma?
FR	Avez-vous été piqué(e) par un insecte?
DE	Wurden Sie von einem Insekt gestochen?
VI	Quý vị có bị côn trùng cắn không?
IT	È stato / a punto / a da un insetto?
KO	곤충에 쏘이셨습니까? Gon-chung-e sso-i-syeot-seum-ni-kka?
RU	Вас ужалило насекомое? Vas uzhalilo nasekomoe?
PL	Czy ukąsił Pana(Panią) owad?
AR	هل اصبت بلدغة حشرة من الحشرات؟ Hal usibt bi-ladghah hasharah min al-hasharaat?
PT	Foi picado(a) por um insecto?
FK	Ki bèt ki pike w?
EL	Σας τσίμπησε έντομο; sas tsEEpeese Edomo?
HI	क्या आपको किसी कीट ने दंश मारा है? kya aapko kisi keet ne dansh mara hai?

When did this occur?

ES ¿Cuándo pasó esto?

ZH 什么时间发生的？
shén me shí jiān fā shēng de?

FR Quand cela s'est-il produit?

DE Wann ist das passiert?

VI Việc này xảy ra khi nào?

IT Quando è successo?

KO 언제 일어난 일입니까?
Eon-je i-reo-nan i-rim-ni-kka?

RU Когда это случилось?
Kogda eto sluchilos'?

PL Kiedy to się wydarzyło?

AR متى حصل هذا؟
Mattaa hasal hadhaa?

PT Quando é que isto aconteceu?

FK Ki lè sa pase?

EL Πότε συνέβη αυτό;
pOte seenEvee aftO?

HI यह कब हुआ?
yeh kab hua?

How long have you been sick? For hours / days / weeks / years

ES ¿Cuánto tiempo se ha sentido mal? Horas / días / semanas / años

ZH 你病多久了？几小时 / 几天 / 几周 / 几年？
nǐ bìng duō jiǔ le? jǐ xiǎo shí? jǐ tiān? jǐ zhōu? jǐ nián?

FR Il y a combien de temps que vous êtes malade? Heures / jours / semaines / années

DE Wie lange sind Sie schon krank? seit Stunden / Tagen / Wochen / Jahren

VI Quý vị bị ốm bao lâu rồi? Tính theo giờ / ngày / tuần / năm

IT Da quanto tempo sta male? Da ore / giorni / settimane / anni

KO 아프신 지 얼마나 되셨습니까? 수 시간 / 수 일 / 수 주 / 수 년
A-peu-sin ji eol-ma-na doe-syeot-seum-ni-kka? Su si-gan / su il / su ju / su nyeon

RU Как долго вы болеете? Часов / дней / недель / лет
Kak dolgo vy boleyete? Chasov / dney / nedel' / let

PL Od jak dawna Pan(i) choruje? Od kilku godzin / dni / tygodni / lat

AR كم مدة عانيت من المرض؟ كم ساعة \ يوم \ أسبوع \ سنة
Kam muddah "aanayt min al-maradh? Kam saa"ah? / Youm / Usbou" / Sanah

PT Há quanto tempo está doente? Há quantas horas / quantos dias / quantas semanas / quantos anos

FK Konbyen tan ou genyen depi ou malad? Plizye hètan / jou / semèn / ane

EL Πόσο καιρό είστε άρρωστοι; Για ώρες / ημέρες / εβδομάδες / χρόνια
pOso kerO EEste Arostee? geea Ores / eemEres / evdomAdes / hrOneea

HI आप कितने समय से बीमार हैं? घंटे / दिन / हफ्ते / वर्षों से
aap kitne samaya se beemaar hain? ghante / din / hafte / varshno se

Are you vaccinated against tetanus? When did you receive your last vaccination?

ES
¿Está vacunado contra el tétanos? ¿Cuando le aplicaron la última vacuna?

ZH
打过破伤风针吗？最后一次打破伤风针是什么时间？
dá guò pò shāng fēng zhēn ma? zuì hòu yī cì dǎ pò shāng fēng zhēn shì shén me shí jiān?

FR
Avez-vous été vacciné(e) contre le tétanos? Quand avez-vous été vacciné(e) pour la dernière fois?

DE
Sind Sie gegen Tetanus geimpft? Letzte Impfung?

VI
Quý vị có chủng ngừa bệnh uốn ván không? Lần chủng ngừa gần đây nhất là khi nào?

IT
È stato / a vaccinato / a contro il tetano? Quando ha fatto l'ultimo richiamo?

KO
파상풍 예방주사를 맞으셨습니까? 예방주사를 언제 마지막으로 맞으셨습니까?
Pa-sang-pung ye-bang-ju-sa-reul ma-jeu-syeot-seum-ni-kka? Ye-bang-ju-sa-reul eon-je ma-ji-ma-geu-ro ma-jeu-syeot-seum-ni-kka?

RU
Вы привиты против столбняка? Когда вам делали последнюю прививку?
Vy privity protiv stolbnyaka? Kogda vam delali poslednyuyu privivku?

PL
Czy był(a) Pani szczepiony(a) na tężec? Kiedy dostał(a) Pan(i) ostatnią szczepionkę?

AR
هل انت حاصل \ حاصلة على التطعيم المضاد لمرض الكزاز؟ متى حصلت على تطعيمك الأخير؟
Hal kunta (male) / kunti (female) haasil / haasilah "alaa at-tat"eem al-mudhaad li-maradh il-kazaaz? Mattaa hasalt "alaa tat"eemaatak al-akheerah?

PT
Já foi vacinado contra o tétano? Quando é que lhe foi administrada a última vacina?

FK
Eske ou te resevwa vaksin kont tetanus? Sou ki dat ou te resevwa denye vaksin an?

EL
Έχετε εμβολιαστεί κατά του τετάνου; Πότε λάβατε το τελευταίο εμβόλιό σας;
Ehete emvoleeastEE katA tu tEtanu? pOte lAvate to teleftEo emvOleeO sas?

HI
क्या आपको टिटनेस का टीका लगा? आपको अंतिम बार टीका कब लगा था?
kya aapko tetanus ka teeka laga? aapko antim baar teeka kab laga tha?

Do you feel sick / weak / tired / exhausted / depressed?

ES ¿Se siente enfermo / débil / cansado / agotado / deprimido?

ZH 你又没有感到恶心 / 虚弱 / 疲劳 / 精疲力竭 / 抑郁？
nǐ yòu méi yǒu gǎn dào ě xīn / xū ruò / pí láo / jīng pí lì jié / yì yù?

FR Vous sentez-vous malade / faible / fatigué(e) / épuisé(e) / déprimé(e)?

DE Fühlen Sie sich krank / schwach / müde / erschöpft / depressiv?

VI Quý vị có cảm thấy ốm / yếu / mệt mỏi / kiệt sức / suy nhược không?

IT Si sente male / debole / stanco / a / esausto / a / depresso / a?

KO 아프십니까 / 힘이 없으십니까 / 피곤하십니까 / 탈진하셨습니까 / 우울하십니까?
A-peu-sim-ni-kka / Hi-mi eop-seu-sim-ni-kka / Pi-gon-ha-sim-ni-kka / Tal-jin-ha-syeot-sem-ni-kka / U-ul-ha-sim-ni-kka?

RU Вы чувствуете себя больным / слабым / уставшим / истощенным / подавленным?
Vy chuvstvuete sebia bol'nym / slabym / ustavshim / istoshchennym / podavlennym?

PL Czy czuje się Pan(i) chory(a) / słaby(a) / wycieńczony(a) / przygnębiony(a)?

AR هل تشعر \ تشعرين بالمرض \ بالضعف \ بالتعب \ بالإرهاق \ بالاكتئاب؟
Hal tash"ur / tash"ureen bil-maradh / bidh-dha"f / bit-ta"b / bil-irhaaq / bil-ikti'aab?

PT Sente-se doente / fraco(a) / cansado(a) / exausto(a) / deprimido(a)?

FK Eske ou santi ou malad / fèb / bouke / tre fatige / deprime ?

EL Νιώθετε άρρωστοι / αδύναμοι / κουρασμένοι / εξαντλημένοι / κατάθλιψη;
neeOthete Arostee / adEEnamee / kurasmEnee / exadleemEnee / katAthleepsee?

HI क्या आप बीमार / कमजोर / थका हुआ / निढाल / दबाव महसूस करते हैं?
kya aap beemaar / kamjor / thaka hua / niddhal / dabav mahsoos karte hain?

Do you have any discomfort? In which area?

ES
¿Tiene alguna molestia? ¿En qué parte?

ZH
你有什么不舒服吗？在哪里？
nǐ yǒu shén me bù shū fú ma? zài nǎ li?

FR
Avez-vous la moindre gêne? Dans quelle région?

DE
Haben Sie Beschwerden? Wo?

VI
Quý vị có thấy khó chịu không? Ở vùng nào?

IT
Ha fastidi? In quale zona?

KO
불편한 데가 있으십니까? 어디 입니까?
Bul-pyeon-han de-ga i-seu-sim-ni-kka? Eo-di im-ni-kka?

RU
Испытываете ли вы какой-нибудь дискомфорт? В каком месте?
Ispytyvaete li vy kakoi-nibud' diskomfort? V kakom meste?

PL
Czy odczuwa Pan / i jakieś dolegliwości? W którym miejscu?

AR
هل تعاني \ تعانين من مضايقة او عدم راحة من نوع ما؟ وفى أي مكان؟
Hal tu"aani / tu"aaneen min mudhaayaqah au "adam raahah min nau"in maa? Wa fi ayyi makaan?

PT
Sente algum mal-estar? Em que parte do corpo?

FK
Eske ou santi ou mal alez? Nan ki kote ?

EL
Έχετε δυσφορία; Σε ποια περιοχή;
Ehete deesforEEa? se peea pereeohEE?

HI
क्या आपको कोई तकलीफ है? किस भाग में?
kya aapko koi takleef hai? kis bhaag mein?

While breathing / lung / chest / heart / head / neck / nose / ears / eyes

ES Al respirar / pulmón / pecho / corazón / cabeza / cuello / nariz / oídos / ojos

ZH 当呼吸时 / 肺部 / 胸部 / 心脏 / 头 / 颈部 / 鼻子 / 耳朵 / 眼
dāng hū xī shí / fèi bù / xiōng bù / xīn zàng / tóu / jǐng bù / bí zi / ěr duǒ / yǎn

FR Quand vous respirez / poumon / thorax / coeur / tête / cou / nez / oreilles / yeux

DE Beim Atmen / Lunge / Brust / Herz / Kopf / Hals / Nase / Ohren / Augen

VI Khi thở / phổi / ngực / tim / đầu / cổ / mũi / tai / mắt

IT Quando respiro / polmone / petto / cuore / testa / collo / naso / orecchie / occhi

KO 숨을 쉴 때 / 폐 / 가슴 / 심장 / 머리 / 목 / 코 / 귀 / 눈
su-meul swil-ttae / pye / ga-seum / sim-jang / meo-ri / mok / ko / gwi / nun

RU Во время дыхания / в легких / в груди / в сердце / в голове / в шее / в носу / в ушах / в глазах
Vo vremia dykhaniya / v legkikh / v grudi / v serdtse / v golove / v shee / v nosu / v ushakh / v glazakh

PL Podczas oddychania / w płucach / w klatce piersiowej / w głowie / w nosie / w uszach / w oczach

AR عند التنفس / بالرئة / بالصدر / بالقلب / بالرأس / بالعنق / بالأنف / بالأذنين / بالعينين
"Ind at-tanaffus / bir-ri'ah / bis-sadr / bil-qalb / bir-ra's / bil-"unuq / bil-anf / bil-udhneyn / bil-"aynayn

PT Enquanto respira / nos pulmões / no tórax / no coração / na cabeça / no pescoço / no nariz / nos ouvidos / nos olhos

FK Pandan ke ou ap respire / poumon / lestomak / kè / nin / zye

EL Κατά την αναπνοή / πνευμόνια / στήθος / καρδιά / κεφάλι / λαιμός / μύτη / αυτιά / μάτια
katA teen anapnoEE / pnevmOneea / stEEthos / kardiA / lemOs / mEEtee / afteeA / mAteea

HI सांस लेने के दौरान / फेफड़े / छाती / हृदय / सिर / गर्दन / नाक / कान / आंखों में ...
sans lene ke dauraan / fefde / chhati / hyrdaya / sir / gardan / naak / kaan / ankhon mein

Nerves / abdomen / stomach / intestines / urinal bladder / kidneys / urethra / genitals

ES nervi / addome / stomaco / intestino / vvescica / reni / uretra / genitali

ZH 神经 / 腹腔 / 胃 / 肠 / 膀胱 / 肾 / 尿道 / 生殖器
Shen jing / fu qiang / wei / chang / pang guang / shen / niao dao / sheng zhi qi

FR Nerfs / abdomen / estomac / intestins / vessie / reins / urètre / organes génitaux

DE Nerven / Bauch / Magen / Darm / Blase / Nieren / Harnröhre / Genitalien

VI XXX

IT nervi / addome / stomaco / intestino / vvescica / reni / uretra / genitali

KO 신경 과민 / 하복부 / 위 / 장(전체) / 소변방광 / 신장 / 요도 / 성기(생식기)
Sin-kyeong-gwa-min / ha-bok-bu / wi / jang(jeon-chae) / so-beon-bang-gwang / sin-jang / yo-do / seung-gi (saeng-sik-gi)

RU Нервы / брюшная полость / желудок / кишечник / мочевой пузырь / почки / мочеиспускательный канал / половые органы
Nervy / bryushnaya polost' / zheludok / kishechnik / mochevoy puzyr' / pochki / mocheispuskatel'nyi kanal / polovye organy

PL Nerwy / brzuch / żołądek / jelita / pęcherz / nerki / cewka moczowa / genitalia

AR الأعصاب / البطن / المعدة / الأمعاء / المتانة البولية / الكلى / مسلك البول / الأعضاء التناسلية
Al-A"saab / Al-batn / Al-Ma"idah / Al-Am"aa' / Al-Mathaanah Al-Bauliyah / Al-Kilaa / Maslak Al-Baul / Al-A"dhaa' at-tanaasuliyah

PT Nervos / abdómen / estômago / intestinos / bexiga urinária / rins / uretra / órgãos genitais

FK Nerfs / abdomen / estomac / intestins / vessie urinaire / reins / urètre / organes génitaux

EL Νεύρα / κοιλιά / στομάχι / έντερα / ουροδόχος κύστη / νεφρά / ουρήθρα / γεννητικά όργανα
nEvra / keeleeA / stomAhee / Edera / urodOhos kEEstee / nefrA / urEEthra / genetikA Organa

HI नस / पेट / क्षुधा / अंतड़ी / पेशाब मूत्राशय / गुर्दे / मूत्रमार्ग / जननांग
Nas / PeT / Kshudhaa / Antarhi / Peshaab moutraashaya / Gurde / Mootramaarga / Jananaang

Joints / arms / legs / pelvic area / hips / teeth

ES Articulaciones / brazos / piernas / región pélvica / caderas / dientes

ZH 关节 / 胳膊 / 腿 / 骨盆处 / 髋部 / 牙齿
guān jié / gē bo / tuǐ / gǔ pén chù / kuān bù / yá chǐ

FR Articulations / bras / jambes / région du bassin / les hanches / les dents

DE Gelenke / Arme / Beine / Becken / Hüfte / Zähne

VI Khớp / tay / chân / vùng xương chậu / hông / răng

IT Articolazioni / braccia / gambe / zona pelvica / anche / denti

KO 관절 / 팔 / 다리 / 골반 부위 / 엉덩이 / 치아
gwan-jeol / pal / dari / gol-ban bu-wi / eong-deong-i / chi-a

RU В суставах / в руках / в ногах / внизу живота / в бедрах / в зубах
V sustavakh / v rukakh / v nogakh / vnizu zhivota / v bedrakh / v zubakh

PL Stawy / ramiona / nogi / miednica / biodra / zęby

AR في المفاصل \ في الذراعين \ في الرجلين \ في المنطقة الحوضية \ في الردفين \ في الأسنان
Fil-mafaasil / fidh-dhiraa"ayn / fir-rijlayn / fil-mantiqah al-haudhiyyah / fir-rudfayn / fil-asnaan

PT articulações / braços / pernas / zona pélvica / ancas / dentes

FK jwenti / bra / janb / zon basin ou / hanch / dan

EL αρθρώσεις / άνω άκρα / κάτω άκρα / πυελική περιοχή / ισχίο / δόντια
arhtOsees / Ano Akra / kAto Akra / pee-eleekEE pereeohEE / eeshEEo / dOdeea

HI जोड़ों / भुजाओं / टांगों / पेड़ू वाले क्षेत्र / नितंब / दांतों में
jodon / bhujaon / tangon / pedu wale kshetron / nitamb / danton mein

Have you noticed any changes in yourself that are of concern to you?

ES ¿Ha notado en usted algún cambio que le preocupe?

ZH 有没有身体的异常变化?
yǒu méi yǒu shēn tǐ de yì cháng biàn huà?

FR Avez-vous remarqué le moindre changement en vous-même qui vous préoccupe?

DE Haben Sie Veränderungen an sich bemerkt, die Ihnen Sorgen machen?

VI Quý vị có nhận thấy thay đổi nào trong cơ thể khiến quý vị cảm thấy lo lắng không?

IT Ha notato cambiamenti in Lei che La preoccupano?

KO 본인한테 걱정스러운 변화가 일어난 것을 느끼셨습니까?
Bon-in-han-te geok-jeong-seu-reo-un byeon-hwa-ga i-reo-nan geo-seul neu-kki-syeot-seum-ni-kka?

RU Заметили ли вы какие-нибудь изменения в себе, которые беспокоят вас?
Zametili li vy kakie-nibud' izmeneniya v sebe, kotorye bespokoyat vas?

PL Czy zauważył(a) Pan(i) u siebie jakieś niepokojące zmiany?

AR هل لاحظت اية تغييرات فى نفسك تثير القلق عندك؟
Hal laahadht ayyati taghyeeraatin fi nafsik tutheer il-qalaq "indak?

PT Notou em si, algumas alterações que o(a) preocupam?

FK Eske ou remake okinn chanjman nan ou menm ki konsenin w?

EL Παρατηρήσατε οποιεσδήποτε αλλαγές στον εαυτό σας που σας απασχολούν;
parateerEEsate opee-esdEEpote alagEs ston eaftO sas pu sas apasholUn?

HI क्या आपने स्वयं में कोई परिवर्तन नोट किया है जो आपकी चिंता का कारण है?
kya aapne swayam mei koi parivartan note kiya hai jo aapki chinta ka kaaran hai?

Please show me these changes

ES	Por favor muéstreme esos cambios
ZH	给我看一看这些变化？ gěi wǒ kàn yī kàn zhè xie biàn huà?
FR	S'il vous plaît, montrez-moi ces changements
DE	Zeigen Sie mir diese Veränderungen
VI	Xin cho tôi xem những thay đổi đó
IT	Mi faccia vedere questi cambiamenti, per favore
KO	이 변화들을 제게 보여주십시오 I-byeon-hwa-deu-reul je-ge bo-yeo-ju-sip-si-o
RU	Пожалуйста, покажите мне эти изменения Pozhaluysta, pokazhite mne eti izmeneniya
PL	Proszę mi je pokazać One
AR	الرجاء بيان لي هذه التغييرات Ar-rajaa' bayaan li hadhihi at-taghyeeraat
PT	Mostre-me essas alterações por favor
FK	Tanpri montre m chanjman sa yo?
EL	Παρακαλώ δείξτε μου αυτές τις αλλαγές parakalO dEExte mu aftEs tees alagEs
HI	कृपया मुझे ये परिवर्तन दिखाएं kripya mujhe ye parivartan dikhayein

When did you become aware of these changes?

ES	¿Cuándo se dio cuenta de estos cambios?
ZH	你什么时候注意到这些变化的？ nǐ shén me shí hòu zhù yì dào zhè xie biàn huà de?
FR	Quand avez-vous eu conscience de ces changements?
DE	Wann haben Sie diese Veränderungen bemerkt?
VI	Quý vị nhận thấy những thay đổi này từ khi nào?
IT	Quando si è accorto / a di questi cambiamenti?
KO	이 변화들을 언제 알게 되셨습니까? I byeon-hwa-deu-reul eon-je al-ge doe-syeot-seum-ni-kka?
RU	Когда вы заметили эти изменения? Kogda vy zametili eti izmeneniya?
PL	Kiedy Pan(i) zauważył(a) te zmiany?
AR	متى ادركت بهذه التغييرات ؟ Mattaa adrakt bi-hadhihi at-taghyeeraat?
PT	Quando é que se deu conta destas alterações?
FK	Ki lè ou vin gen konesans chanjman sa yo?
EL	Πότε λάβατε επίγνωση αυτών των αλλαγών; pOte lAvate epEEgnosee aftOn ton alagOn?
HI	आपको इन परिवर्तनों की जानकारी कब हुई? ... aapko in parivartnon ki jaankari kab hui?

... hours / days / weeks / years ago

ES ... hace horas / días / semanas / años

ZH ... 几小时 / 几天 / 几周 / 几年前
jǐ xiǎo shí / jǐ tiān / jǐ zhōu / jǐ nián qián

FR ... il y a des heures / des jours / des semaines / des années

DE ... Stunden / Tage / Wochen / Jahre

VI cách đây ... giờ / ngày / tuần / năm

IT ... ore / giorni / settimane / anni fa

KO ... 시간 / 일 / 주 / 년 전
... si-gan / il / ju / nyeon jeon

RU ... часов / дней / недель / лет тому назад
... chasov / dney / nedel' / let tomu nazad

PL ... parę godzin / dni / tygodni / lat temu

AR ... ساعات \ أيام \ اسابيع \ سنوات قبل
Saa"at / ayah / asaabee" / sanawaat qabl ...

PT Há ... horas / dias / semanas / ... anos

FK ... hètan / jou / semen / plizye ane de sa

EL ... ώρες / ημέρες / εβδομάδες / χρόνια πριν
... Ores / eemEres / evdomAdes / hrOnia preen

HI ... घंटे / दिन / हफ्ते / वर्ष पहले
... ghante / din / hafte / varsha pehle

What kind of changes are you observing?

ES ¿Qué tipo de cambios ha notado?

ZH 你看到哪一种变化？
nǐ kàn dào nǎ yī zhǒng biàn huà?

FR Quel genre de changement avez-vous observé?

DE Was für Veränderungen sind das?

VI Quý vị đang nhận thấy có dạng thay đổi nào?

IT Che tipo di cambiamenti ha notato?

KO 어떤 변화들이 눈에 띕니까?
Eo-tteon byeon-hwa-deu-ri nu-ne ttuim-ni-kka?

RU Какого рода изменения вы наблюдаете?
Kakogo roda izmeneniya vy nablyudaete?

PL Jakiego rodzaju są to zmiany?

AR ما هي نوع التغيرات التي تلاحظها \ تلاحظيها؟
Maa hiya nau" at-taghyeeraat alati tulaahidhhaa / tulaahidheehaa?

PT Que tipo de alterações tem observado?

FK Ki kalite chanjman ou remake?

EL Τι είδους αλλαγές παρατηρείτε;
tee EEdus alagEs parateerEEte?

HI आप किस प्रकार के परिवर्तनों पर गौर कर रहे हैं? ...
aap kis prakaar ke parivartnon par gaur kar rahe hain?

anxiety / bruises / bleeding tendency (increased) / depression

ES angustia / moretones / (mayor) tendencia a sangrar / depresión

ZH 紧张 / 淤斑 / 易出血（加重的） / 抑郁
jǐn zhāng / yū bān / yì chū xiě (jiā zhòng de) / yì yù

FR Anxiété / contusion / tendance au saignement (augmentée) / dépression

DE Ängste / blaue Flecken / Blutung (vermehrt) / Depression

VI sự lo âu / các vết bầm tím / dễ bị chảy máu (tăng) / suy nhược

IT ansia / lividi / tendenza a sanguinare (aumentata) / depressione

KO 불안 / 멍 / 출혈 경향(증가된) / 우울증
bu-ran / meong / chul-hyeol gyeong-hyang(jeung-ga-doen) / u-ul-jeung

RU страх / синяки / (повышенная) склонность к кровотечению / депрессия
strakh / sinyaki / (povyshennaya) sklonnost' k krovotecheniyu / depressiya

PL Lęk / sińce / skłonność do krwawienia (większa) / depresję

AR التخوف \ الكدمات \ (الزيادة في) نزيف الدم \ الكآبة
At-takhawwuf / al-kadmat / (az-ziyadah fi) nazif ad-damm / al-ka'aabah

PT ansiedade / contusões / tendência a sangramento (aumentada) / depressão

FK anksye / venn foule / tandans pou ou senyen(ogmante) / depresyon

EL άγχος / μώλωπες / τάση για αιμορραγία (αυξημένη) / κατάθλιψη
Aghos / mOlopes / tAsee geea emoragEEa (afxeemEnee) / katAthleepsee

HI चिंता / खरोंच / रक्तस्राव प्रवृत्ति (बढ़ी हुई) / डिप्रेशन ...
chinta / khronch / raktsraav pravratti(badhi hui) / depression

exhaustion / color changes / fever / spots / tumorous swellings

ES agotamiento / cambios de color / fiebre / manchas / tumoraciones

ZH 精疲力竭 / 颜色变化 / 发烧 / 出斑点 / 包块样肿大
jīng pí lì jié / yán sè biàn huà / fā shāo / chū bān diǎn / bāo kuài yàng zhǒng dà

FR épuisement / changements de couleur / fièvre / taches / gonflement tumoral

DE Erschöpfung / Farbveränderungen / Fieber / Flecken / Geschwulste

VI kiệt sức / thay đổi màu sắc da / ốm / có các nốt nhỏ / bướu sưng

IT spossatezza / cambiamenti di colore / febbre / macchie / rigonfiamenti tumorali

KO 탈진 / 색깔 변화 / 열 / 반점 / 종양 같이 부어 오르는 것
tal-jin / saek-kkal byeon-hwa / yeol / ban-jeom / jong-yang ga-chi bu-eo o-re-neun geot

RU истощение / изменение цвета / повышенная температура / пятна / опухание
istoshchenie / izmenenie tsveta / povyshennaya temperatura / pyatna / opukhanie

PL wycieńczenie / zmiany w kolorze / gorączkę / plamy / nowotworowe obrzęki

AR الإرهاق \ تغيرات لونية \ الحمى \ البقعات \ التضخمات الورمية
Al-irhaaq / taghyeeraat launiyyah / al-hummaa / al-buq"aat / at-tadhakhkhumaat al-waramiyyah

PT exaustão / alterações de coloração / febre / manchas / inchaços tumorosos

FK bouke / chanjman koulè / lafyèv / plak / anflamasyon kouwè time

EL εξάντληση / αλλαγές χρώματος / πυρετός / στίγματα / διογκώσεις σχετιζόμενες με όγκο
exAntleesee / alagEs hrOmatos / peeretOs / stEEgmata / deeogOsees sheteezOmenes me Ogo

HI निढाल / रंग परिवर्तन / बुखार / ढब्बे / गांठीय सूजन .
niddhal / rang parivartan / bukhaar / dhabbe / gantheeya soojan

weight loss, weight gain / skin changes / intolerance to heat or cold

ES baja de peso, aumento de peso / cambios de la piel / intolerancia al calor o frío

ZH 体重减轻，增加 / 皮肤改变 / 怕热怕冷
tǐ zhòng jiǎn qīng, zēng jiā / pí fū gǎi biàn / pà rè pà lěng

FR perte de poids, gain de poids / changements cutanés / intolérance à la chaleur ou au froid

DE Gewichtsverlust, -zunahme / Hautveränderungen / Intoleranz: Hitze, Kälte

VI giảm cân, tăng cân / thay đổi về da / không chịu được nóng hoặc lạnh

IT perdita di peso, aumento di peso / cambiamenti della pelle / intolleranza al calore o al freddo

KO 체중 감소, 체중 증가 / 피부 변화 / 고온이나 저온을 못견디는 것
che-jung gam-so, che-jung jeung-ga / pi-bu byeon-hwa / go-o-ni-na jeo-o-neul mot-gyeon-di-neun geot

RU увеличение, уменьшение массы тела / изменения кожи / непереносимость жары или холода
uvelichenie, umen'shenie massy tela / izmeneniya kozhi / neperenosimost' zhary ili kholoda

PL utrata wagi / przybranie na wadze / zmiany skórne / nietolerancja na ciepło lub zimno

AR خفض الوزن، زيادة الوزن \ تغيرات جلدية \ عدم تحمل الحرارة والبرد
Khafdh al-wazn, ziyaadah al-wazn / taghyeeraat jildiyyah / "adam tahammul al-haraarah au al-bard

PT perda de peso, aumento de peso / alterações na pele / intolerância ao calor ou ao frio

FK megri, gwosi / chanjman nan po w / paka tolere ni chale ni fredi

EL απώλεια βάρους, αύξηση βάρους / δερματικές αλλαγές / δυσανεξία στη θερμότητα ή το κρύο
apOleea vArus, Afxeesee varus / dermateekEs alagEs / deesanexEEa stee thermOteeta ee to krEEo

HI वजन घटना, वजन बढ़ना / त्वचा परिवर्तित होना / गर्मी या ठंड बर्दाश्त न कर पाना ...
vajan ghatna, vajan badhana / tvacha parivatran / garmi ya thand bardast na kar paanan

itching / night sweats / pain / shaking chills / swelling

ES picazón / sudores nocturnos / dolor / escalofríos / hinchazón

ZH 搔癢 / 夜间出汗 / 痛 / 打寒战 / 肿胀
são yǎng / yè jiān chū hàn / tòng / dǎ hán zhàn / zhǒng zhàng

FR démangeaisons / sueurs nocturnes / douleur / frissons / gonflements

DE Juckreiz / Nachtschweiß / Schmerzen / Schüttelfrost / Schwellung

VI ngứa / đổ mồ hôi về đêm / đau / những cơn lạnh run / sưng

IT prurito / sudorazione notturna / dolori / brividi di freddo / gonfiore

KO 가려움 / 밤에 땀 흘리기 / 통증 / 오한으로 떨림 / 붓기
ga-ryeo-um / ba-me ttam heul-li-gi / tong-jeung / o-ha-neu-ro tteol-lim / but-gi

RU зуд / ночная потливость / боль / лихорадочный озноб / опухоль
zud / nochnaya potlivost' / bol' / likhoradochnyi oznob / opukhol'

PL swędzenie / nocne poty / ból / dreszcze / obrzęk

AR الحك \ التعرق بالليل \ الألم \ الرعشات \ التضخم
Al-hakk / at-ta"arruq bil-layl / al-alam / ar-ra"shaat / at-tadhakhkhum

PT comichão / suores nocturnos / dor / calafrios com tremores / inchaço

FK gratèl / swye lannwit / doulè / gwo fisyon / enflamasyon

EL φαγούρα / νυχτερινή εφίδρωση / πόνος / ρίγος / οίδημα
fagUra / neehtereenEE efEEdrosee / pOnos / rEEgos / EEdeema

HI खारिश होना / रात में पसीना आना / दर्द / कंपकंपाती ठंड / सूजन ...
kharish hona / raat mei pasheena aana / dard / kanpkanpati thand / soojan

sadness / changes in urination

ES	tristeza / cambios en la micción (orina)
ZH	情绪低落 / 小便变化 qíng xù dī luò / xiǎo biàn biàn huà
FR	tristesse / changements dans la miction
DE	Traurigkeit / Veränderungen beim Wasserlassen
VI	buồn chán / thay đổi về tiểu tiện
IT	tristezza / cambiamenti della minzione
KO	슬픔 / 소변보는 데 변화 생김 seul-peum / so-byeon-bo-neun de byeon-hwa saeng-gim
RU	грусть / нарушения мочеиспускания grust' / narusheniya mocheispuskaniya
PL	smutek / zmiany w oddawaniu moczu
AR	الحزن \ تغيرات في التبول Al-huzn / taghyeeraat fit-tabawwul
PT	tristeza / alterações da micção
FK	Tris / chanjman nan pipi
EL	λύπη / αλλαγές στην ούρηση IEEpee / alagEs steen Ureesee
HI	गमगीन होना / मूत्र में परिवर्तन ... gamgin hona / mutra mein parivartan

changes in the appearance of the nails / changes in hair growth

ES	cambios en el aspecto de las uñas / en el crecimiento del pelo
ZH	指甲改变 / 毛发生长异常 zhī jiǎ gǎi biàn / máo fà shēng zhǎng yì cháng
FR	changements dans l'aspect des ongles / dans la croissance des cheveux
DE	Veränderungen der Nägel / des Haarwuchses
VI	thay đổi về hình dạng móng / thay đổi về tình trạng mọc tóc
IT	cambiamenti nell'aspetto delle unghie / cambiamenti nella crescita dei capelli
KO	손(발)톱 외양의 변화 / 털(머리) 자라는 데 변화 생김 son(bal)-top oe-yang-ui byeon-hwa / teol(meori) ja-ra-neun de byeon-hwa saeng-gim
RU	изменения структуры ногтей / нарушения роста волос izmeneniya struktury nogtei / narusheniya rosta volos
PL	zmiany w wyglądzie paznokci / zmiany w poroście włosów
AR	تغييرات في شكل الأظفار \ تغييرات في نمو الشعر Taghyeeraat fi shakl al-adhfaar / taghyeeraat fi numouw ash-sha"r
PT	alterações na aparência das unhas / alterações no crescimento do cabelo
FK	chanjman nan zong ou / chanjman nan fason cheve w pouse
EL	αλλαγές στην εμφάνιση των νυχιών / αλλαγές στην τριχοφυΐα alagEs steen emfAneesee ton neeheeOn / alagEs steen treehofeeEEa
HI	नाखून की बनावट में परिवर्तन / बालों के विकास में परिवर्तन ... naakhoon ki banavat mein parivartan / baloin ke vikas mein parivartan

digestive problems (diarrhea, constipation) / enlargement

ES problemas digestivos (diarrea, estreñimiento) / distensión abdominal

ZH 消化性问题（拉肚子，便秘）/ 增大
xiāo huà xìng wèn tí (lā dù zǐ, biàn mì) / zēng dà

FR problèmes digestifs (diarrhée, constipation) / gonflement abdominal

DE Verdauungsstörungen (Durchfall, Verstopfung) / Vergrößerung

VI các vấn đề về tiêu hóa (tiêu chảy, táo bón) / nở lớn

IT problemi digestivi (diarrea, stipsi) / distensione addominale

KO 소화 문제 (설사, 변비) / 확대
so-hwa mun-je (seo-lsa, byeon-bi) / hawk-dae

RU проблемы пищеварения (понос, запоры) / увеличение
problemy pishchevareniya (ponos, zapory) / uvelichenie

PL problemy w trawieniu (biegunka, obstrukcja) / powiększenie

AR اضطرابات هضمية (الإسهال، الإمساك) \ التضخم
Idhtiraabaat hadhmiyyah (al-is'haal, al-imsaak) / at-tadhakhkhum

PT Problemas digestivos (diarreia, prisão de ventre) / aumento

FK pwoblèm dijessyon (dyare / konstipasyon) / dilatasyon

EL πεπτικά προβλήματα (διάρροια, δυσκοιλιότητα) / μεγέθυνση
pepteekA provlEEmata (deeAreea, deeskeeleeOteeta) / megEEtheensee

HI हाजमे की परेशानी (अतिसार, कब्ज) /विस्तरण ...
hajme ki pareshani (atisaar, kabj) / vistaran

decreased (increased) appetite or thirst / wounds

ES	aumento (disminución) del apetito o la sed / heridas
ZH	食欲下降（上升）或口渴 / 伤口 shí yù xià jiàng (shàng shēng) huò kǒu kě / shāng kǒu
FR	diminution (augmentation) de l'appétit ou de la soif / blessures
DE	wenig (mehr) Appetit oder Durst / Wunden
VI	khẩu vị giảm (tăng) hoặc khát nước ít (nhiều) hơn / các vết thương
IT	riduzione (aumento) dell'appetito o della sete / ferite
KO	식욕 혹은 목마름 감소(증가) / 상처 si-gyok ho-geun mong-ma-reum gam-so(jeung-ga) / sang-cheo
RU	пониженный (повышенный) аппетит или жажда / раны ponizhennyi (povyshennyi) appetit ili zhazhda / rany
PL	mniejszy (większy) apetyt lub pragnienie / rany
AR	شهية متناقصة (او متزايدة) للأكل، او العطش \ الجروح Shahiyyah mutanaaqisah (au mutazaayidah) lil-akl, au al-"atash / al-jurouh
PT	diminuição (aumento) do apetite ou da sede / ferimentos
FK	rediksyon (ogmantasyon) apeti oswa swaf / blesi
EL	μειωμένη (αυξημένη) όρεξη ή δίψα / τραύματα meeomEnee (afxeemEnee) Orexee ee dEEpsa / trAvmata
HI	भूख या प्यास घटना (बढ़ना) / घाव bhoonkh ya prayas ghatana (badhna) / ghav

Have you experienced this before?

ES	¿Ya había tenido esto antes?
ZH	以前有过这样的问题吗？ yǐ qián yǒu guò zhè yàng de wèn tí ma?
FR	Avez-vous remarqué cela avant?
DE	Hat sich so etwas schon einmal ereignet?
VI	Quý vị đã bao giờ gặp phải vấn đề này chưa?
IT	Ha provato queste cose prima d'ora?
KO	이전에도 이것을 경험하신 적 있습니까? I-jeo-ne-do i-geo-seul gyeon-gheom-ha-sin jeok it-seum-ni-kka?
RU	Было ли это у вас раньше? Bylo li eto u vas ran'she?
PL	Czy doświadczał(a) Pan(i) tego już wcześniej?
AR	هل تعرضت لمثل هذا من قبل؟ Hal ta"arradhta / ta"arradhti li-mithl hadha min qabl?
PT	Já tinha sentido isto antes?
FK	Eske ou te gen gen sa a deja?
EL	Το έχετε βιώσει αυτό πριν; to Ehete viOsee aftO preen?
HI	क्या आपने पहले इसका अनुभव किया था? kya aapne pehle iska anubhav kiya tha?

Did you previously visit a doctor because of this?

ES ¿Ya había consultado al médico por esta razón?

ZH 来这之前看过医生吗？
lái zhè zhī qián kàn guò yī shēng ma?

FR Avez-vous déjà consulté un médecin pour cette raison?

DE Waren Sie deswegen schon einmal bei einem Arzt?

VI Trước đây, quý vị có đi khám bác sĩ về vấn đề này không?

IT È stato / a dal medico in passato per questo motivo?

KO 이것 때문에 의사한테 가신 적이 이전에도 있습니까?
I-geot ttae-mu-ne ui-sa-han-te ga-sin jeo-gi i-jeo-ne-do it-seum-ni-kka?

RU Посещали ли вы ранее врача по этому поводу?
Poseshchali li vy ranee vracha po etomu povodu?

PL Czy w związku z tym był(a) Pan(i) już wcześniej u lekarza?

AR هل قمت بزيارة طبيب من قبل بهذا الشأن؟
Hal qumt bi-ziyaarah tabeeb min qabl bi-hadha ash-sha'n?

PT Já visitou anteriormente um médico por causa disto?

FK Eske ou te wè yon doktè pou sa a deja ?

EL Επισκεφτήκατε γιατρό στο παρελθόν εξαιτίας αυτού;
epeeskeftEEkate geeatrO sto parelthOn exetEEas aftU?

HI क्या आपने इस कारण पहले डॉक्टर का दौरा किया था?
kya aapne is karaN pehle doctor ka daura kiya tha?

Did you receive treatment for your ailment? Was the treatment successful?

ES
¿Le dieron tratamiento para ese problema? ¿Resultó útil el tratamiento?

ZH
以前是否对这些问题做过治疗？效果好吗？
yǐ qián shì fǒu duì zhè xie wèn tí zuò guò zhì liáo? xiào guǒ hǎo ma?

FR
Avez-vous déjà reçu un traitement pour ce trouble? Le traitement a-t-il été efficace?

DE
Wurden Sie dagegen behandelt? Erfolgreich?

VI
Quý vị có được điều trị cho căn bệnh đó không? Biện pháp điều trị đó có hiệu quả không?

IT
Ha ricevuto una cura per questo disturbo? La cura ha avuto successo?

KO
이 질병에 대해 치료를 받으셨습니까? 치료가 성공적이었습니까?
I jil-byeong-e dae-hae chi-ryo-reul ba-deu-syeot-seum-ni-kka? Chi-ryo-ga seong-gong-jeo-gi-eot-seum-ni-kka?

RU
Лечились ли вы по поводу болезни? Было ли это лечение успешным?
Lechilis' li vy po povodu bolezni? Bylo li eto lechenie uspeshnym?

PL
Czy był(a) Pan(i) leczony(a) na tę chorobę? Czy został Pan(i) wyleczony(a)?

AR
هل تلقيت العلاج لمشكلتك؟ هل كان العلاج ناجحاً؟
Hal talaqqait bil-"ilaaj li-mushkiltak? Hal kaan al-"ilaaj naajihan?

PT
Recebeu tratamento para o seu padecimento? O tratamento foi bem sucedido?

FK
Eske ou te resevwa tretman pou maladi a ? Eske tretman an te mache ?

EL
Λάβατε θεραπεία για αυτήν την ασθένειά σας; Ήταν επιτυχής η θεραπεία;
lAvate therapEEa geea aftEEn teen asthEneeA sas? EEtan epeeteeehEEs ee therapEEa?

HI
क्या आपने अपनी तकलीफ का इलाज करा लिया? क्या इलाज सफल रहा था?
kya aapne apni takleef ka ilaaj kara liya? kya ilaaj safal raha tha?

4 Medical Anamnesis

Have you been previously hospitalized? When? Why?

ES	¿Ya ha estado hospitalizado antes? ¿Cuándo? ¿Por qué motivo?

ZH
你以前住过院吗？什么时间？为什么？
nǐ yǐ qián zhù guò yuàn ma? shén me shí jiān? wèi shěn me?

FR
Avez-vous été hospitalisé(e) dans le passé? Quand? Pourquoi?

DE
Waren Sie im Krankenhaus? Wann? Warum?

VI
Quý vị đã bao giờ phải nằm viện chưa? Khi nào? Tại sao?

IT
È stato / a ricoverato / a in ospedale in passato? Quando? Perché?

KO
과거에 입원하신 적이 있습니까? 언제? 왜?
Gwa-geo-e i-bwon-ha-sin jeo-gi it-seum-ni-kka? Eon-je? Wae?

RU
Вас раньше госпитализировали? Когда? По какому поводу?
Vas ran'she gospitalizirovali? Kogda? Po kakomu povodu?

PL
Czy leżał(a) Pan(i) już kiedyś w szpitalu? Kiedy? Z jakiego powodu?

AR
هل سبق أن كنت فى المستشفى؟ متى؟ لماذا؟
Hal sabaq an kunta (male) \ kunti (female) fil-mustashfaa? Mattaa? Limaadhaa?

PT
Já foi hospitalizado(a) anteriormente? Quando? Porquê?

FK
Eske ou te janm entenin lopital? Ki lè? Poukisa?

EL
Έχετε νοσηλευτεί στο παρελθόν; Πότε; Γιατί;
Ehete noseeleftEE sto parelthOn? pOte? geeatEE?

HI
क्या आपको पहले कभी अस्पताल में रखा गया था? कब? क्यों? ...
kya aapko pehle kabhi aspataal mein rakha gaya tha? kab? kyon?

(minor) surgery / drug therapy / examination / observation

ES	cirugía (menor) / tratamiento farmacológico / exámenes / observación
ZH	（小的）手术 / 药物治疗 / 检查身体 / 留院观察 (xiǎo de) shǒu shù / yào wù zhì liáo / jiǎn chá shēn tǐ / liú yuàn guān chá
FR	chirurgie (mineure) / traitement médicamenteux / examen / observation
DE	(kleine) Operation / medikamentöse Behandlung / Untersuchung / Beobachtung
VI	(tiểu) phẫu / trị liệu bằng thuốc / khám nghiệm / theo dõi
IT	operazione chirurgica (di piccola entità) / terapia farmacologica / visita / osservazione
KO	(경미한) 수술 / 약물 치료 / 진단 / 관찰 (gyeong-mi-han) su-sul / yak-mul chi-ryo / jin-dan / gwan-chal
RU	(малая) операция / курс лечения / обследование / наблюдение (malaya) operatsiya / kurs lecheniya / obsledovanie / nablyudenie
PL	(drobnej) operacji / terapii lękowej / badania / obserwacji
AR	عملية جراحية (خفيفة) \ علاج دوائي \ فحص \ مراقبة "Amaliyah jaraahiyyah (khafeefah) \ "ilaaj dawaa'ei \ fahs \ muraaqabah
PT	(pequena) cirurgia / terapia medicamentosa / exame médico / observação
FK	(Ti) operasyon / terapi dwog / egzamin / obsevasyon
EL	(μικρή) χειρουργική επέμβαση / φαρμακευτική αγωγή / εξέταση / παρακολούθηση (meekrEE) heerurgeekEE epEmvasee / farmakefteekEE agogEE / exEtasee / parakolUtheesee
HI	(लघु) सर्जरी / ड्रग इलाज / जांच / निरीक्षण (laghu)surgery / drug ilaaz / jaanch / nirikShaN

Have you ever received a blood transfusion?

ES ¿Alguna vez ha recibido transfusión de sangre?

ZH 你以前输过血吗？
nǐ yǐ qián shū guò xiě ma?

FR Avez-vous reçu une transfusion de sang?

DE Haben Sie jemals eine Bluttransfusion erhalten?

VI Quý vị có bao giờ phải truyền máu không?

IT Ha mai ricevuto una trasfusione sanguigna?

KO 수혈 받은 적이 있습니까?
Su-hyeol ba-deun jeo-gi it-seum-ni-kka?

RU Вам когда-нибудь делали переливание крови?
Vam kogda-nibud' delali perelivanie krovi?

PL Czy otrzymał Pan(i) kiedykolwiek transfuzję krwi?

AR هل سبق إجراء عملية نقل الدم عليك؟
Hal sabaq ijraa' "amaliyyah naql ad-damm "alayk?

PT Já alguma vez recebeu uma transfusão de sangue?

FK Eske ou janm resevwa yon trasnfisyon san?

EL Λάβατε ποτέ μετάγγιση αίματος;
lAvate potE metAgeesee Ematos?

HI क्या आपने कभी रक्ता दान प्राप्त किया है?
kya aapne kabhi raktadhaan prapt kiya hai?

Did you have the following childhood diseases?

ES ¿Tuvo usted las siguientes enfermedades de la niñez?

ZH 你得过以下儿童病吗？
nǐ dé guò yǐ xià ér tóng bìng ma?

FR Avez-vous présenté les maladies suivantes au cours de votre enfance?

DE Hatten Sie eine der folgenden Kinderkrankheiten?

VI Quý vị có bao giờ mắc căn bệnh trẻ nhỏ nào sau đây hay chưa?

IT Ha avuto le seguenti malattie infantili?

KO 다음의 유년기 질환을 앓으셨습니까?
Da-eu-mui yu-nyeon-gi jil-hwa-neul a-reu-syeot-seum-ni-kka?

RU Болели ли вы следующими детскими болезнями?
Boleli li vy sleduyushchimi detskimi boleznyami?

PL Czy przechodził(a) Pan(i) następujące choroby wieku dziecięcego?

AR هل اصبت بالأمراض التالية أثناء الطفولة؟
Hal usibt bil-amraadh it-taaliyah athnaa' at-tufoulah?

PT Teve as seguintes doenças da infância?

FK Eske ou te gen maladi swivan yo lè ou te timoun?

EL Είχατε τις ακόλουθες παιδικές ασθένειες;
EEhate tees akOluthes pedeekEs asthEnee-es?

HI क्या आपको निम्नलिखित बचपन की बीमारियां थी? ...
kya aapko nimnlikhit bachpan ki bemariyan thi?

Diphtheria / German measles / poliomyelitis (polio)

ES Difteria / rubéola (sarampión alemán) / poliomielitis (polio)

ZH 白喉 / 风疹 / 脊髓灰质炎
bái hóu / fēng zhěn / jí suǐ huī zhì yán

FR Diphtérie / rubéole / poliomyélite (polio)

DE Diphtherie / Röteln / Poliomyelitis (Kinderlähmung)

VI Bệnh bạch hầu / bệnh sởi Đức / bệnh bại liệt

IT Difterite / rosolia / poliomelite (polio)

KO 디프테리아 / 풍진 / 소아마비
di-peu-te-ria / pun-gjin / so-a-ma-bi

RU Дифтерия / краснуха / полиомиелит
Difteriya / krasnukha / poliomielit

PL Błonicę / różyczkę / paraliż dziecięcy (chorobę Heinego- Mediny)

AR الدفتيريا \ الحصبة الألمانية \ شلل الأطفال
Diftiriyaa \ al-hasbah al-almaaniyah \ shalal il-atfaal

PT difetria / rubéola / poliomielite (polio)

FK Difteri / woubewòl (lawoujòl alman) / poliomyelitis (polyo)

EL διφθερίτιδα / ερυθρά / πολιομυελίτιδα
deeftherEEteeda / ereethrA / poleeoome-elEEteeda

HI कंठरोग / जर्मन खसरा / पोलियोमाइलाइटिस (पोलियो) ...
kanthrog / German khasra / poliomyelitis (polio)

measles / chickenpox / whooping cough / mumps

ES sarampión / varicela / tos ferina / paperas (parotiditis)

ZH 麻疹 / 水痘 / 白日咳 / 流行性腮腺炎
má zhěn / shuǐ dòu / bǎi rì ké / iú xíng xìng sāi xiàn yán

FR rougeole / varicelle / coqueluche / oreillons

DE Masern / Windpocken / Keuchhusten / Mumps

VI bệnh sởi / bệnh đậu mùa / ho gà / bệnh quai bị

IT morbillo / varicella / pertosse / parotite

KO 홍역 / 수두 / 백일해 / 볼거리
hong-yeok / su-du / bae-gil-hae / bol-geo-ri

RU корь / ветрянка / коклюш / свинка
kor' / vetryanka / kokliush / svinka

PL odrę / ospę / koklusz / świnkę

AR الحصبة \ جُديري الماء \ السعال الديكي \ النكاف
Al-hasbah \ judayri al-maa' \ as-su"aal ad-deeki \ an-nikaaf

PT sarampo / varíola / tosse convulsa / papeira

FK lawoujòl / woubewòl (lawoujòl alman) / koklich / malmouton

EL ιλαρά / ανεμοβλογιά / κοκκίτης / μαγουλάδες
eelarA / anemovlogeeA / kokEEtees / magulAdes

HI खसरा / चेचक / काली खांसी / गलसुआ
khasra / chechak / kaali khansi / galsua

Do you have / have you ever had ...

ES ¿Tiene / ha tenido ...

ZH 你是否有 / 曾经有过？...
nǐ shì fōu yǒu / céng jīng yǒu guò? ...

FR Avez-vous / avez-vous jamais eu? ...

DE Haben / hatten Sie (ein / e) ...

VI Quý vị có đang / đã từng mắc ...

IT Ha / ha mai avuto ...

KO ... 현재 있습니까 / 이전에 있은 적이 있습니까?
... hyeon-jae it-seum-ni-kka / i-jeo-ne i-seun jeo-gi it-seum-Ni-kka?

RU У вас есть / когда-нибудь были ...
U vas est' / kogda-nibud' byli ...

PL Czy choruje Pan(i) / czy kiedykolwiek chorował(a) Pan(i) na ...

AR ... ـِﺑ ﺔﺑﺎﺻﻹﺍ ﻚﻟ ﻖﺑﺳ ﻞﻫ \ ﺎًﻴﻟﺎﺣ ﺔﺑﺎﺻﻣ \ ﺏﺎﺻﻣ ﺖﻧﺍ ﻞﻫ
Hal inta (male) \ inti (female) musaab \ musaabah (female) haaliyan \ hal sabaq lak al-isaabah bi-

PT Sofre de / já alguma vez sofreu de ...

FK Eske ou genyen / te janm genyen ...

EL Έχετε / Είχατε ...
Ehete / EEhate ...

HI क्या आपको निम्नलिखित में से कोई बीमारी है / हुई थी ...
kya aapko nimnlikhit mein se koi beemari hai / hui thee ...

Alzheimer's Disease / AIDS / Angina pectoris / asthma / bladder inflammation

ES enfermedad de Alzheimer / SIDA / angina de pecho / asma / inflamación de la vejiga

ZH 老年痴呆症 / 艾滋病 / 胸痛 / 哮喘 / 膀胱炎
lǎo nián chī dāi zhèng / ài zī bìng / xiōng tòng / xiào chuǎn / páng guāng yán

FR Maladie d'Alzheimer / sida / angine de poitrine / asthme / inflammation de la vessie

DE Alzheimer / AIDS / Angina pectoris / Asthma / Blasenentzündung

VI Bệnh Alzheimer / AIDS / Chứng đau thắt ngực / bệnh suyễn / viêm bàng quang

IT Il morbo di Alzheimer / AIDS / angina pectoris / asma / infiammazione della vescica

KO 알츠하이머 병 / 에이즈 / 협심증 / 천식 / 방광 염증
Al-cheu-ha-i-meo- byeong / e-i-jeu / hyeop-sim-jeung / cheon-sik / bang-gwang yeom-jeung

RU Болезнь Альцгеймера / СПИД / стенокардия / астма / воспаление мочевого пузыря
Bolezn' Al'tsgeymera / SPID / stenokardiya / astma / vospalenie mochevogo puzyrya

PL Chorobę Alzheimera / AIDS / duszniçę bolesną / astmę / zapalenie pęcherza

AR مرض الألتسهايمر \ مرض الأيدز \ الربو \ التهاب المثانة
Maradh al-Alzheimer \ maradh al-AIDS \ Ar-rabou \ iltihaab il-mathaanah

PT Doença de Alzheimer / SIDA / Angina de peito / asma / inflamação da bexiga

FK Maladi Alzheimer / SIDA / Anjin Pwatrin (pwatrinin) / opresyon / enflamasyon vesi

EL νόσο του Αλζχέιμερ / EITZ / στηθάγχη / άσθμα / φλεγμονή ουροδόχου κύστης
nOso tu Alzheimer / AIDS / steethAghee / Asthma / flegmonEE urodOhu kEEstees

HI एल्ज़िमर की बीमारी / एड्स / कंठशूल / दमा / मूत्राशय में जलन ...
Alzheimer ki beemari / Aids / kanThashool / damaa / mutraashay mein jalan

anemia / blood clot / high blood pressure / bronchitis / breast cancer

ES anemia / embolia / trombosis / hipertensión / bronquitis / cáncer de mama

ZH 贫血 / 血凝块 / 高血压 / 气管炎 / 乳腺癌
pín xiě / xiě níng kuài / gāo xuè yā / qì guǎn yán / rǔ xiàn ái

FR anémie / trouble de la coagulation du sang / pression sanguine élevée / bronchite / cancer du sein

DE Blutarmut / Blutgerinnsel / Bluthochdruck / Bronchitis / Brustkrebs

VI thiếu máu / máu đóng cục / huyết áp cao / viêm phế quản / ung thư vú

IT anemia / coaguli di sangue / pressione alta / bronchite / cancro al seno

KO 빈혈 / 응혈(혈병) / 고혈압 / 기관지염 / 유방암
bin-hyeol / eung-hyeol(hyeol-byeong) / go-hyeo-rap / gi-gwan-ji-yeom / yu-bang-am

RU анемия / тромб / повышенное кровяное давление / бронхит / рак молочной железы
anemiya / tromb / povyshennoe krovyanoe davlenie / bronkhit / rak molochnoy zhelezy

PL anemię / skrzepy krwi / nadciśnienie / zapalenie oskrzeli / raka piersi

AR فقر الدم \ جلطة دم \ ضغط دمّ عالي \ التهاب القصبات الهوائية \ سرطان الثدي
Faqr ad-damm \ jultah damm \ dhaght damm aali \ iltihaab al-qabdhaat al-hawaa'iyah \ sirataan ath-thadiy

PT anemia / coágulo sanguíneo / tensão arterial alta / bronquite / cancro da mama

FK anemi / kayo san / tansyon / bwonchit / kansè tete

EL αναιμία / θρόμβο αίματος / υψηλή αρτηριακή πίεση / βρογχίτιδα / καρκίνο του μαστού
anemEEa / thrOmvo Ematos / eepseelEE arteereeakEE pEEesee / broghEEteeda / karkEEno tu mastU

HI खून की कमी / खून का थक्का / उच्च रक्तचाप / श्वसनली में सूजन / स्तन कैंसर ...
khoon ki kami / khoon ka thakka / uchch raktachaap / shwasnali mein soojan / stan cancer

chronic intestinal disease / ulcerative colitis / depression

ES enfermedad intestinal crónica / colitis ulcerosa / depresión

ZH 慢性肠道疾病 / 溃疡性结肠炎 / 抑郁症
màn xìng cháng dào jí bìng / kuì yáng xìng jiē cháng yán / yì yù zhèng

FR maladie intestinale chronique / colite ulcéreuse / dépression

DE chronische Darmerkrankung / Colitis ulcerosa / Depression

VI bệnh đường ruột mãn tính / viêm loét đại tràng / suy nhược

IT malattia intestinale cronica / colite ulcerosa / depressione

KO 만성 장 질환 / 궤양성대장염 / 우울증
man-seong jang jil-hwan / gwe-yang-seong-dae-jang-yeom / u-ul-jeung

RU хроническое заболевание кишечника / язвенный колит / депрессия
khronicheskoe zabolevanie kishechnika / yazvennyi kolit / depressiya

PL przewlekłą chorobę jelit / wrzodziejące zapalenie okrężnicy / depresję

AR المرض المعوي المُزمن \ إلتهاب قولون تقرّحي \ الكآبة
Al-maradh al-mi"awi al-muzmin \ iltihaab qoloun taqarruhiy \ al-ka'aabah

PT doença intestinal crónica / colite ulcerosa / depressão

FK maladi entestin grav / kolit ulsewez (enflamasyon kolon) / depresyon

EL χρόνια εντερική νόσος / ελκώδη κολίτιδα / κατάθλιψη
hrOneea edereekEE nOsos / elkOdee kolEEteeda / katAthleepsee

HI पुराना आंत्र रोग / नासूर जठरशोथ / तनाव...
purana aantra rog / nasoor jaTharshoth / tanaav

diabetes / emphysema / epilepsy / genital disease

ES diabetes / enfisema / epilepsia / enfermedad de los genitales

ZH 糖尿病 / 肺气肿 / 颠痫 / 生殖性疾病
táng niào bìng / fèi qì zhǒng / diān xián / shēng zhí xìng jí bìng

FR diabète / emphysème / épilepsie / maladie génitale

DE Diabetes / Emphysem / Epilepsie / Erkrankung der Geschlechtsorgane

VI bệnh tiểu đường / khí thũng / chứng động kinh / bệnh liên quan tới cơ quan sinh dục

IT diabete / enfisema / epilessia / malattia genitale

KO 당뇨병 / 폐기종 / 간질 / 생식기 질환
dang-nyo-byeong / pye-gi-jong / gan-jil / saeng-sik-gi jil-hwan

RU диабет / эмфизема / эпилепсия / заболевание половых органов
diabet / emfizema / epilepsiya / zabolevanie polovykh organov

PL cukrzycę / rozedmę / padaczkę / schorzenie genitaliów

AR مرض السكّر \ مرض النفاخ \ مرض الصرع \ مرض تناسلي
Maradh as-sukkar \ maradh an-nifaakh \ maradh as-sar" \ maradh tanaasuli

PT diabetes / enfisema / epilepsia / doença genital

FK sik / anfizem / epilipsi / maladi jenital

EL διαβήτης / εμφύσημα / επιληψία / ασθένεια γεννητικών οργάνων
deeavEEtees / emfEEseema / epeeleepsEEa / asthEneea geneeteekOn orgAnon

HI म ऽ ुमेह / वातस्फीति / मिरगी / जननइन्द्रिय...
madhumeh / vatsphiti / mirgi / jananindriya

gallstones / jaundice / gout / hepatitis (liver inflammation)

ES	cálculos biliares / ictericia / gota / hepatitis (inflamación del hígado)
ZH	胆结石 / 黄疸 / 痛风 / 肝炎（肝部发炎） dǎn jié shí / huáng dǎn / tòng fēng / gān yán (gān bù fā yán)
FR	calculs biliaires / ictère / goutte / hépatite (inflammation du foie)
DE	Gallensteine / Gelbsucht / Gicht / Hepatitis (Leberentzündung)
VI	sỏi mật / bệnh vàng da / bệnh gút (thống phong) / bệnh viêm gan
IT	calcoli / itterizia / gotta / epatite (infiammazione del fegato)
KO	담석 / 황달 / 통풍 / 간염(간 염증) dam-seok / hwang-dal / tong-pung / gan-nyeom(gan yeom-jung)
RU	желчные камни / желтуха / подагра / гепатит (воспаление печени) zhelchnye kamni / zheltukha / podagra / gepatit (vospalenie pecheni)
PL	kamienie żółciowe / żółtaczkę / podagrę / zapalenie wątroby
AR	حصى كيس الصفراء \ اليرقان \ مرض النقرس \ إلتهاب الكبد Hasaa kees as-safraa' \ al-yarqaan \ maradh an-naqras \ iltihaab al-kabad
PT	cálculos biliares / icterícia / gota / hepatite (inflamação do fígado)
FK	woch nan vesikil bilye / la jonis / goutt / hepatitis (enflamasyon nan fwa)
EL	χολόλιθος / ίκτερος / ποδάγρα / ηπατίτιδα (ηπατική φλεγμονή) holOleethos / EEkteros / podAgra / eepatEEteeda (eepateekEE flegmonEE)
HI	गलस्टोन / पीलिया / गठिया / हेपेटाइटिस (यकृत जलन)... gallstones / peeliya / gathiya / hepatitis (yakrit jalan)

heart disease / heart defect (cardiac pacemaker) / heart attack

ES enfermedad cardíaca / defectos del ritmo (marcapasos) / ataque cardíaco

ZH 心脏病 / 心功能不全(心脏起搏器) / 心肌梗塞
xīn zàng bìng / xīn gōng néng bù quán (xīn zàng qǐ bó qì) / xīn jī gěng sè

FR maladie du coeur, déficience cardiaque (pacemaker) / attaque cardiaque

DE Herzerkrankung / Herzfehler (Herzschrittmacher) / Herzinfarkt

VI bệnh tim / loạn nhịp tim (máy điều hòa nhịp tim) / nhồi máu cơ tim

IT malattia cardiaca / difetto del ritmo cardiaco (pacemaker) / attacco cardiaco

KO 심장 질환 / 심장 결함(인공 심박 조율기) / 심장 발작
sim-jang jil-hwan / sim-jang gyeol-ham(in-gong sim-bak jo-yul-gi) / sim-jang bal-jak

RU заболевание сердца / порок сердца (кардиостимулятор) / инфаркт миокрада
zabolevanie serdtsa / porok serdtsa (kardiostimulyator) / infarkt miokrada

PL chorobę serca / wadę serca (rozrusznik serca) / zawał serca

AR مرض القلب \ عيب قلب (منظّم قلب) \ نوبة قلبية
Maradh il-qalb \ "ayb qalb (munadhdhim qalb) \ naubah qalbiyyah

PT doença cardíaca / defeito cardíaco (pacemaker cardíaco) / ataque cardíaco

FK maladi kè / pwoblèm kè (aparèy pace maker) / kriz kadyak

EL καρδιοπάθεια / καρδιακή ανωμαλία (καρδιακό βηματοδότη) / καρδιακή προσβολή
kardeeopAtheea / kardeeakEE anomalEEa (kardeeakO veematodOtee) / kardeeakEE prosvolEE

HI दिल की बीमारी / दिल मैं दोष (दिल के लिये पैस मैकर) / दिल का दौरा
Dil ki biimaari / Dil meyn dosh (dil ke liye peys mekar) / Dil ka douraa

heart failure / pulse irregularities / HIV / colorectal polyps

ES insuficiencia cardíaca / pulso irregular / VIH / pólipos colorrectales

ZH 心脏衰竭 / 脉搏不齐 / 艾滋病毒阳性 / 直结肠息肉
xīn zàng shuāi jié / mài bó bù qí / ài zī bìng dú yáng xìng / zhí jié cháng xī ròu

FR insuffisance cardiaque / pouls irrégulier / HIV / polypes colo-rectaux

DE Herzinsuffizienz / Herzrhythmusstörungen / HIV / kolorektale Polypen

VI suy tim / nhịp mạch đập bất thường / HIV / u kết tràng

IT collasso cardiaco / irregolarità del polso / HIV / polipi colorettali

KO 심장 마비 / 맥박 이상 / 인체 면역 결핍 바이러스(HIV) / 결장직장의 폴립
sim-jang ma-bi / maek-bak i-sang / in-che myeon-nyeok gyeol-pip ba-i-reo-seu(HIV) / gyeol-jang-jik-jang-ui pol-lip

RU сердечная недостаточность / нарушения ритма сердца / ВИЧ / полипы ободочной и прямой кишок
serdechnaya nedostatochnost' / narusheniya ritma serdtsa / VICh / polipy obodochnoy i pryamoy kishok

PL niewydolność serca / nieregularne tętno / HIV / polipy jelita grubego

AR عجز القلب \ مخالفات نبض \ إتش آي في \ زوائد لحمية قولونية مستقيمة
"Ajz il-qalb \ mukhaalafaat nabdh \ HIV \ zawaa'id lahmiyyah qoloniyyah mustaqeemiyyah

PT insuficiência cardíaca / irregularidades das pulsações / VIH / pólipos no cólon e no recto

FK kriz kadyak / batman kè w pa nòmal / polip (che) nan kolon

EL καρδιακά ανεπάρκεια / ακανόνιστο παλμό / HIV / πολύτοπόδας παχέως εντέρου
kardeeakEE anepArkeea / akanOneesto palmO / HIV / polEEpodas pahEos edEru

HI हृदय गति रूकना / अनियमित नब्ज / एच्आईवी / कोलोरेक्टल पोलिस...
hridya gati rukna / aniyamit nabz / HIV / colorectal polyps

liver cirrhosis / pulmonary embolism / pneumonia / migraine

ES cirrosis hepática / embolia pulmonar / neumonía / migraña

ZH 肝硬化 / 肺拴塞 / 肺炎 / 偏头痛
gān yìng huà / fèi shuān sāi / fèi yán / piān tóu tòng

FR cirrhose du foie / embolie pulmonaire / pneumonie / migraine

DE Leberzirrhose / Lungenembolie / Lungenentzündung / Migräne

VI bệnh xơ gan / tắc mạch phổi / viêm phổi / chứng đau nửa đầu

IT cirrosi epatica / embolia polmonare / polmonite / emicrania

KO 간경화 / 폐 색전증 / 폐렴 / 편두통
gan-gyeong-hwa / pye saek-jeon-jeung / pye-ryeom / pyeon-du-tong

RU цирроз печени / легочная эмболия / пневмония / мигрень
tsirroz pecheni / legochnaya emboliya / pnevmoniya / migren'

PL marskość wątroby / zator tętnicy płucnej / zapalenie płuc / migrenę

AR تليف الكبد \ جلطة رئوية \ مرض ذات الرئة \ صداع مرض شقيقة
Talayyuf al-kabad \ jultah ri'awiyyah \ maradh dhaat ir-ri'ah \ sudaa' maradh shaqeeqah

PT cirrose do fígado / embolismo pulmonar / pneumonia / enchaqueca

FK siwòz di fwa / anboli pulmonè / nimoni / migrenn

EL κίρρωση ήπατος / πνευμονική εμβολή / πνευμονία / ημικρανία
kEErosee EEpatos / pnevmoneekEE emvolEE / pnevmonEEa / eemeekranEEa

HI यकृत सूत्रणरोग / तपेदिक रक्तशो ६ ान–अवरो ६ ा / निमोनिया / तपेदिक / माइग्रेन...
yakrit sootraNrog / tapedik raktashodhan-avrodh / pneumonia / tapedic / migraine

Crohn's disease / inflammation of the kidney pelvis / kidney stones

ES Enfermedad de Crohn / inflamación de pelvis renal / cálculos (piedras) renales

ZH 克隆病 / 肾盂肾炎 / 肾结石
kè lóng bìng / shèn yú shèn yán / shèn jié shí

FR Maladie de Crohn / inflammation du bassinet du rein / calculs rénaux

DE Morbus Crohn / Nierenbeckenentzündung / Nierensteine

VI Bệnh Crohn / viêm xương chậu vùng thận / sỏi thận

IT Morbo di Crohn / infiammazione della pelvi renale / calcoli renali

KO 크론씨 병 / 신우 염증 / 신장 결석
keu-ron-ssi byeong / sin-u yeom-jeung / sin-jang gyeol-seok

RU Болезнь Крона / воспаление почечной лоханки / почечные камни
Bolezn' Krona / vospalenie pochechnoy lokhanki / pochechnye kamni

PL Chorobę Leśniowskiego-Crohna / zapalenie miedniczek nerkowych / kamicę nerkową

AR مرض كرون \ إلتهاب حوض الكلية \ أحجار الكلية
Maradh Crohn \ iltihaab haudh al-kilyah \ ahjaar al-kilyah

PT doença de Crohn / inflamação do rim ou do pélvis / pedras no rim

FK Maladi Crohn / enflamasyon basin ren an / wòch nan ren

EL νόσος του Crohn / φλεγμονή νεφρικής κοιλότητας ούρων / πέτρες στα νεφρά
nOsos tu Crohn / flegmonEE vefreekEEs keelOteetas Uron / pEtres sta nefrA

HI क्रोन की बीमारी / वृक्क गुर्दे की जलन / गुर्दे की पथरी...
Crohen's ki beemari / vrikk gurde ki jalan / gurde ki pathri

pancreatic disease / prostate disease / rheumatic disease / thyroid disease

ES enfermedad de páncreas / próstata / reumatismo / enfermedad tiroidea

ZH 胰腺疾病 / 前列腺疾病 / 风湿性疾病 / 甲状腺疾病
yí xiàn jí bìng / qián liè xiàn jí bìng / fēng shī xìng jí bìng / jiǎ zhuàng xiàn jí bìng

FR maladies du pancréas / maladies de la prostate / maladies rhumatismales / maladies de la glande thyroïde

DE Pankreas- / Prostataerkrankung / Rheuma / Schilddrüsenerkrankung

VI bệnh tụy / bệnh tiền liệt tuyến / bệnh thấp khớp / bệnh tuyến giáp

IT malattia pancreatica / malattia prostatica / malattia reumatica / malattia della tiroide

KO 췌장 질환 / 전립선 질환 / 류마티스성 질환 / 갑상선 질환
chew-jang jil-hwan / jeol-lip-seon jil-hwan / ryu-ma-ti-seu-seong jil-hwan / gap-sang-seon jil-hwan

RU заболевание поджелудочной железы / заболевание предстательной железы / ревматизм / заболевание щитовидной железы
zabolevanie podzheludochnoy zhelezy / zabolevanie predstatel'noy zhelezy / revmatizm / zabolevanie shchitovidnoy zhelezy

PL chorobę trzustki / chorobę gruczołu krokowego / reumatyzm / chorobę tarczycy

AR مرض البنكرياس \ مرض البروستات \ مرض روماتزمي \ مرض درقّي
Maradh al-bankreas \ maradh al-brostaat \ maradh roumatizmi \ maradh daraqiy

PT doença do pâncreas / doença da próstata / doença reumática / doença da tireóide

FK maladi pankreyas / maladi pwostat / maladi rimatis / maladi tiwòyid

EL παγκρεατική νόσος / νόσος προστάτη / ρευματοπάθεια / νόσος του θυρεοειδούς
pagreateekEE nOsos / nOsos prostAtee / revmatopAtheea / nOsos tu theereoeedUs

HI मल संबंधी बीमारियां / शक्तिक्षय बीमारियां / वातरोग / गलग्रंथि बीमारी...
mall sambandhi beemariyan / shaktikshay beemariyan / vaatrog / galgranthi beemari

stroke / thrombosis / tuberculosis / tumor

ES	embolia / trombosis / tuberculosis / tumores
ZH	中风 / 血栓形成 / 结核病 / 肿瘤 zhòng fēng / xiě shuān xíng chéng / jiē hé bìng / zhǒng liú
FR	apoplexie / thrombose / tuberculose / tumeur
DE	Schlaganfall / Thrombose / Tuberkulose / Tumorerkrankung
VI	đột quỵ / chứng huyết khối / bệnh lao / khối u
IT	ictus / trombosi / tubercolosi / tumore
KO	뇌졸증 / 혈전증 / 결핵 / 종양 noe-jol-jeung / hyeol-jeon-jeung / gyeol-haek / jong-yang
RU	инсульт / тромбоз / туберкулёз / опухоль insul't / tromboz / tuberkulyoz / opukhol'
PL	udar / zakrzepicę / gruźlicę / nowotwór
AR	جلطة دماغية \ التخثّر \ السلّ \ ورم Jultah dimaaghiyah \ at-takhayyur \ as-sull \ waram
PT	acidente vascular cerebral / trombose / tuberculose / tumor
FK	estwok / bòul san / tibekilòz / time
EL	εγκεφαλικό επεισόδιο / θρόμβωση / φυματίωση / όγκος egefaleekO epeesOdeeo / thOmvosee / feematEEosee / Ogos
HI	दौरा पड़ना / घनासता / तपेदिक / फोड़ा daura paDna / ghanasrata / tapedik / phoDa

Do you have a malignant disease? In which area?

ES ¿Tiene alguna enfermedad maligna? ¿En qué parte?

ZH 你有恶性疾病吗？在哪个部位？
nǐ yǒu è xìng jí bìng ma? zài nǎ gè bù wèi?

FR Avez-vous une maladie maligne? Dans quelle région?

DE Haben Sie eine bösartige Erkrankung? Wo?

VI Quý vị có mắc căn bệnh ác tính nào không? Ở vùng nào?

IT Ha una malattia maligna? In quale area?

KO 악성 질환이 있습니까? 어디에 있습니까?
Ak-seong jil-hwan-i it-seum-ni-kka? Eo-di-e it-seum-ni-kka?

RU У вас есть злокачественное заболевание? В какой области?
U vas est' zlokachestvennoe zabolevanie? V kakoy oblasti?

PL Czy ma Pan(i) nowotwór złośliwy? W którym miejscu?

AR هَلْ تعاني \ تعانين من مرض خبيث؟ في أي جزء من جسمك؟
Hal tu"aani \ tu"aaneen min maradh khabeeth? Fi ayyi jiz' min jismak?

PT Sofre de uma doença maligna? Em que sítio?

FK Eske ou gen yon malidi ki grav? Nan ki zon?

EL Έχετε κακοήθη νόσο; Σε ποια περιοχή;
Ehete kakoEEthee nOso? se peeA pereeohEE?

HI क्या आपको कोई गंभीर बीमारी है? किस भाग में ?
kya aapko koi gambheer beemari hai? kis bhaag mein?

Medical Anamnesis

What type of treatment have you received?

ES ¿Qué tipo de tratamiento le han dado?

ZH 你都接受过什么样的治疗？
nǐ dōu jiē shòu guò shén me yàng de zhì liáo?

FR Quel type de traitement avez-vous reçu?

DE Wie sind Sie behandelt worden?

VI Quý vị đã được điều trị bằng phương pháp nào?

IT Che tipo di trattamento ha ricevuto?

KO 어떤 치료를 받으셨습니까?
Eo-tteon chi-ryo-reul ba-deu-syeot-seum-ni-kka?

RU Какое лечение вы получили?
Kakoe lechenie vy poluchili?

PL W jaki sposób był Pan(i) leczony(a)?

AR أي نوع من علاج تلقيته؟
Ayyi nou" min "ilaaj talaqqayteh?

PT Que tipo de tratamento já recebeu?

FK Ki kalite tretman ou te resevwa?

EL Τι είδους θεραπεία λάβατε;
tee EEdus therapEEa lAvate?

HI आपने किस तरह का इलाज करवाया?
aapne kis tarah ka ilaaz karvaya?

surgery / radiation therapy / chemotherapy / naturopathic treatment

ES	cirugía / radioterapia / quimioterapia / medicina naturista
ZH	手术 / 放射治疗 / 化疗 / 自然疗法 shǒu shù / fàng shè zhì liáo / huà liáo / zì rán liáo fǎ
FR	chirurgie / radiothérapie / chimiothérapie / traitement homéopathique
DE	Operation / Bestrahlung / Chemotherapie / Naturheilkunde
VI	phẫu thuật / phóng xạ trị liệu / hóa học trị liệu / nhiên liệu pháp
IT	operazione chirurgica / radioterapia / chemioterapia / trattamento naturopatico
KO	수술 / 방사능 치료 / 화학요법 / 자연 요법 치료 su-sul / bang-sa-neung chi-ryo / hwa-hang-nyo-beop / ja-yeon yo-beop chi-ryo
RU	операция / лучевая терапия / химиотерапия / натуропатическое лечение operatsiya / luchevaya terapiya / khimioterapiya / naturopaticheskoe lechenie
PL	(poprzez) operację / radioterapię / chemoterapię / naturopatię
AR	عملية جراحية \ علاج إشعاع \ علاج كيمياوي \ طب دوائي طبيعي "Amaliyyah jaraahiyyah \ "ilaaj ish"aa" \ "ilaaj kimiyaawi / tibb dawaa'ei tabi'ei
PT	cirurgia / terapia de radiação / quimioterapia / tratamento naturopático
FK	operasyon / terapi radyasyon / terapi kimo / tretman natirel
EL	χειρουργική επέμβαση / ακτινοθεραπεία / χημειοθεραπεία / θεραπεία με τη χρήση φυσικών μεθόδων heerurheekEE epEmvasee / akteenotherapEEa / heemeeotherapEEa / therapEEa me tee hrEEsee feeseekOn methOdon
HI	शल्य चिकित्सा / विकरणीय चिकित्सा / रासायनी चिकित्सा / प्राकृतिक चिकित्सा shalya chikitsa / vikiraniye chikitsa / rasayani chikitsa / prakratik chikitsa

Have you ever had any of the following contagious diseases?

¿Ha tenido alguna de las siguientes enfermedades contagiosas?

CH
你得过以下的传染病吗？
nǐ dé guò yǐ xià de chuán rǎn bìng ma?

FR Avez-vous jamais eu aucune des maladies contagieuses suivantes?

DE Hatten Sie jemals eine der folgenden ansteckenden Krankheiten?

VI Quý vị đã bao giờ mắc căn bệnh truyền nhiễm nào sau đây chưa?

IT Ha mai avuto qualcuna delle seguenti malattie contagiose?

KO
다음의 전염성 질환을 앓으신 적이 있습니까?
Da-eu-mui jeon-yeom-seong jil-hwa-neul a-reu-sin jeo-gi it-seum-ni-kka?

RU
Вы когда-нибудь болели следующими заразными болезнями?
Vy kogda-nibud' boleli sleduyushchimi zaraznymi boleznyami?

PL Czy chorował(a) Pan(i) kiedykolwiek na którąś z następujących chorób zakaźnych?

AR
هل سبق أن اصبت بأية من الأمراض المعدية التالية؟
Hal sabaq an usibt bi-ayyatin min al-amraadh al-mu"diyyah at-taaliyah?

PT Já alguma vez teve qualquer uma das doenças contagiosas seguintes?

FK Eske ou te janm gen yon nan maladi kontaje sa yo?

EL
Είχατε οποιαδήποτε από τις ακόλουθες μεταδοτικές νόσους;
EEhate opeeadEEpote apO tees akOluthes metadoteekEs nOsus?

HI
क्या आपको कभी निम्नलिखित में से कोई छूत की बीमारी हुई है?
kya aapko kabhi nimnlikhit mein se koi Chhoot ki beemaari hui hain?

HIV / AIDS / hepatitis A,B,C,D / tuberculosis / typhus / cholera

ES VIH / SIDA / hepatitis A, B, C, D / tuberculosis / tifus / cólera

ZH 艾滋病毒阳性 / 艾滋病 / 甲肝,乙肝, 丙肝,丁肝 / 结核病 / 斑疹伤寒 / 霍乱
ài zī bìng dú yáng xìng / ài zī bìng / jiǎ gān, yǐ gān, bǐng gān, dīng gān / jié hé bìng / bān zhěn shāng hán / huò luàn

FR VIH / sida / hépatite A, B, C, D / tuberculose / typhus / choléra

DE HIV / AIDS / Hepatitis A,B,C,D / Tuberkulose / Typhus / Cholera

VI HIV / AIDS / viêm gan A,B,C,D / bệnh lao / sốt phát ban / bệnh tả

IT HIV / AIDS / epatite A,B,C,D / tubercolosi / tifo / colera

KO 인체 면역 결핍 바이러스(HIV) / 에이즈 / 간염, A, B, C, D / 결핵 / 발진티푸스 /
콜레라
in-che myeon-yeok gyeol-pip ba-i-reo-seu(HIV) / e-i-jeu / gan-nyeom, A, B, C, D /
gyeol-haek / bal-jin-ti-pu-seu / kol-le-ra

RU ВИЧ / СПИД / гепатит А, В, С, D / туберкулёз / тиф / холера
VICh / SPID / gepatit A, B, C, D / tuberkulyoz / tif / kholera

PL HIV / AIDS / zapalenie wątroby typu A,B,C,D / gruźlicę / dur plamisty / cholerę?

AR مرض الإنش آي في \ الأيدز \ إلتهاب الكبد أ, بي, سي, دي \ مرض السلّ \ مرض التيفوس \ مرض
الكوليرا
Maradh al-HIV / AIDS / iltihaab al-kabad A, B, C, D / maradh as-sull / maradh at-
typhus / maradh al-cholera

PT VIH / SIDA / hepatite A, B, C, D / tuberculose / tifo / cólera

FK VIH / SIDA / hepatit A,B,C,D / tibekilòz / tifoyid / kolera

EL HIV / EITZ / ηπατίτιδα A,B,C,D / φυματίωση / τύφο / χολέρα
HIV / AIDS / eepatEEteeda A,B,C,D / feematEEosee / tEEfo / holEra

HI एचआईवी / एडस / हेपेटाइटिस ए,बी,सी,डी / तपेदिक / टाइफस ज्वर / हैजा...
HIV / AIDS / hepatitis A,B,C,D / tapedik / typhus jwar / haiza

amoebic dysentery / malaria / sleeping sickness / syphilis / gonorrhea

disentería amibiana / malaria / trastornos del sueño / sífilis / gonorrea

阿米巴痢疾 / 疟疾 / 昏睡病 / 梅毒 / 淋病
ā mǐ bā lì jí / nüè jí / hūn shuì bìng / méi dú / lìn bìng

FR dysenterie amibienne / malaria / maladie du sommeil / syphilis / gonorrhée

DE Amöbenruhr / Malaria / Schlafkrankheit / Syphilis / Gonorrhö

VI bệnh kiết lỵ do amíp / bệnh sốt rét / bệnh ngủ / bệnh giang mai / bệnh lậu

IT dissenteria amebica / malaria / malattia del sonno / sifilide / gonorrea

KO 아메바성 적리 / 말라리아 / 수면병 / 매독 / 임질
a-me-ba-seong jeong-ni / mal-la-ria / su-myeon-byeong / mae-dok / im-jil

RU амебная дизентерия / малярия / сонная болезнь / сифилис / гонорея
amebnaya dizenteriya / malyariya / sonnaya bolezn' / sifilis / gonoreya

PL dyzenterię pełzakową / malarię / śpiączkę / syfilis / rzeżączkę

AR الزحار الأميبي \ مرض الملاريا \ مرض النوم \ مرض الزهري \ مرض السيلان
As-zuhaar al-Ameebi / maradh al-malaria / maradh an-naum / maradh az-zuhari /
maradh as-saylaan

PT disenteria amebiana / malária / doença do sono / sífilis / gonorreia

FK move dyare / malaria / maladi domi / siflis (vewòl) / ekoulman

EL αμοιβαδοειδή δυσεντερία / ελονοσία / ασθένεια ύπνου / σύφιλη / βλεννόρροια
ameevadoeedEE deesenderEEa / elonosEEa / asthEneea EEpnu / sEEfeelee /
vlenOreea

HI अमीबाजन्य पेचिस / मलेरिया / अनिद्रा / उपदंश / सुजाक
amibajanya pechis / malaria / anidra / updansh / suzaak

Which vaccinations have you received?

ES ¿Qué vacunas le han aplicado?

ZH 你打过什么疫苗？
nǐ dǎ guò shén me yì miáo?

FR Quels vaccins avez-vous déjà reçus?

DE Welche Impfungen haben Sie erhalten?

VI Quý vị đã được chủng ngừa loại bệnh nào?

IT Che vaccinazioni ha fatto?

KO 어떤 예방주사를 맞으셨습니까?
Eo-tteon ye-bang-ju-sa-reul ma-jeu-syeot-seum-ni-kka?

RU Какие прививки вы получили?
Kakie privivki vy poluchili?

PL Jakie szczepionki Pan(i) przyjmował(a)?

AR ما هي التطعيمات التي تلقيتها؟
Maa hiya at-tat"eemaat ilati talaqqayt'haa?

PT Que vacinas já recebeu?

FK Ki vaksin ke ou resevwa?

EL Ποια εμβόλια λάβατε;
peea emvOleea lAvate?

HI आपने कौन से टीके लगवाए हैं?...
aapne kaunse teeke lagvaye hain?

tetanus / polio / diphtheria / whooping cough / measles / German measles / mumps

tétanos / poliomielitis / difteria / tos ferina / sarampión / rubéola / parotiditis

破伤风 / 脊髓灰质炎 / 白喉 / 百日咳 / 麻疹 / 风疹 / 流行性腮腺炎
pò shāng fēng / jí suǐ huī zhì yán / bái hóu / bǎi rì ké / má zhěn / fēng zhěn / liú xíng xing sāi xiàn yán

FR tétanos / polio / diphtérie / coqueluche / rougeole / rubéole / oreillons

DE Tetanus / Polio / Diphtherie / Keuchhusten / Masern / Röteln / Mumps

VI bệnh uốn ván / bệnh bại liệt / bệnh bạch hầu / ho gà / bệnh sởi / bệnh ban đào / bệnh quai bị

IT tetano / polio / difterite / pertosse / morbillo / rosolia / parotite

KO 파상풍 / 소아마비 / 디프테리아 / 백일해 / 홍역 / 풍진 / 볼거리
pa-sang-pung / so-a-ma-bi / di-peu-te-ri-a / bae-gil-hae / hong-yeok / pung-jin / bol-ge-ri

RU столбняк / полиомиелит / дифтерия / коклюш / корь / краснуха / свинка
stolbnyak / poliomielit / difteriya / koklyush / kor' / krasnukha / svinka

PL przeciw tężcowi / przeciw chorobie Heine-Medina / przeciw błonicy / przeciw kokluszowi / przeciw odrze / przeciw różyczce / przeciw śwince

AR مرض الكزاز \ شلل الأطفال \ دفتريا \ السعال الديكي \ الحصبة \ الحصبة الألمانية \ النكاف
Maradh al-kazaaz / shalal al-atfaal / diftiriya / as-su"aal ad-deeki / al-hasbah / al-hasbah al-'almaaniyah / an-nakaaf

PT tétano / polio / difteria / tosse convulsa / sarampo / rubéola / papeira

FK Tetanos / polio / difteri / koklich / lawoujòl / ti ;awoujòl [woubewòl] / malmouton

EL τέτανος / πολιομυελίτιδα / διφθερίτιδα / κοκκίτις / ιλαρά / ερυθρά / μαγουλάδες
tEtanos / poleeomee-elEEteeda / deeftherEEteeda / kokEEtees / eelarA / ereethrA / magulAdes

HI टिटनस / पोलियो / डिफ्थीरिया / काली खांसी / खसरा / जर्मन खसरा / कनपेड...
tetanus / polio / diphtheria / kaali khansi / khasra / german khasra / kanped

meningitis / hepatitis A,B / yellow fever / cholera

ES	meningitis / hepatitis A, B / fiebre amarilla / cólera
ZH	脑膜炎 / 甲肝，乙肝 / 黄热病 / 霍乱 nǎo mó yán / jiǎ gān, yǐ gān / huáng rè bìng / huò luàn
FR	méningite / hépatite A, B / fièvre jaune / choléra
DE	Meningitis / Hepatitis A,B / Gelbfieber / Cholera
VI	viêm màng não / viêm gan A,B / sốt vàng da / bệnh tả
IT	meningite / epatite A,B / febbre gialla / colera
KO	뇌막염 / 간염 A, B / 황열병 / 콜레라 noe-mag-yeom / gan-nyeom A, B / hwang-yeol-byeong / kol-le-ra
RU	менингит / гепатит А, В / желтая лихорадка / холера meningit / gepatit A, B / zheltaya likhoradka / kholera
PL	przeciw zapaleniu opon mózgowych / przeciw zapaleniu wątroby typu A,B / przeciw żółtej febrze / przeciw cholerze
AR	التهاب السحايا \ التهاب الكبد أ و بى \ الحمى الصفراء \ الكوليرا Iltihaab as-sahaayaa / iltihaab al-kabad A wa B / al-hummaa as-safraa' / al-cholera
PT	meningite / hepatite A, B / febre amarela / cólera
FK	Menenjit / epatit A, B / lafyèv jòn / kolera
EL	μηνιγγίτιδα / ηπατίτιδα A,B / κίτρινος πυρετός / χολέρα meeneegEEteeda / eepatEEteeda A,B / kEEtreenos peeretOs / holEra
HI	गर्दन तोड़ बुखार / हेपेटाइटिस ए,बी / पीला बुखार / हैजा gardan toD bukhaar / hepatitis A,B / peela bukhaar / haiza

Medication

Are you presently taking any medication?

¿Toma medicamentos actualmente?

你目前使用什么药呢？
nǐ mù qián shǐ yòng shén me yào ne?

FR Prenez-vous des médicaments pour le moment?

DE Nehmen Sie derzeit irgendein Medikament?

VI Quý vị hiện có đang dùng thuốc men gì không?

IT Al momento presente sta assumendo farmaci?

KO 현재 드시는 약이 있습니까?
Hyeon-jae deu-si-neun ya-gi it-seum-ni-kka?

RU Вы сейчас принимаете какое-либо лекарство?
Vy seychas prinimaete kakoe-libo lekarstvo?

PL Czy przyjmuje Pan(i) obecnie jakiekolwiek leki?

AR هل تأخذ \ تأخذين اي دواء في الوقت الحاضر؟
Hal ta'khudh / ta'khudeen ayyi dawaa' fil-waqt il-haadhir?

PT Actualmente, está a tomar algum medicamento?

FK Eske ou ap pran medikan kounye la?

EL Λαμβάνετε επί του παρόντος φάρμακα;
lamvAnete epEE tu parOdos fArmaka?

HI क्या अभी आप कोई दवा ले रहे हैं?
kya Abhi aap koi davaa le rahe hain?

Please show me the medication packaging

ES	Por favor muéstreme las cajitas o envases
ZH	请让我看一下药的包装 qǐng ràng wǒ kàn yī xià yào de bāo zhuāng
FR	S'il vous plaît, montrez-moi l'emballage de ce médicament
DE	Zeigen Sie mir die Packung
VI	Xin cho tôi xem bao gói thuốc
IT	La prego di mostrarmi la confezione del farmaco
KO	약 포장지를 보여주십시오 yak po-jang-ji-reul bo-yeo-ju-sip-si-o
RU	Покажите, пожалуйста, упаковку лекарства Pokazhite, pozhaluysta, upakovku lekarstva
PL	Proszę mi pokazać opakowanie leku
AR	رجاءاً ارني \ اريني غلاف الدواء Rajaa'an arini / areeni ghilaaf ad-dawaa'
PT	Mostre-me, por favor, a embalagem do medicamento
FK	Tanpri montre m anbalaj medikaman an
EL	Παρακαλώ δείξτε μου τη συσκευασία φαρμάκου parakalO dEExte mu tee seeskevasEEa farmAku
HI	कृपया मुझे दवा का पैकेट दिखाएं kripya mujhe davaa ka packet dikhaein

Please write down the name of the medication

Por favor anóteme el nombre del medicamento

请写下该药的名称
qǐng xiě xià gāi yào de míng chēng

FR S'il vous plaît, écrivez le nom du médicament.

DE Schreiben Sie bitte den Namen des Medikaments auf

VI Xin viết cho tôi tên của loại thuốc đó

IT La prego di scrivere il nome del farmaco

KO 약 이름을 적어 주십시오
Yak i-reu-meul jeo-geo ju-sip-si-o

RU Пожалуйста, напишите название лекарства
Pozhaluysta, napishite nazvanie lekarstva

PL Proszę zapisać nazwę leku

AR رجاءاً إكتب \ اكتبي اسم الدواء
Rajaa'an iktib / iktibee ism ad-dawaa'

PT Escreva, por favor, o nome do medicamento

FK Tanpri ekri non medikaman an

EL Παρακαλώ γράψτε την ονομασία φαρμάκου
parakalO grApste teen onomasEEa farmAku

HI कृपया दवा का नाम लिखें
kripya davaa ka naam likhein

How do you take this medication? When? How often?

ES ¿Cómo toma el medicamento? ¿Cuándo? ¿Con qué frecuencia?

ZH 你是怎么用药的？ 什么时间？多久一次？
nǐ shì zěn me yòng yào de? shén me shí jiān? duō jiǔ yī cì?

FR Comment prenez-vous ce médicament? Depuis quand? Combien de fois?

DE Wie nehmen Sie dieses Medikament? Wann? Wie oft?

VI Quý vị dùng loại thuốc này như thế nào? Khi nào? Bao nhiêu lâu dùng một lần?

IT Come prende questo farmaco? Quando? Quanto spesso?

KO 어떻게 이 약을 드십니까? 언제? 얼마나 자주?
Eo-tteo-ke i ya-geul deu-sim-ni-kka? Eon-je? Eol-ma-na ja-ju?

RU Как вы принимаете это лекарство? Когда? Как часто?
Kak vy prinimaete eto lekarstvo? Kogda? Kak chasto?

PL Jak Pan(i) przyjmuje ten lek? Kiedy? Jak często?

AR كيفَ تَأخذ \ تأخذين هذا الدواء؟ متى؟ كم مرة؟
Kayf ta'khudh / ta'khudheen hadhaa ad-dawaa'? Mattaa? Kam marrah?

PT Como toma este medicamento? Quando? Quantas vezes?

FK Kijan ou pran medikaman sa a? A kil è ? Konbyen fwa?

EL Πώς λαμβάνετε αυτά τα φάρμακα; Πότε; Πόσο συχνά;
pos lamvAnete aftA ta fArmaka? pOte? pOso seehnA?

HI आप यह दवा किस प्रकार लेते हैं? कब? कितनी बार? ...
Aap yeh davaa kis prakaar lete haïn? Kab? Kitni bar?

tables / drops / capsules / suppositories / ointment / injection / infusion

| ES | pastillas / gotas / cápsulas / supositorios / pomada / inyección / solución intravenosa |

ES pastillas / gotas / cápsulas / supositorios / pomada / inyección / solución intravenosa

ZH 片剂 / 滴剂 / 胶囊 / 栓剂 / 膏剂 / 针剂 / 浸剂
piàn jì / dī jì / jiāo náng / shuān jì / gāo jì / zhēn jì / jìn jì

FR comprimés / gouttes / capsules / suppositoires / onguent / injection / infusion

DE Tabletten / Tropfen / Kapseln / Zäpfchen / Salbe / Injektion / Infusion

VI thuốc viên / thuốc rò / viên con nhộng / thuốc đạn / thuốc mỡ / tiêm / truyền

IT compresse / gocce / capsule / supposte / pomata / iniezione / infusione

KO 정제 / 방울 / 캡슐 / 좌약 / 연고 / 주사 / 링겔
jeong-je / bang-ul / kaep-syul / jwa-yak / yeon-go / ju-sa / ring-gel

RU таблетки / капли / капсулы / свечи / мазь / инъекция / инфузия
tabletki / kapli / kapsuly / svechi / maz' / in"ektsiya / infuziya

PL tabletki / krople / kapsułki / czopki / maść / zastrzyki / napar

AR بالمناضد / بالقطرات / بالكبسولات / بالتحاميل / بالمرهم / بالحقن / بالصبّ
Bil-manaadhid / bil-qutraat / bil-kabsoulaat / bit-tahaamil / bil-marham / bil-huqan / bis-sabb

PT comprimidos / drageias / cápsulas / supositórios / pomada / injecção / infusão

FK Tab / gout / kapsil (grenn) / sipozitwa / pomade / piki / infizyon

EL δισκία / σταγόνες / κάψουλες / υπόθετα / αλοιφή / ένεση / έγχυση
deeskEEa / stagOnes / kApsules / eepOtheta / aleefEE / Enesee / Egheesee

HI गोलियां / बूंदें / कैप्सूल / सपॉजिटरीज / मरहम / इंजेक्शन / निषेचन...
Goliyan / bunde / capsules / suppositories / marham / injection / niShechan

1 / 2 / 3 times daily / every ... hours

ES 1 / 2 / 3 veces al día / cada ... horas

ZH 一天一次 / 一天两次 / 一天三次 / 几小时一次
yī tiān yī cì / yī tiān liǎng cì / yī tiān sān cì / jǐ xiǎo shí yī cì

FR 1 / 2 / 3 fois par jour / toutes les ... heures

DE 1 / 2 / 3 mal täglich / alle ... Stunden

VI 1 / 2 / 3 lần hàng ngày / ... giờ một lần

IT 1 / 2 / 3 / volte al giorno / ogni ... ore

KO 매일 1 / 2 / 3 번 / ... 시간 마다 한번
mae-il han / du / se beon / ... si-gan ma-da han-beon

RU 1 / 2 / 3 раза в день / каждые ... часа(часов)
1 / 2 / 3 raza v den' / kazhdye ... chasa(chasov)

PL 1 / 2 / 3 / razy dziennie / co ... godzin

AR مرة \ مرتان \ ٣١ مرات يومياً \ كُلّ __ ساعة
Marrah / marrataan / thalaath marraat yaumiyyan / kulli __ saa"ah

PT 1 /2 / 3 vezes por dia / cada ... horas

FK 1 / 2 / 3 fwa pa jou / chak ... hètan

EL 1 / 2 / 3 φορές την ημέρα / κάθε ... ώρες
mEEa / dEEo / trees forEs teen eemEra / kAthe ... Ores

HI 1 / 2 / 3 बार प्रतिदिन / प्रत्येक...घंटे
1 / 2 / 3 baar pratidin / pratyek ... ghante

Have you taken the medication today?

ES ¿Hoy tomó el medicamento?

ZH 你今天吃这些药了吗？
nǐ jīn tiān chī zhè xie yào le ma?

FR Avez-vous pris ce médicament aujourd'hui?

DE Haben Sie das Medikament heute genommen?

VI Hôm nay, quý vị đã dùng thuốc chưa?

IT Oggi ha preso il farmaco?

KO 오늘 약 드셨습니까?
On-eul yak deu-syeot-seum-ni-kka?

RU Вы принимали сегодня лекарство?
Vy prinimali segodnya lekarstvo?

PL Czy przyjmował(a) Pan(i) dzisiaj ten lek?

AR هل أخذت الدواء اليوم؟
Hal akhadht ad-dawaa' al-youm?

PT Já tomou o medicamento hoje?

FK Eske ou pran medikaman an jodia?

EL Λάβατε τα φάρμακα σήμερα;
lAvate ta fAarmaka sEEmera?

HI क्या आपने आज दवा ली?
kya aapne aaj davaa lee?

Have you taken your medication on a regular basis?

ES ¿Ha tomado el medicamento regularmente?

ZH 这是你的常规药吗？
zhè shì nǐ de cháng guī yào ma?

FR Prenez-vous ce médicament régulièrement?

DE Haben Sie Ihr Medikament regelmäßig genommen?

VI Quý vị có dùng thuốc đều đặn không?

IT Ha preso il Suo farmaco regolarmente?

KO 정기적으로 약을 드셨습니까?
Jeong-gi-jeo-geu-ro ya-geul deu-syeot-seum-ni-kka?

RU Вы регулярно принимаете ваше лекарство?
Vy regulyarno prinimaete vashe lekarstvo?

PL Czy przyjmuje Pan(i) ten lek regularnie?

AR هَلْ أخذت دوائك بشكل متكرر؟
Hal akhadht dawaa'ak bishakl mutakarrir?

PT Tem tomado o seu medicamento com regularidade?

FK Eske ou pran medikaman w lan sou yon baz regilye?

EL Λαμβάνετε τα φάρμακά σας τακτικά;
lamvAnete ta fArmakA sas takteekA?

HI क्या आपने नियमित रूप से अपनी दवा ली है?
Kya aapne niyamit roop se apni davaa lee hai?

Have you ever experienced drug intolerance? Specify

ES	¿Ha tenido intolerancia a algún medicamento? Especifique
ZH	以前用药有没有副作用发生？请说明是什么 yǐ qián yòng yào yǒu méi yǒu fù zuò yòng fā shēng? qǐng shuō míng shì shén me
FR	Avez-vous fait l'expérience d'une intolérance à un médicament? Veuillez spécifier.
DE	Haben Sie ein Medikament einmal nicht vertragen? Welches?
VI	Quý vị đã bao giờ gặp phải tình trạng không dung nạp được thuốc chưa? Xin trình bày cụ thể
IT	Ha mai sofferto di intolleranza ad un farmaco? Specificare
KO	약 부작용을 경험한 적이 있습니까? 구제척으로 명시하십시오 Yak bu-ja-gyong-eul gyeong-heom-han jeo-gi it-seum-ni-kka? Gu-che-je-geu-ro myeong-si-ha-sip-si-o
RU	Проявилась ли у вас непереносимость к какому-нибудь лекарству? Уточните Proyavilas' li u vas neperenosimost' k kakomu-nibud' lekarstvu? Utochnite
PL	Czy doświadczał(a) Pan(i) kiedykolwiek nietolerancji jakiegoś leku? Proszę to bliżej opisać
AR	هل سبق لك تعصب جسمك لدواء من الأدوية؟ بين \ بيني بالتفصيل Hal sabaq lak ta"assub jismak li-dawaa' min al-adwiyyah? Bayyin / bayyinee at-tafaaseel
PT	Já alguma vez sentiu intolerância a um medicamento? Especifique
FK	Eske ou janm santi yon intolerans medikaman? Spesifye
EL	Είχατε ποτέ δυσανεξία σε φάρμακο; Καθορίστε EEhate potE deesanexEEa se fArmako? kathorEEste
HI	क्या आपने कभी दवा की असहनशीलता का अनुभव किया? वर्णन करें kya aapne kabhi davaa ki asahansheelta ka anubhav kiya? varNan karein

6 Allergies

Are you allergic to something?

ES	¿Es usted alérgico a algo?
ZH	你对什么东西过敏吗？ nǐ duì shén me dōng xī guò mǐn ma?
FR	Etes-vous allergique à quelque chose?
DE	Sind Sie gegen irgendetwas allergisch?
VI	Quý vị có dị ứng với thứ gì không?
IT	Lei è allergico a qualcosa?
KO	알레르기가 있으십니까? al-le-reu-gi-ga i-seu-sim-ni-kka?
RU	У вас есть аллергия на что-либо? U vas est' allergiya na chto-libo?
PL	Czy jest Pan(i) na cokolwiek uczulony(a)?
AR	هل عندك حساسية لشيء؟ Hal "indak / indik hassaasiyyah li-shey'?
PT	É alérgico(a) a algo?
FK	Eske ou fè aleji ak okenn bagay?
EL	Είστε αλλεργικοί σε κάτι; EEste alergeekEE se kAtee?
HI	क्या आपको किसी चीज से एलर्जी है? ... Kya aapko kisi cheez se alarzi hai?

Medications / penicillin / food products / pollen / animals / latex / band-aids

ES Medicamentos / penicilina / alimentos / polen / animales / látex / banditas adhesivas (curitas)

ZH 药品 / 青霉素 / 食品 / 花粉 / 动物 / 乳胶品 / 绷带
yào pǐn / qīng méi sù / shí pǐn / huā fěn / dòng wù / rǔ jiāo pǐn / bēng dài

FR à des médicaments / à la pénicilline / à des produits alimentaires / à du pollen / à des animaux / à du latex / à du sparadrap

DE Medikament / Penicillin / Lebensmittel / Pollen / Tiere / Latex / Pflaster

VI Thuốc men / penicillin / thực phẩm / phấn hoa / thú vật / cao su / băng dán y tế

IT Farmaci / penicillina, alimenti / polline / animali / lattice / cerotti

KO 약 / 페니실린 / 식품 / 꽃가루 / 동물 / 라텍스 / 반창고
yak / pe-ni-sil-lin / sik-pum / kkot-ga-ru / dong-mul / ra-tek-seu / ban-chang-go

RU Лекарства / пенициллин / продукты питания / пыльца / животные / латекс / лейкопластырь
Lekarstva / penitsillin / produkty pitaniya / pyl'tsa / zhivotnye / lateks / leikoplastyr'

PL Leki / penicylinę / potrawy / pyłek kwiatowy / zwierzęta / lateks / plastry

AR الأدوية \ البنسلين \ المنتوجات الغذائية \ حبوب اللقاح \ الحيوانات \ مادة اللاتيكس \ الضمادات
Al-adwiyah \ al-penicillin \ al-mantoujaat al-ghadhaa'iyah \ huboob al-liqaah \ al-haywaanaat \ maadah al-latex \ adh-dhamaadaat

PT Medicamentos / penicilina / produtos alimentares / pólen / animais / látex / pensos adesivos

FK Medikaman / penisilinn / pwodwi manje / pollen / bèt / lateks / pansman

EL Φάρμακα / πενικιλίνη / τροφίμα / γύρη / ζώα / λάτεξ / λευκοπλάστ
fArmaka / peneekeelEEnee / trOfeema / gEEree / zOa / lAtex / lefkoplAst

HI औषि ८ करण / पेंसिलीन / भोजन उत्पाद / पराग / जंतु / वानस्पतिक दु र ८ ८ / बैंड–एड ...
AushdhikaraN / penicillin / bhojanutpaad / parag / jantu / vanispatikdugdh / band-aid

Insect stings / iodine / x-ray contrast agents / preservatives

ES Picaduras de insectos / yodo / agentes radiopacos / conservadores

ZH 虫叮 / 碘 / x 光照影剂 / 保鲜剂
chóng dīng / diǎn / x guāng zhào yǐng jì / bǎo xiān jì

FR à des piqûres d'insectes / à l'iode / aux agents de contraste pour la radiologie / à des agents de conservation

DE Insektenstiche / Jod / Röntgenkontrastmittel / Konservierungsstoffe

VI Vết côn trùng cắn / Iot / chất làm tương phản khi chụp X quang / các chất bảo quản

IT Punture di insetti / iodio / mezzi di contrasto per raggi X / conservanti

KO 곤충에 물린 데 / 요오드 / 엑스레이 조영제 / 방부제
gon-chung-e mul-lin de / yo-o-deu / ek-seu-re-i jo-yeong-je / bang-bu-je

RU Укусы насекомых / йод / рентгеноконтрастные вещества / консерванты
Ukusy nasekomykh / yod / rentgenokontrastnye veshchestva / konservanty

PL Ukąszenia owadów / jodynę / odczynniki kontrastu rentgena / konserwanty

AR لدغات الحشرات \ اليود \ مواد التباين الكيمياوية للتصوير الشعاعي \ المواد الواقية من الفساد
Ladghaat al-hasharaat / al-yod / mawwaad at-tabaayun al-kimyaawiyah lit-tasweer ash-shu'aa'iy / al-mawwaad al-waaqiyah min al-fasaad

PT Picadas de insectos / iodo / agentes de contraste de raios X / conservantes

FK Lè ensekt pike w / iyod / ajan kontras radyografi / pwodwo presevasyon

EL Τσιμπήματα εντόμων / ιώδιο / σκιαγραφικές ουσίες ακτινογραφίας / συντηρητικά
tseebEEmata edOmon / eeOdeeo / skeeagrafeekEs usEEes

HI कीट दंश / आयोडीन / एक्स-रे कंट्रास्ट एजेंट / रासायनिक पदार्थ
Keetdans / iodine / x-ray conatrast agents / rasaynik padartha

What are the resulting symptoms?

ES	¿Qué síntomas se producen?
ZH	会是什么变化？ huì shì shén me biàn huà?
FR	Quels sont les symptômes qui en ont résulté?
DE	Welche Symptome haben Sie dann?
VI	Bệnh đó gây ra các triệu chứng nào?
IT	Quali sono i sintomi?
KO	결과되는 증상은 무엇입니까? gyeol-gwa-doe-neun jeung-sang-eun mu-eo-sim-ni-kka?
RU	Какими симптомами это проявляется? Kakimi simptomami eto proyavlyaetsya?
PL	Jakie powodują objawy?
AR	ما هي الأعراض الناتجة عن الحساسية؟ Maa hiya al-a'araadh an-naatijah 'an al-hassaasiyah?
PT	Quais são os sintomas resultantes?
FK	Ki sentòm ou genyen?
EL	Τι συμπτώματα προκύπτουν; tee seemptOmata prokEEptun?
HI	इसके परिणामी लक्षण क्या हैं? ... Iske pariNami lakshaN kya hai?

Rash / itching / breathing problems / asthma / hay fever

ES Erupción / comezón / dificultad para respirar / asma / fiebre del heno

ZH 皮肤红疹 / 痒 / 呼吸困难 / 哮喘 / 花粉热
pí fū hóng zhěn / yǎng / hū xī kùn nán / xiào chuǎn / huā fěn rè

FR une éruption / des démangeaisons / des problèmes respiratoires / de l'asthme / un rhume des foins

DE Hautausschlag / Juckreiz / Atemprobleme / Asthma / Heuschnupfen

VI Nổi mẩn / ngứa / các vấn đề về hô hấp / bệnh suyễn / sốt phát ban

IT Arrossamento / prurito / problemi respiratori / asma / febbre da fieno

KO 발진 / 가려움 / 호흡 곤란 / 천식 / 건초열
bal-jin / ga-ryeo-um / ho-heup gol-lan / cheon-sik / geon-cho-yeol

RU Сыпь / зуд / проблемы с дыханием / астма / сенная лихорадка
Syp' / zud / problemy s dykhaniem / astma / sennaya likhoradka

PL Wysypkę / swędzenie / trudności z oddychaniem / astmę / gorączkę sienną

AR الطفح الجلدي \ الحك \ إضطرابات في التنفس \ الربو \ حمى القش
At-tafah al-jildi / al-hakk / idhtiraabaat fit-tanaffus / ar-rabou / hummaa al-qashsh

PT Erupção cutânea / comichão / problemas respiratórios / asma / febre dos fenos

FK Erupsyon po / pwoblem respirasyon / opresyon / rim nan nen

EL Εξάνθημα / φαγούρα / αναπνευστικά προβλήματα / άσθμα / αλλεργική ρινίτιδα
exAnteema / fagUra / anapnefsteekA provlEEmata / Asthma / allergeekEE reenEEteeda

HI चकत्ता / खारिश / सांस लेने में परेशानी / दमा / परागज बुखार ...
Chakatta / kharish / sans lene me pareshani / dama / paragaj bukhaar

Collapse / shock / nausea / vomiting / abdominal pain / diarrhea

ES Colapso / choque / náusea / vómito / dolor abdominal / diarrea

ZH 崩溃感 / 休克 / 恶心 / 呕吐 / 腹痛 / 腹泻
bēng kuì gǎn / xiū kè / ě xīn / ǒu tù / fù tòng / fù xiè

FR Un collapsus / un choc / des nausées / un vomissement / des douleurs abdominales / de la diarrhée

DE Kollaps / Schock / Übelkeit / Erbrechen / Bauchschmerzen / Durchfall

VI Suy sụp / sốc / buồn nôn / ói mửa / đau bụng / tiêu chảy

IT Collasso / shock / nausea / vomito / dolore addominale / diarrea

KO 쓰러짐 / 쇼크 / 매스꺼움 / 구토 / 복통 / 설사
sseu-reo-jim / syo-keu / mae-seu-kkeo-um / gu-to / bok-tong / seol-sa

RU Коллапс / шок / тошнота / рвота / боль в животе / понос
Kollaps / shok / toshnota / rvota / bol' v zhivote / ponos

PL Zapaść / szok / mdłości / wymioty / ból brzucha / biegunkę

AR الإنهيار العصبي \ الصدمة \ الغثيان \ القيء \ الأوجاع البطنية \ الإسهال
Al-inhiyaar al-asabi / as-sadmah / al-ghathayaan / al-qay' / al-awjaa' al-batniyah / al-is'haal

PT Colapso / choque / náusea / vómitos / dores abdominais / diarreia

FK Tonbe / chok / noze / vomisman / doulè nan vant / dyare

EL Κατάρρευση / καταπληξία / ναυτία / εμετός / κοιλιακός πόνος / διάρροια
katArefsee / katapleexEEa / naftEEa / emetOs / keeleeakOs pOnos / deeAreea

HI हिम्मत हारना / सदमा / नज़ला / उल्टी / पेट दर्द / अतिसार
Himmat harna / sadma / najala / ulti / petdard / atisaar

7 Social Anamnesis

Are you married?

ES ¿Es usted casado (m) / casada (f)?

ZH 你结婚了吗？
nǐ jié hūn le ma?

FR Etes-vous marié(e)?

DE Sind Sie verheiratet?

VI Quý vị đã lập gia đình chưa?

IT È sposato / a?

KO 결혼하셨습니까?
Gyeol-hon-ha-syeot-seum-ni-kka?

RU Вы женаты / замужем?
Vy zhenaty / zamuzhem?

PL Czy jest Pan(i) żonaty (zamężna)?

AR هل أنت متزوج \ متزوجة؟
Hal inta (male) / inti (female) mutazawwij / mutazawwijah?

PT É casado(a)?

FK Eske ou marye?

EL Είστε παντρεμένος / η;
EEste pandremEnos / ee?

HI क्या आप विवाहित हैं?
Kya aap vivahit hain?

Do you have children? How many? How old?

ES ¿Tiene hijos? ¿Cuántos? ¿De qué edad?

ZH 你有孩子吗？几个？几岁了？
nǐ yǒu hái zi ma? jǐ ge? jǐ suì le?

FR Avez-vous des enfants? Combien? Quel âge?

DE Haben Sie Kinder? Wieviele? Wie alt?

VI Quý vị có con không? Bao nhiêu người con? Tuổi?

IT Ha figli? Quanti? Che età hanno?

KO 자녀가 있으십니까? 몇 명입니까? 몇 살입니까?
Ja-nyeo-ga i-seu-sim-ni-kka? Myeot myeong-im-ni-kka? Myeot sa-rim-ni-kka?

RU У вас есть дети? Сколько? Сколько им лет?
U vas est' deti? Skol'ko? Skol'ko im let?

PL Czy ma Pan(i) dzieci? Ile? W jakim wieku?

AR هل عندك أطفال؟ كم منهم؟ كم عمرهم؟
Hal "indak atfaal? Kam minhum? Kam "umrhum?

PT Tem filhos? Quantos? Que idade têm?

FK Eske ou gen pitit? Konbyen? Ki laj yo?

EL Έχετε παιδιά; Πόσα; Πόσο χρονών;
Ehete pedeeA? pOsa? pOso hronOn?

HI क्या आपके बच्चे हैं? कितने? कितनी उम्र के?
Kya aapke bachche hain? kitne? Kitni umra ke?

Do you live alone / in a nursing home

.S ¿Vive solo / sola / en una clínica de reposo?

.H 你是自己住 / 住在养老院？
nǐ shì zì jǐ zhù / zhù zài yǎng lǎo yuàn?

.R Vivez-vous seul(e)? dans une institution de soins?

DE Leben Sie alleine / im Altersheim?

VI Quý vị sống một mình / tại nhà điều dưỡng

IT Vive solo / a / in una casa di riposo?

KO 혼자 / 유료 양로원에서 사십니까?
Hon-ja / yu-ryo yang-nyo-won-e-seo sa-sim-ni-kka?

RU Вы живете сами / в доме престарелых
Vy zhivete sami / v dome prestarelykh

PL Czy mieszka Pan(i) sam(a) / w domu opieki społecznej

AR هل تعيش \ تعيشين لوحدك \ في دار عناية الكبار
Hal ta"eesh / ta"eesheen li-wahdak / fi daar "inaayah al-kibaar

PT Vive só / num lar para a terceira idade

FK Eske ou viv pou kont ou / nan yon sant retret

EL Ζείτε μόνος / η / σε οίκο ευγηρίας
zEEte mOnos / ee / se EEko evgeerEEas

HI क्या आप अकेले / नर्सिंग होम में रहते हैं
Kya aap akele / nursing home mein rahte hain

What is your profession? Are you ...

ES ¿A qué se dedica? ¿Es usted ... ?

ZH 你的职业是什么？你是 ...
nǐ de zhí yè shì shén me? nǐ shì ...

FR Quelle est votre profession? Etes-vous ... ?

DE Was arbeiten Sie? Sind Sie ...

VI Quý vị làm nghề gì? Quý vị là ...

IT Quale è la Sua professione? È ...

KO 직업이 무엇입니까? ... 이십니까?
Ji-geo-bi mu-eo-sim-ni-kka? ... i-sim-ni-kka?

RU Кто вы по профессии? Вы ...
Kto vy po professii? Vy ...

PL Jaki jest Pana(i) zawód? Czy jest Pan(i) ...

AR ما هو مهنتك؟ هل انت ...
Maa huwa mehnatak? Hal inta (male) / inti (female) ...

PT Qual é a sua profissão? É ...

FK Ki pwofesyon w? Eske ou se ...

EL Ποιο είναι το επάγγελμά σας; Είστε ...
peeO EEne to epAgelmA sas; EEste ...

HI आपका पेशा क्या है? क्या आप ...
Aapka pesha kya hai? Kya aap ...

Does your work primarily consist of ... ?

ES   Su trabajo consiste principalmente en ... ?

ZH   你的工作性质属于 ... ?
nǐ de gōng zuò xìng zhì shǔ yú ... ?

FR   Votre travail consiste principalement en ... ?

DE   Besteht Ihre Arbeit hauptsächlich aus ... ?

VI   Có phải là công việc của quý vị chủ yếu liên quan tới ?

IT   Il Suo lavoro consiste soprattutto di ... ?

KO   직장에서 하시는 일이 주로 ... 입니까?
Jik-jang-e-seo ha-si-neun i-ri ju-ro ... im-ni-kka?

RU   Ваша работа в основном заключается в ... ?
Vasha rabota v osnovnom zaklyuchaetsya v ... ?

PL   Czy Pana(i) praca głównie polega na ...

AR   هل شغلك إلى اكبر حد عبارة عن ... ؟
Hal shughlak ilaa akbar hadd "ibaarah "an ... ?

PT   O seu trabalho consta principalmente de ... ?

FK   Eske travay ou konsiste de ... ?

EL   Η εργασία σας περιλαμβάνει κυρίως ... ;
ee ergasEEa sas pereelamvAnee keerEEos ... ?

HI   क्या आपके काम में प्राथमिक रूप से ... शामिल है?
Kya aapke kaam mein prathmic roop se shamil hai?

hard physical work / seated work

ES	trabajo físico pesado / trabajar sentado
ZH	强体力型 / 坐办公室的 qiáng tǐ lì xíng / zuò bàn gōng shì de
FR	travail physique lourd / en position assise
DE	harter körperlicher / sitzender Tätigkeit
VI	lao động nặng nhọc / công việc văn phòng
IT	lavoro fisico pesante / lavoro in posizione seduta
KO	힘든 육체 노동 / 앉아서 하는 일 him-deun yuk-che no-dong / an-ja-seo ha-neun il
RU	тяжелом физическом труде / сидячей работе tyazhelom fizicheskom trude / sidyachey rabote
PL	ciężkiej pracy fizycznej / pracy w pozycji siedzącej
AR	شغل شاق \ شغل جالس Shughl shaaq / shughl jaalis
PT	trabalho físico árduo / trabalho sentado
FK	travay ki mande anpil egzesis / travay ki chita
EL	σκληρή σωματική εργασία / καθιστική δουλειά skleerEE somateekEE ergasEEa / katheesteekEE duleeA
HI	कठोर शारीरिक काम / बैठने का काम ... KaThor sharirik kaam / BaiThne ka kaam

working with paints / varnishes / solvents / in a dusty environment

ES trabajo con pinturas / barnices / solventes / en un ambiente polvoriento

ZH 工作用油漆 / 清漆 / 溶剂 / 有尘埃的环境
gōng zuò yòng yóu qī / qīng qī / róng jì / yǒu chén āi de huán jìng

FR travail avec des peintures / des vernis / des solvants / dans un environnement poussiéreux

DE Arbeit mit Farben / Lacken / Lösungsmitteln / in staubigem Umfeld

VI làm việc có liên quan tới sơn / véc-ni / chất dung môi / môi trường bụi bậm

IT lavoro con vernici / lacche / solventi / in un ambiente polveroso

KO 페인트 칠하기 / 니스 칠하기 / 용제(신나) 가지고 하는 일 / 먼지 많은 작업 환경
pe-in-teu chil-ha-gi / ni-seu chil-ha-gi / yong-je(sin-na) ga-ji-goha-neun il / meon-ji ma-neun jag-eop hwan-gyeong

RU работе с красками / лаками / растворителями / в пыльной атмосфере
rabote s kraskami / lakami / rastvoritelyami / v pyl'noy atmosfere

PL pracy przy farbach / lakierach / rozpuszczalnikach / w środowisku zakurzonym

AR العمل مع الصبغات \ الطلاءات الكيمياوية \ المذيبات \ في بيئة ذات كثرة من الغبار
Al-"amal ma" as-sibghaat / at-talaa'aat al-kimyaawiyyah / al-mudheebaat / fi bee'ah dhaati kathrah min al-ghubaar

PT trabalho com tinta / vernizes / dissolventes / num ambiente poeirento

FK travay ak penti / venis / solvan / nan yon anviwonman ki gen anpil pousye

EL εργασία με βαφές / βερνίκια / διαλύτες / σε περιβάλλον με σκόνη
ergasEEa me vafEs / vernEEkeea / deealEEtes / se pereevAlon me skOnee

HI पेंट / वार्निश / घुलनशील पदार्थों के साथ / ८ धूलभरे वातावरण में काम करना
paint / varnish / ghulansheel padarthon ke saath / dhoolbhare vaataavaraN mein kaam karna

Are special safety measures required for your work?

ES ¿Su trabajo requiere medidas de seguridad especiales?

ZH 你的工作需要什么安全保护措施吗？
nǐ de gōng zuò xū yào shén me ān quán bǎo hù cuò shī ma?

FR Des mesures de sécurité spéciales sont-elles requises pour votre travail?

DE Müssen Sie in der Arbeit Sicherheitsmaßnahmen treffen?

VI Công việc của quý vị có bắt buộc phải áp dụng các biện pháp an toàn đặc biệt không?

IT Sono richieste misure speciali di sicurezza per il Suo lavoro?

KO 특별한 안전 조치가 필요한 일을 하십니까?
Teuk-byeol-han an-jeon jo-chi-ga pi-ryo-han i-reul ha-sim-ni-kka?

RU Нужны ли особые меры безопасности на вашей работе?
Nuzhny li osobye mery bezopasnosti na vashey rabote?

PL Czy Pana(i) praca wymaga specjalnych środków bezpieczeństwa?

AR هل يستلزم إجراءات خاصة للسلامة في عملك؟
Hal yastalzim ijraa'aat khaasah lis-salaamah fi "amalak?

PT Para o seu trabalho são necessárias medidas de segurança especial?

FK Eske li egzije pou pran anpil mezi sekirite nan travay ou an?

EL Απαιτούνται ειδικά μέτρα ασφάλειας για τη δουλειά σας;
apetUde eedeekA mEtra asfAleeas geea tee duleeA sas?

HI क्या आपके काम के लिए विशेष सुरक्षा सा 6 नों की जरूरत होती है? ...
Kya aapke kaam ke liye visheSh surakSha sadhanon ki jarurat hoti hai?

mask / (protective) glasses / gloves / protective suit / ear protector

ES mascarilla / gafas protectoras / guantes / traje protector / protector de oído

ZH 面罩 / 护目镜 / 手套 / 隔离衣 / 耳朵保护器
miàn zhào / hù mù jìng / shǒu tào / gé lí yī / ěr duǒ bǎo hù qì

FR masque / verres (protecteurs) / gants / vêtement protecteur / protection acoustique

DE Maske / (Schutz)Brille / Handschuhe / Schutzanzug / Gehörschutz

VI mặt nạ / kính (bảo hộ) / găng tay / bộ quần áo bảo hộ / dụng cụ bảo vệ tai

IT maschera / occhiali (protettivi) / guanti / tuta protettiva / protezione per le orecchie

KO 마스크(보호용) / 안경 / 장갑 / 보호복 / 귀마개
mask(bo-ho-yong) / an-gyeong / jang-gap / bo-ho-bok / gwi-ma-gae

RU маска / (защитные) очки / перчатки / защитный костюм / средства защиты органов слуха
maska / (zashchitnye) ochki / perchatki / zashchitnyi kostyum / sredstva zashchity organov slukha

PL maski / (ochronnych) okularów / rękawic / ubrania ochronnego / ochrony uszu?

AR القناع \ نظارات (للحماية) \ القفازات \ بذلة حماية \ الحماية للأذنين
Al-qanaa" / nadhdhaaraat (lil-himaayah) / al-quffaazaat / badhlah himaayah / al-himaayah lil-udhneyn

PT máscara / óculos (de protecção) / luvas / fato protector / protector dos ouvidos

FK mask / linèt pwoteksyon / gan / rad pwoteksyon / pwoteksyon pou zorey ou

EL μάσκα / (προστατευτικά) γυαλιά / γάντια / προστατευτική στολή / ωτοασπίδες
mAska / (prostatefteekA) geealeeA / gAndeea / prostatefteekEE stolEE / otoaspEEdes

HI नकाब / (रक्षक) चश्में / दस्ताने / रक्षक सूट / कान रक्षक
Nakaab / (rakShak) chashmein / dastaane / rakShak suit / kaan rakShak

Do you smoke regularly? How much per day? For how many years?

ES ¿Fuma usted normalmente? ¿Qué tanto al día? ¿Por cuántos años?

ZH 你经常抽烟吗？一天抽多少？抽几年了？
nǐ jīng cháng chōu yān ma? yī tiān chōu duō shǎo? chōu jǐ nián le?

FR Fumez-vous régulièrement? Combien par jour? Depuis combien d'années?

DE Rauchen Sie regelmäßig? Wie viel am Tag? Wie viele Jahre?

VI Quý vị có hay hút thuốc không? Bao nhiêu điếu một ngày? Quý vị hút thuốc được bao nhiêu năm rồi?

IT Fuma regolarmente? Quanto al giorno? Da quanti anni?

KO 정기적으로 담배를 피우십니까? 하루에 얼마나? 몇 년 동안이나?
Jeong-gi-jeo-geu-ro dam-bae-reul pi-u-sim-ni-kka? Ha-ru-e eol-ma-na? Myeot nyeon dong-a-ni-na?

RU Вы курите постоянно? Сколько в день? Сколько лет?
Vy kurite postoyanno? Skol'ko v den'? Skol'ko let?

PL Czy pali Pan(i) papierosy regularnie? Ile dziennie? Od ilu lat?

AR هل تدخن \ تدخنين بالعادة؟ كم باليوم الواحد؟ ولكم سنة؟
Hal tudakhkhin / tudakhkhineen bil-"aadah? Kam bil-youm al-waahid? Wa li-kam sanah?

PT Fuma com regularidade? Quanto fuma por dia? Durante quantos anos?

FK Eske ou fimin sou yon baz regilye? Konbyen ke ou fimin pa jou? Pandan konbyen ane ?

EL Καπνίζετε τακτικά; Πόσο την ημέρα; Για πόσα χρόνια;
kapnEEzete takteekA? pOso teen eemEra? geea pOsa hrOneea?

HI क्या आप नियमित रूप से धूम्रपान करते हैं? दिन में कितनी बार? कितने वर्षों से?
Kya aap niyamit roop se dhumrapaan karte hain? Din mein kitni baar? Kitne varShon se?

Do you regularly drink alcohol?

ES ¿Toma alcohol normalmente?

ZH 你经常喝酒吗？
nǐ jīng cháng hē jiǔ ma?

FR Buvez-vous régulièrement de l'alcool?

DE Trinken Sie regelmäßig Alkohol?

VI Quý vị có thường uống rượu không?

IT Beve regolarmente alcol?

KO 정기적으로 술을 드십니까?
Jeong-gi-jeo-geu-ro su-reul deu-sim-ni-kka?

RU Вы употребляете алкоголь регулярно?
Vy upotreblyaete alkogol' regulyarno?

PL Czy regularnie pije Pan(i) alkohol?

AR هل تشرب / تشربين الكحول بشكل متكرر؟
Hal tishrab / tishrabeen al-kohoul bi-shakl mutakarrir?

PT Bebe álcool regularmente?

HK Eske ou bouwe tafya?

EL Πίνετε τακτικά αλκοόλ;
pEEnete takteekA alkoOl?

HI क्या आप प्रतिदिन शराब पीते हैं?
Kya aap pratidin sharaab peete hain?

Do you drink more than 1–2 bottles of beer / glasses of wine per day?

ES ¿Bebe más de 1 o 2 botellas de cerveza / vasos de vino al día?

ZH 你是否每天超过1-2瓶啤酒 / 1-2杯葡萄酒？
nǐ shì fǒu měi tiān chāo guò 1-2 píng pí jiǔ / 1-2 bēi pú táo jiǔ?

FR Buvez-vous plus d'une ou deux bouteilles de bière / combien de verres de vin par jour?

DE Trinken Sie mehr als 1-2 Flaschen Bier / Gläser Wein täglich?

VI Quý vị có uống nhiều hơn 1-2 chai bia / cốc rượu vang một ngày không?

IT Beve più di 1-2 bottiglie di birra / bicchieri di vino al giorno?

KO 하루에 맥주1-2 병 / 포도주 1-2잔 이상 드십니까?
Ha-ru-e maek-ju han-du byeong / po-do-ju han-du-jan i-sang deu-sim-ni-kka?

RU Вы пьете больше одной-двух бутылок пива / одного-двух стаканов вина в день?
Vy p'ete bol'she odnoy-dvukh (1-2) butylok piva / odnogo-dvukh (1-2) stakanov vina v den'?

PL Czy wypija Pan(i) więcej niż 1–2 butelki piwa / kieliszki wina dziennie?

AR هل تشرب \ تشربين اكثر من علية واحدة من البيرة \ كأس واحد من النبيذ فى اليوم الواحد؟
Hal tishrab / tishrabeen akthar min "ilbah waahidah min al-beerah / ka's waahid min an-nabeedh fil-youm il-waahid?

PT Bebe mais do que uma ou duas garrafas de cerveja / copos de vinho por dia?

FK Eske ou bouwe plis ke 1-2 boutey bye / ve divin pa jou?

EL Πίνετε περισσότερο από 1 έως 2 μπουκάλια μπύρας / ποτήρια κρασί την ημέρα;
pEEnete pereesOtero apO Ena Eos dEEo bukAleea bEEras / potEEreea krasEE teen eemEra?

HI क्या आप प्रतिदिन 1 से 2 बोतल बीयर / गिलास शराब पीते हैं?
Kya aap pratidin 1 se 2 botal beer / glass sharaab peete hain?

Do you regularly take medications / drugs?

ES ¿Toma regularmente medicamentos / drogas?

ZH 你平常是否吃药 / 吸毒？
nǐ píng cháng shì fǒu chī yào / xī dú?

FR Prenez-vous régulièrement des médicaments / des drogues?

DE Nehmen Sie regelmäßig Medikamente / Drogen?

VI Quý vị có thường xuyên dùng thuốc / chất kích thích không?

IT Prende regolarmente farmaci / droghe

KO 정기적으로 약 / 마약을 드십니까?
Jeong-gi-jeo-geu-ro yak / ma-ya-geul deu-sim-ni-kka?

RU Вы регулярно принимаете лекарства / наркотики?
Vy regulyarno prinimaete lekarstva / narkotiki?

PL Czy regularnie przyjmuje Pan(Pan) leki?

AR هل تأخذ \ تأخذين أدوية \ تتعاطى \ تتعاطين مخدرات بشكل متكرر؟
Hal ta'khudh / ta'khudheen adwiyah / tit"aati / tit"aateen mukhaddiraat bi-shaklin mutakarrir?

PT Toma medicamentos / consome drogas?

FK Eske ou ap pran okinn medikaman / dwoug?

EL Λαμβάνετε τακτικά φάρμακα / ναρκωτικά;
lamvAnete takteekA fArmaka / narkoteekA?

HI क्या आप नियमित रूप से दवा / ड्रग्स लेते हैं? ...
Kya aap niyamit roop se davaa / drugs lete hain?

headache tablets / pain killers / tranquilizers / sleeping pills / diet pills

ES para el dolor de cabeza / analgésicos / tranquilizantes / para dormir / para adelgazar

ZH 抗头痛药 / 去痛药 / 镇静剂 / 安眠药 / 减肥药
Kàng tóu tòng yào / qù tòng yào / zhèn jìng jì / ān mián yào / jiǎn féi yào

FR comprimés pour les maux de tête / des antidouleurs / des tranquillisants / des somnifères / des pilules pour maigrir

DE Kopfschmerz- / Schmerz- / Beruhigungs- / Schlafmittel / Diätpillen

VI thuốc viên chữa đau đầu / thuốc giảm đau / thuốc an thần / thuốc ngủ / thuốc viên dành cho người ăn kiêng

IT pasticche contro il mal di testa / analgesici / tranquillanti / pillole di sonnifero / pillole dimagranti

KO 두통약 / 진통제 / 신경 안정제 / 수면제 / 다이어트 약
du-tong-yak / jin-tong-je / sin-gyeong an-jeong-je / su-myeon-je / da-i-eo-teu yak

RU таблетки от головной боли / болеутоляющие / транквилизаторы / снотворное / таблетки для похудения
tabletki ot golovnoy boli / boleutolyayushchie / trankvilizatory / snotvornoe / tabletki dlya pokhudeniya

PL tabletki od bólu głowy / środki przeciwbólowe / środki uspokajające / pigułki nasenne / pigułki odchudzające

AR حبات للصداع \ حبات مضادة للألم \ المسكنات \ حبات للنوم \ حبات تخفيف الوزن
Habbaat lis-sudaa" / habbaat mudhaaddah lil-alam / al-musakkinaat / habbaat lin-noum / habbaat takhfeef al-wazn

PT comprimidos para a dor de cabeça / analgésicos / calmantes / comprimidos para dormir / comprimidos para emagrecer

FK aspirin / kont doulè / kalman / grenn pou ede ou domi / gren pou ede ou megri

EL δισκία για πονοκέφαλο/παυσίπονα / ηρεμιστικά / υπνωτικά / χαπάκια δίαιτας
deeskEEa geea ponokEfalo/pafsEEpona/eeremeesteekA / eepnoteekA / hapAkeea dEEetas

HI सिरदर्द की गोलियां / दर्दनिवारक / शान्तिकारी / नींद की गोलियां / भूखव ६ कि गोलियां ...
Sirdard ki goliyan / dardnivaarak / shantikari / neend ki goliyan / bhukhvardhak goliyan

Methadone / hashish / marijuana / cocaine / heroin

ES Metadona / hachís / marihuana / cocaína / heroína

ZH 美散痛 / 印度大麻 / 大麻 / 可卡因 / 海洛因
měi sǎn tòng / yìn dù dà má / dà má / kě kǎ yīn / hǎi luò yīn

FR Méthadone / hashish / marijuana / cocaïne / héroïne

DE Methadon / Haschisch / Marihuana / Kokain / Heroin

VI Methadone (thuốc ngủ gây tê) / hashis / cần sa / cocaine / bạch phiến

IT Metadone / hascisc / marijuana / cocaina / eroina

KO 메타돈 / 하시시 / 마리화나 / 코카인 / 헤로인
me-ta-don / ha-si-si / ma-ri-hwa-na / ko-ka-in / he-ro-in

RU Метадон / гашиш / марихуана / кокаин / героин
Metadon / gashish / marikhuana / kokain / geroin

PL Metadon / haszysz / marihuanę / kokainę / heroinę

AR الميثادون \ الهشيش \ الماريوانا \ الكوكايين \ الهيروين
Al-methadone / al-hasheesh / al-mariyuwana / al-kokaaeen / al-heroeen

PT Metadona / haxixe / marijuana / cocaína / heroína

FK Methadone / hashish / mariwana / kokayin / hewoin

EL μεθαδόνη / χασίς / μαριχουάνα / κοκαΐνη / ηρωίνη
methadOnee / hasEEs / mareeguAna / kokaEEnee / eeroEEnee

HI मीथाडॉन / हशीश / मेरीजुआना / कोकेन / हीरोइन
methadone / hashish / marijuana / cocaine / heroin

Amphetamine (speed) / ecstasy / LSD / alcohol

ES	Anfetaminas ("speed") / éxtasis / LSD / alcohol
ZH	安非他明（速效的）/ 狂喜 / 麦角二乙胺 / 酒精 ān fēi tā míng (sù xiào de) / kuáng xǐ / mài jiǎo èr yǐ àn / jiǔ jīng
FR	Amphétamine (speed) / ecstasy / LSD / alcool
DE	Amphetamine (Speed) / Ecstasy / LSD / Alkohol
VI	Amphetamine (thuốc kích thích) / thuốc gây hưng phấn / LSD (ma túy mạnh tạo ảo giác) / rượu
IT	Anfetamina (speed) / ecstasy / LSD / alcol
KO	암페타민 (스피드) / 엑스타시 / LSD / 술 am-pe-ta-min (seu-pi-deu) / ek-seu-ta-si / LSD / sul
RU	Амфетамин(спид) / экстази / ЛСД / алкоголь Amfetamin(spid) / ekstazi / LSD / alkogol'
PL	Amfetaminę / ekstasy / LSD / alkohol
AR	الأمفيتامين (ما يسمى بال"سبيد") \ الإكستاسي \ الأيل ايس دي \ الكحول Al-amfetameen (maa yusammaa bis-"speed") / al-ecstasy / al-eyl es dee / al-kuhool
PT	Anfetaminas (speed) / ecstasy / LSD / álcool
FK	Amfetamin / ekstasi / LSD / tafya
EL	αμφεταμίνη (σπιντ) / έκταση / ελ-σι-ντι / αλκοόλ amfetamEEnee (speed) / Ektasee / LSC / alkoOl
HI	एमफेटामाइन (गति) / उत्तेजना / एलएसडी / शराब amphetamine (gati) / uttejana / LSD / Sharaab

Do you exercise?

ES ¿Hace usted ejercicio?

ZH 你做体育锻炼吗？
nǐ zuò tǐ yù duàn liàn ma?

FR Faites-vous de l'exercice?

DE Treiben Sie Sport?

VI Quý vị có tập thể dục không?

IT Fa sport?

KO 운동하십니까?
Un-dong-ha-sim-ni-kka?

RU Вы выполняете физические упражнения?
Vy vypolnyaete fizicheskie uprazhneniya?

PL Czy gimnastykuje się Pan(i)?

AR هل تمارس \ تمارسين الرياضة البدنية؟
Hal tumaaris / tumaariseen ar-riyaadhat il-badaniyyah?

PT Faz exercício físico?

FK Eske ou fè egzesis?

EL Ασκείστε;
AskEEste?

HI क्या आप व्यायाम करते हैं?
Kya aap vyayaam karte hain?

Do you travel frequently? To which areas?

ES ¿Viaja a menudo? ¿A qué partes?

ZH 你经常旅游吗？去哪些地区？
nǐ jīng cháng lǚ yóu ma? qù nǎ xiē dì qū?

FR Voyagez-vous beaucoup? vers quels pays?

DE Reisen Sie viel? Wohin?

VI Quý vị có thường đi du lịch không? Tới khu vực nào?

IT Viaggia di frequente? In quali zone?

KO 여행을 자주 하십니까? 어떤 지역으로?
Yeo-haeng-eul ja-ju ha-sim-ni-kka? Eo-tteon ji-yeo-geu-ro?

RU Вы часто путешествуете? Куда?
Vy chasto puteshestvuete? Kuda?

PL Czy często Pan(i) podróżuje? Dokąd?

AR هل تسافر \ تسافرين كثيراً؟ إلى أية مناطق؟
Hal tusaafir / tusaafireen kathiiran? Ilaa ayy manaatiq?

PT Viaja com frequência? Para que regiões?

FK Eske ou vwayaje anpil? Nan ki zon?

EL Ταξιδεύετε συχνά; Σε ποιες περιοχές;
taxeedEvete seehnA? se peeEs pereeohEs?

HI क्या आप बार–बार यात्रा करते हैं? किन क्षेत्रों की? ...
Kya aap baar-baar yatra karte hain? Kin Shetron ki?

America / South America / Europe / Asia / Africa / Australia

ES Estados Unidos / América Latina / Europa / Asia / África / Australia

ZH 美国 / 南美洲 / 欧洲 / 亚洲 / 非洲 / 澳大利亚
měi guó / nán měi zhōu / ōu zhōu / yà zhōu / fēi zhōu / ào dà lì yà

FR Amérique / Amérique du Sud / Europe / Asie / Afrique / Australie

DE Amerika / Südamerika / Europa / Asien / Afrika / Australien

VI Hoa Kỳ / Nam Mỹ / Châu Âu / Châu Á / Châu Phi / Châu Úc

IT America / Sudamerica / Europa / Asia / Africa / Australia

KO 미국 / 남미 / 유럽 / 아시아 / 아프리카 / 호주
mi-guk / nam-mi / yu-reop / a-si-a / a-peu-ri-ka / ho-ju

RU Америка / Южная Америка / Европа / Азия / Африка / Австралия
Amerika / Yuzhnaya Amerika / Evropa / Aziya / Afrika / Avstraliya

PL Do Ameryki / Ameryki Południowej / Europy / Azji / Afryki / Australii

AR امريكا \ امريكا الجنوبية \ اوروبا \ آسيا \ افريقيا \ استراليا
America / America al-janoubiyah / Oropaa / Aasyaa / Ifreeqiyaa / Ostraaliya

PT América / América do Sul / Europa / Ásia / África / Austrália

FK Amerik / Amerik di Sid / Ewop / Azi / Afik / Ostrali

EL Αμερική / Νότια Αμερική / Ευρώπη / Ασία / Αφρική / Αυστραλία
AmereekEE / nOtea AmereekEE / evrOpee / asEEa / afreekEE / afstralEEa

HI अमेरिका / दक्षिणी अमेरिका / यूरोप / एशिया / अफ्रीका / आस्ट्ेलिया
America / dakShiNi America / Europe / Asia / Africa / Australlia

8 Family History

Are your father and mother still alive?

ES ¿Viven su padre y su madre?

ZH 你的父母亲还活着吗？
nǐ de fù mǔ qīn hái huó zhe ma?

FR Votre père et votre mère sont-ils toujours en vie?

DE Leben Ihr Vater und Ihre Mutter noch?

VI Cha mẹ quý vị có còn sống không?

IT Suo padre e Sua madre sono ancora in vita?

KO 부모님이 아직 살아 계십니까?
Bu-mo-ni-mi a-jik sa-ra gye-sim-ni-kka?

RU Ваши мама и папа живы?
Vashi mama i papa zhivy?

PL Czy Pani(i) ojciec i matka jeszcze żyją?

AR هل ما زال والديك على قيد الحياة؟
Hal maa zaal waalidayk "alaa qayd il-hayaah?

PT O seu pai e a sua mãe ainda estão vivos?

FK Eske manman w ak papa w vivan toujou?

EL Ζουν ακόμη ο πατέρας και η μητέρα σας;
zun akOmee o patEras ke ee meetEra sas?

HI क्या आपके माता व पिता जीवित हैं?
kyaa aapke maataa va pitaa jiivit hain?

Does / did he / she have a serious illness?

ES ¿Tiene / tuvo él / ella alguna enfermedad grave?

ZH 他 / 她 有没有 / 过去有没有得过大病？
tā / tā yǒu méi yǒu / guò qù yǒu méi yǒu dé guò dà bìng?

FR A-t-il (elle) (eu) une maladie grave?

DE Hat / hatte er / sie eine ernste Erkrankung?

VI Cha / mẹ quý vị hiện có đang / đã từng mắc bệnh nặng không?

IT Lei / lui ha / ha avuto una malattia grave?

KO 아버지 / 어머니가 중병이 있으십니까? / 있으셨습니까?
A-beo-ji / eo-meo-ni-ga jung-byeong-i it-seu-sim-ni-kka / it-seu-syeot-seum-ni-kka?

RU У него / неё есть / были серьёзные болезни?
U nego / neyo est' / byli ser'yoznye bolezni?

PL Czy on(a) chorował(a) / choruje na jakąś poważną chorobę?

AR هل يعاني \ تعانين حالياً او سبق أن عاني \ عانت من مرض شديد؟
Hal yu"aani / tu"aani haaliyan au sabaq an "aanaa / "aanat min maradh shaded?

PT Ele ou ela sofre / sofreu de uma doença grave?

FK Eske li gen / te gen yon maladi grav?

EL Έχει / Είχε αυτός / αυτή σοβαρή ασθένεια;
Ehee / EEhe aftOs / aftEE sovarEE asthEneea?

HI क्या वे कोई गंभीर बीमारी के शिकार थे / थीं?
kyaa vey koi gambhir beemaarii ke shikaar the / thiin?

What was his / her cause of death?

ES	¿De qué murió él / ella?
ZH	他 / 她的死因是什么？ tā / tā de sǐ yīn shì shén me?
FR	Quelle est la cause de leur mort?
DE	Woran ist er / sie gestorben?
VI	Vì sao cha / mẹ quý vị qua đời?
IT	Quale è stata la causa del suo decesso?
KO	아버지 / 어머니는 어떻게 돌아가셨습니까? A-beo-ji / eo-meo-ni-neun eo-tteo-ke do-ra-ga-syeot-seum-ni-kka?
RU	От чего он / она умер(ла)? Ot chego on / ona umer(la)?
PL	Jaka była przyczyna jego / jej zgonu?
AR	ماذا كان سبب وفاؤه؟ / وفاتها؟ Maadhaa kaan sabab wafaa'uh? \ wafaa'iha?
PT	Qual foi a causa da morte dele / dela?
FK	De kisa ke li mouri?
EL	Ποια ήταν η αιτία του θανάτου του / της; peea EEtan ee etEEa tu thanAtu tu / tees?
HI	उनकी मौत का कारण क्या था? ...... unki maut ka kaaraN kyat ha?

Did / does anyone in your family have the following disease?

¿Tuvo / tiene alguien de su familia la enfermedad siguiente?

在你家里有没人得过 / 在 得以下疾病?
zài nǐ jiā lǐ yǒu méi rén dé guò / zài dé yǐ xià jí bìng?

Est-ce que quelqu'un dans votre famille a ou a eu les maladies suivantes?

Gibt / gab es eine der folgenden Erkrankungen in Ihrer Familie?

Gia đình quý vị có ai hiện đang / đã từng mắc căn bệnh sau đây không?

Qualcuno nella Sua famiglia è stato affetto / è affetto dalla seguente malattia?

가족 중에 다음의 병이 있는 사람이 있습니까 / 있었습니까?
Ga-jok jung-e da-eu-mui byeong-i in-neun sa-ram-i it-seum-ni-kka / it-seot-seum-ni-kka?

У кого-нибудь в вашей семье была / есть следующая болезнь?
U kogo-nibud' v vashei sem'e byla / est' sleduyushchaya bolezn'?

Czy ktoś z Pana(i) rodziny chorował / choruje na następujące choroby?

هل يعاني \ سبق أن عانى احد من أفراد عائلتك من المرض التالي؟
Hal yu"aani / sabaq an "aanaa ahad min afraad "aa'ilatak min al-maradh at-taali?

Algum familiar seu sofre da doença seguinte?

Eske gen okinn moun nan fanmi ki te gen / genyen yon de maladi swivan yo?

Είχε / Έχει κάποιος στην οικογένειά σας την ακόλουθη νόσο;
EEhe / Ehee kApeeos steen eekogEneeA sas teen akOluthee nOso?

क्या आपके परिवार में किसी को यह बीमारी थी / है?......
kyaa aapke parivaar mein kisii ko yeh beemaarii thii / hai?

If yes, which family member?

ES	En tal caso, ¿que miembro de la familia?
ZH	如果有，是谁呢？ rú guǒ yǒu, shì shéi ne?
FR	Si oui, quel membre de la famille?
DE	Wenn ja, welches Familienmitglied?
VI	Nếu có, đó là ai trong gia đình quý vị?
IT	Se sì, chi?
KO	대답이 긍정일 경우, 누구입니까? Dae-da-bi geung-jeong-il gyeong-u, nu-gu-im-ni-kka?
RU	Если да, у кого из членов семьи? Esli da, u kogo iz chlenov sem'i?
PL	Jeśli tak, to kto z rodziny?
AR	إذا كان الجواب نعم، اي فرد من أفراد العائلة؟ Idhaa kaan al-jawaab na"m, ayyi fard min afraad al-"aa'ilah?
PT	Se responder sim, qual é grau de parentesco do familiar?
FK	Si wi, ki moun nan fanmi w?
EL	Εάν ναι, ποιο οικογενειακό μέλος; eAn ne, peeO eekogeneeakO mElos?
HI	अगर हां, तो परिवार के किस सदस्य को? …… agar haan, to parivaar ke kis sadasya ko?

Father / mother / grandparents / brother / sister / children

ES Padre / madre / abuelos / hermano / hermana / hijos

ZH 父亲 / 母亲 / 祖父母 / 兄弟 / 姐妹 / 孩子
fù qīn / mǔ qīn / zǔ fù mǔ / xiōng dì jiě mèi / hái zǐ

FR Père / mère / grands-parents / frère / soeur / enfants

DE Vater / Mutter / Großeltern / Bruder / Schwester / Kinder

VI Cha / mẹ / ông bà / anh (em) trai / chị (em) gái / con

IT Padre / madre / nonni / fratello / sorella / figli

KO 아버지 / 어머니 / 조부모 / 남자 형제 / 여자 형제 / 자녀
a-beo-ji / eo-meo-ni / jo-bu-mo / nam-ja hyeong-je / yeo-ja hyeong-je / ja-nyeo

RU Отец / мать / дедушка и бабушка / брат / сестра / дети
Otets / mat' / dedushka i babushka / brat / sestra / deti

PL Ojciec / matka / dziadkowie / brat / siostra / dzieci?

AR الأب \ الأم \ الأجداد \ الأخ \ الأخت \ الأطفال
Al-abb / al-umm / al-ajdaad / al-akh / al-ukht / al-atfaal

PT Pai / mãe / avós / irmão / irmã / filhos

FK Papa.manman / grandparan w / frè / sè / pitit

EL Πατέρας / Μητέρα / Παπποὺς ή γιαγιά / Αδελφός / Αδελφή / Παιδιά
patEras / meetEra / papUs ee geeageeA / adelfOs / adelfEE / pedeeA

HI पिता / माता / दादा दादी या नाना नानी / भाई / बहन / बच्चे
pita / maataa / daadaa-daadii yaa naanaa-naanii / bhaii / bahan / bachche

9 Head, Neck

Do you have headaches? Constantly / occasionally?

ES ¿Tiene dolores de cabeza? ¿Constantemente / a veces?

ZH 你头痛吗? 持续痛 / 间断痛?
nǐ tóu tòng ma? chí xù tòng / jiān duàn tòng?

FR Avez-vous des maux de tête? Constamment / occasionnellement?

DE Haben Sie Kopfschmerzen? Ständig / gelegentlich?

VI Quý vị có bị đau đầu không? Thường xuyên / thỉnh thoảng? Dây Thần Kinh

IT Soffre di mal di testa? Costantemente / occasionalmente?

KO 두통이 있으십니까? 항상 / 가끔?
Du-tong-i i-seu-sim-ni-kka? Hang-sang / ga-kkeum?

RU Вас беспокоят головные боли? Постоянно / иногда?
Vas bespokoyat golovnye boli? Postoyanno / inogda?

PL Czy ma Pan(i) bóle głowy? Stale / czasami?

AR هل تعاني \ تعانين من الصداعات؟ دائماً \ من حين إلى آخر؟
Hal tu"aani? / tu"aaneen min as-sudaa"aat? Daa'iman / min heyn ila aakhir?

PT Tem dores de cabeça? Constantemente / ocasionalmente?

FK Eske ou gen maltèt? Tout tan / pa fwa?

EL Έχετε πονοκέφαλους; Συνέχεια / Περιστασιακά;
Ehete ponokEfalus? seenEheea / pereestaseeakA

HI क्या आपको सिर दर्द होता है? लगातार / कभी–कभी? ... क्यूक्यू न्यूरो
Kya aapko sir dard hota hai? lagaataar / kabhi-kabhi?

Do you feel pain in the back of your neck?

ES ¿Siente dolor en la nuca (detrás del cuello)?

ZH 你脖子后面痛吗？
nǐ bó zǐ hòu miàn tòng ma?

FR Avez-vous mal dans la nuque?

DE Schmerzt Sie Ihr Nacken?

VI Quý vị có thấy đau ở phía sau cổ không?

IT Ha dolore alla nuca?

KO 목 뒤가 아픕니까?
Mok dwi-ga a-peum-ni-kka?

RU Испытываете ли боль в задней части шеи?
Ispytyvaete li bol' v zadney chasti shei?

PL Czy odczuwa Pan(i) ból w tyle szyi?

AR هل تشعر \ تشعرين بالألم في خلف رقبتك؟
Hal tash"ur / tash"ureen bil-alam fi khalf ruqbatak?

PT Sente dor na parte de trás do pescoço?

FK Eske ou santi doulè nan padeye kou w?

EL Νιώθετε πόνο στο πίσω μέρος του λαιμού σας;
neeOthete pOno sto pEEso mEros tu lemU sas?

HI क्या आप अपनी गर्दन की पिछली तरफ दर्द महसूस करते हैं?
Kya aap apni gardan ki piChhli taraf dard mehsoos karte hain?

Have you been hit on your head? At which location?

ES	¿Se golpeó en la cabeza? ¿En qué parte?

ES ¿Se golpeó en la cabeza? ¿En qué parte?

ZH 头伤着了吗？那个部位？
tóu shāng zháo le ma? nǎ ge bù wèi?

FR Avez-vous été touché(e) à la tête? A quel endroit?

DE Haben Sie einen Schlag auf den Kopf bekommen, Wo?

VI Quý vị có bị đánh vào đầu không? Ở chỗ nào?

IT È stato colpito / a alla testa? Dove?

KO 머리를 맞으셨습니까? 어디입니까?
Meo-ri-reul ma-jeu-syeot-seum-ni-kka? Eo-di-im-ni-kka?

RU Били ли вас когда-нибудь по голове? В какое место?
Bili li vas kogda-nibud' po golove? V kakoe mesto?

PL Czy doznał Pan(i) uderzenia w głowę? W którym miejscu?

AR هل تلقيت ضرباً على رأسك؟ في أي مكان بالضبط؟
Hal talaqqayt dharban "alaa ra'sak? Fi ayyi makaan bidh-dhabt?

PT Bateram-lhe na cabeça? Em que sítio?

FK Eske ou pran kou nan tèt ? Ki bò ?

EL Χτυπήσατε στο κεφάλι; Σε ποιο σημείο;
hteepEEsate sto kefAlee? se peeo seemEEo?

HI क्या आपके सिर में चोट लगी है? किस भाग में?
Kya aapke sir mein chot lagi hai? Kis bhaag mein?

Did you loose consciousness?

ES ¿Perdió el conocimiento?

ZH 你当时有没有昏迷？
nǐ dāng shí yǒu méi yǒu hūn mí?

FR Avez-vous perdu connaissance?

DE Waren Sie bewusstlos?

VI Quý vị có bị ngất không?

IT Ha perso conoscenza?

KO 의식을 잃으셨습니까?
Ui-si-geul i-reu-syeot-seum-ni-kka?

RU Вы теряли сознание?
Vy teryali soznanie?

PL Czy stracił(a) Pani przytomność?

AR هل فقدت الوعي؟
Hal faqadt al-wa"i?

PT Perdeu os sentidos?

FK Eske ou te pedi konesans?

EL Χάσατε τις αισθήσεις σας;
hAsate tees esthEEsees sas?

HI क्या आपने होश खो दिया?
Kya aapne hosh Kho dia?

Do you have an eye problem? Which problem in particular?

ES ¿Tiene algún problema en los ojos? ¿Qué problema en especial?

ZH 你眼睛有问题吗？什么问题？
nǐ yǎn jīng yǒu wèn tí ma? shén me wèn tí?

FR Avez-vous un problème à l'oeil? Quel problème en particulier?

DE Haben Sie Probleme mit Ihren Augen? Welche?

VI Quý vị có bệnh về mắt không? Cụ thể, đó là bệnh gì?

IT Ha problemi agli occhi? Specificamente che problema?

KO 눈에 문제가 있습니까? 구체적으로 어떤 문제 입니까?
Nu-ne mun-je-ga it-seum-ni-kka? Gu-che-jeo-geu-ro eo-tteon mun-je im-ni-kka?

RU У вас есть нарушение зрения? Какое именно?
U vas est' narusheniye zreniya? Kakoe imenno?

PL Czy ma Pan(i) kłopoty z oczami? Na czym on polega?

AR هل تعاني \ تعانين من مشكلة فى العين؟ من أية مشكلة بالضبط؟
Hal tu"aani / tu"aaneen min mushkilah fil-"ayn? Min ayyi mushkilah bidh-dhabt?

PT Tem um problema nos olhos? Que problema em particular?

FK Eske ou gen pwoblèm nan zye? Ki pwoblèm an patikilye ?

EL Έχετε προβλήματα ματιών; Ποιο πρόβλημα συγκεκριμένα;
Ehete provlEEmata mateeOn? peeO prOvleema seegekreemEna?

HI क्या आपको आंख में कुछ परेशानी है? विशेष रूप से क्या परेशानी है? ...
Kya aapko aankh mein kuChh pareshaani hai? Vishesh roop se kya pareshaani hai?

Ophthalmic Problem 151

impaired vision (temporary) / loss of eyesight / double images

ES	visión anormal (temporal) / pérdida de la vista / visión doble
ZH	视力受损（暂时性的）/ 视力下降 / 重影 shì lì shòu sǔn (zàn shí xìng de) / shì lì xià jiàng / chóng yǐng
FR	altération de la vision (temporaire) / perte de la vue / diplopie
DE	Sehstörungen (vorübergehend) / Sehverlust / Doppelbilder
VI	suy giảm thị lực (tạm thời) / không nhìn thấy / hoa mắt
IT	vista indebolita (temporaneamente) / perdita della vista / raddoppiamento delle immagini
KO	시각 장애(일시적) / 시력 손실 / 물체가 두개로 보임 si-gak jang-ae(il-si-jeok) / si-ryeok son-sil / mul-che-ga du-gae-ro bo-im
RU	(временное) нарушение зрения / потеря зрения / двоение в глазах (vremennoe) narushenie zreniya / poterya zreniya / dvoenie v glazakh
PL	osłabiony wzrok (tymczasowo) / utrata wzroku / podwójne widzenie
AR	الضعف فى البصر (مؤقت) \ فقدان البصر \ ازدواج الرؤية Adh-dhu"f fil-basar (mu'aqqat) / fuqdaan al-basar / izdiwaaj ar-ru'yah
PT	visão alterada (temporariamente) / perda da vista / imagens duplas
FK	vizyon twoub(tanporè) / pedi vizyon / vizyon doub
EL	μειωμένη όραση (προσωρινή) / απώλεια όρασης / διπλή όραση meeomEnee Orasee (prosoreenEE) / apOleea Orasees / deeplee Orasee
HI	खराब दृष्टि (अस्थाई) / दृष्टि खोना / दोहरी आकृतियां नज़र आना ... khraab driShti (A-sthayi) / driShti Khona / dohri aakritiyaan nazar aana

blurred vision / watery eyes / pain / inflammation

ES visión borrosa / ojos llorosos / dolor / inflamación

ZH 视力模糊 / 流泪 / 痛 / 发炎
shì lì mó hú / liú lèi / tòng / fā yán

FR vision trouble / yeux humides / douleur / inflammation

DE unscharfes Sehen / wässrige Augen / Schmerz / Entzündung

VI nhìn không rõ / chảy nước mắt / đau / sưng viêm

IT vista offuscata / occhi annacquati / dolore / infiammazione

KO 물체가 흐리게 보임 / 눈물이 고임 / 통증 / 염증
mul-che-ga heu-ri-ge bo-im / nun-mu-ri go-im / tong-jeung / yeom-jeung

RU затуманенное зрение / слезотечение / боль / воспаление
zatumanennoe zrenie / slezotechenie / bol' / vospalenie

PL nieostre widzenie / łzawiące oczy / ból / zapalenie

AR التشوش في البصر \ تدمع العيون \ الألم \ الإلتهاب
At-tashawwush fil-basar / tadammu" al-"uyoon / al-alam / al-iltihaab

PT Visão turva / olhos lacrimejantes / dor / inflamação

FK vizyon twoub / zye ki fè dlo / doulè / enflamasyon

EL θολή όραση / δακρύρροια / πόνος / φλεγμονή
tholEE Orasee / dakrEEreea / pOnos / flegmonEE

HI अस्पष्ट दृष्टि / आंखों में पानी आना / दर्द / जलन ...
A-spaSht driShti / aankhon mein paani aana / dard / jalan -

light flashes / black spots before the eyes / sensitivity to light

ES destellos / puntos negros frente a los ojos / hipersensibilidad a la luz

ZH 眼冒金星 / 眼前有黑点 / 怕光
yǎn mào jīn xīng / yǎn qián yǒu hēi diǎn / pà guāng

FR éclairs lumineux / taches devant les yeux / sensibilité à la lumière

DE Lichtblitze / schwarze Punkte vor den Augen / Lichtempfindlichkeit

VI các tia sáng lóe / nảy đom đóm mắt / nhạy cảm với ánh sáng

IT lampi luminosi / macchie nere davanti agli occhi / sensibilità alla luce

KO 빛 번득임 / 눈 앞에 검은 점들이 보임 / 빛에 예민함
bit beon-deu-gim / nun a-pe geo-meun jeom-deu-ri bo-im / bi-che ye-min-ham

RU вспышки света / черные точки перед глазами / чувствительность к свету
vspyshki sveta / chernye tochki pered glazami / chuvstvitel'nost' k svetu

PL błyski światła / ciemne plamki przed oczami / wrażliwość na światło

AR الومضات الضوئية \ ظهور البقعات السوداء امام العيون \ الحساسية للنور
Al-wamdhaat adh-dhou'iyyah / dhuhoor al-buq"aat as-saudaa' amaan al-"uyoon /
al-hassaasiyyah lin-noor

PT Clarões de luz / manchas negras no campo de visão / sensibilidade à luz

FK limyè kap flache / pwin nwa devan zye w / zye w sansib a limye

EL αναβόσβημα φωτός / μαύρα στίγματα μπροστά από τα μάτια / ευαισθησία στο
φως
anavOsveema fotOs / mAvra stEEgmata brostA apO ta mAteea / evestheesEEa sto fos

HI प्रकाश काैंधना/आंखो के आगे काले धब्बे दिखना/प्रकाश के प्रति संवेदनशीलता ...
Prakash kaundhna / aankhon ke aage kaale Dhabbe dikhnaa / prakash ke prati
samvedanSheelta

burning sensation / sticky eyes at nighttime

ES	ardor de ojos / ojos pegajosos en la noche
ZH	烧灼感 / 夜间眼皮发粘 shāo zhuó gǎn / yè jiān yǎn pí fā nián
FR	sensation de brûlures, les yeux qui collent au cours de la nuit
DE	Brennen / nachts verklebte Augen
VI	cảm giác bỏng rát / mắt rất khó chịu vào ban đêm
IT	bruciore / occhi appiccicosi la notte
KO	따가움 / 밤에 눈이 끈적거림 tta-ga-um / ba-me nu-ni kkeun-jeok-geo-rim
RU	чувство жжения / слипание век после ночи chuvstvo zhzheniya / slipanie vek posle nochi
PL	uczucie pieczenia / wieczorem klejące się oczy
AR	إحساس الإحتراق او الإلتهاب \ التدبق فى العينن فى الأوقات الليلية Ihsaas al-ihtiraaq au al-iltihaab / at-tadabbuq fil-"aynayn fil-auqaat al-layliyyah
PT	sensação de ardor / prurido nos olhos durante a noite
FK	sensasyon boulè / zye w kolan ak lasi pandan lan nwit
EL	αίσθημα καύσου / κολλώδη μάτια τις νυχτερινές ώρες Estheema kAfsu / kolOdee mAteea tees neehtereenEs Ores
HI	जलन संवेदना / रात के समय चिपचिपी आंखें jalan samvedna / raat ke samay chipchipi aankhen

Which eye is affected? Left / right / both eyes

S ¿Cuál es el ojo afectado? El izquierdo / el derecho / los dos

H 哪只眼有问题？左眼 / 右眼 / 双眼
nǎ zhī yǎn yǒu wèn tí? zuǒ yǎn / yòu yǎn / shuāng yǎn

R Quel oeil est affecté? Le gauche / le droit ou les deux

DE Welches Auge? links / rechts / beide

VI Mắt nào bị bệnh? Mắt trái / phải / cả hai mắt

T Quale occhio è interessato? Sinistro / destro / entrambi

KO 어떤 눈이 문제입니까? 왼쪽 / 오른쪽 / 양쪽 눈
Eo-tteon nu-ni mun-je-im-ni-kka? Oen-jjok / o-reun-jjok / yang-jjok nun

RU Какой глаз беспокоит? Левый / правый / оба глаза
Kakoi glaz bespokoit? Levyi / pravyi / oba glaza

PL Którego oka to dotyczy? Lewego / prawego / obydwu oczu

AR اي عين هو العين المصاب؟ العين اليساري \ اليميني \ العينين
Ayyi "ayn huwa al-"ayn al-musaab? Al-"ayn al-yasaari / al-yameeni / al-"aynayn

PT Que olho é afectado? o esquerdo / o direito / os dois olhos

FK Ki les nan ye yo ki afekte? Gòch / dwat / tou de (2) zye yo

EL Ποιο μάτι επηρεάστηκε; Αριστερό / Δεξί / Και τα δύο μάτια
peeo mAtee epeereAsteeke? areesterO / dexEE / ke ta dEEo mAteea

HI कौन सी आंख प्रभावित है? बांयी / दांयी / दोनों आंखें
Kaun si aankh praBhavit hai? baanyi / daanyi / dono aankhen

Did something get caught in your eye?

ES	¿Se le metió algo en el ojo?
ZH	你眼中进什么东西了吗？ nǐ yǎn zhōng jìn shén me dōng xī le ma?
FR	Avez-vous reçu quelque chose dans l'oeil?
DE	Ist etwas in Ihr Auge gekommen?
VI	Quý vị có bị vật gì bay vào mắt không?
IT	Le è entrata qualcosa negli occhi?
KO	눈에 뭐가 들어 갔습니까? Nu-ne mwo-ga deu-reo gat-seum-ni-kka?
RU	Что-нибудь попало вам в глаз? Chto-nibud' popalo vam v glaz?
PL	Czy coś wpadło Panu(i) do oka?
AR	هل دخل شيء في عينك؟ Hal dakhal shay' fi "aynak?
PT	Entrou algo no seu olho?
FK	Eske gen yon bagay ki kole nan zye a?
EL	Μπήκε κάτι στο μάτι σας; bEEke kAtee sto mAtee sas?
HI	क्या आपकी आंख में कुछ गिर गया था? ... Kya aapki aankh mein kuChh gir gaya tha?

Ophthalmic Problem 157

foreign body / liquid / blow to the eye

:S basurilla / líquido / golpe en el ojo

H 异物 / 液体 / 被气或水喷过
yì wù / yè tǐ / bèi qì huò shuǐ pēn guò

R corps étranger / liquide / un coup de vent

E Fremdkörper / Flüssigkeit / Schlag auf das Auge

VI dị vật / chất lỏng / mắt bị chấn động mạnh

NT corpo estraneo / liquido / colpo all'occhio

KO 이물질 / 액체 / 눈을 맞았다
i-mul-jil / aek-che / nu-neul ma-jat-da

RU инородное тело / жидкость / удар в глаз
inorodnoe telo / zhidkost' / udar v glaz

PL obce ciało / płyn / uderzenie w oko

AR شيء او جسم غريب \ سائل \ ضربة للعين
Shay' au jism ghareeb \ saa'il / dharbah lil-"ayn

PT corpo estranho / líquido / pancada no olho

FK yon ko etranje / likid / resevwa yon kou nan zye a

EL ξένο αντικείμενο / υγρό / φύσημα στο μάτι
xEno andeekEEmeno / eegrO / fEEseema sto mAtee

HI बाहरी तत्व / तरल / आंख में फूंकना
Baahri Tatva / taral / aankh mein phunkna

Do you wear glasses / contact lenses?

ES ¿Usa usted lentes / lentes de contacto?

ZH 你戴眼镜 / 隐形眼镜吗？
nǐ dài yǎn jìng / yǐn xíng yǎn jìng ma?

FR Portez-vous des lunettes? des verres de contact?

DE Tragen Sie Brille / Kontaktlinsen?

VI Quý vị có đeo kính / kính áp tròng không?

IT Porta occhiali / lenti a contatto?

KO 안경 / 콘택트 렌즈를 끼십니까?
An-gyeong / kon-taek-teu ren-jeu-reul kki-sim-ni-kka?

RU Вы носите очки / контактные линзы?
Vy nosite ochki / kontaktnye linzy?

PL Czy nosi Pan(i) okulary / szkła kontaktowe?

AR هل تلبس \ تلبسين النظارات او تستعمل \ تستعملين العدسات اللاصقة؟
Hal talbis / talbiseen an-nadhaaraat au tasta"mil / tasta"mileen al-"adasaat al-laasiqah?

PT Usa óculos / lentes de contacto?

FK Eske ou met linett / kontak?

EL Φοράτε γυαλιά / φακούς επαφής;
forAte geealeeA / fakUs epafEEs?

HI क्या आप चश्मा / कॉन्टैक्ट लेंस पहनते हैं?
Kya aap chashmaa / contact lens pahente hain?

Do you work in front of a computer screen? For the entire day?

S ¿Trabaja frente a una computadora / ordenador? ¿Todo el día?

H 你工作用电脑吗？整天用吗？
nǐ gōng zuò yòng diàn nǎo ma? zhěng tiān yòng ma?

R Travaillez-vous devant un écran d'ordinateur? Toute la journée?

E Arbeiten Sie am Computerbildschirm? Den ganzen Tag?

VI Quý vị có làm việc trước màn hình máy điện toán không? Trong cả ngày?

T Lavora davanti allo schermo di un computer? Tutto il giorno?

O 컴퓨터 앞에서 일 하십니까? 하루 종일 하십니까?
Kom-pu-te a-pe-seo il ha-sim-ni-kka? Ha-ru jong-il ha-sim-ni-kka?

U Вы работаете перед экраном компьютера? Целый день?
Vy rabotaete pered ekranom komp'yutera? Tselyi den'?

PL Czy pracuje Pan(i) siedząc przed komputerem? Przez cały dzień?

R هل تعمل \ تعملين امام شاشة كمبيوترية؟ لليوم بكامله؟
Hal ta"mal / ta"maleen amaan shaashah kompyuteriyyah? Lil-youm bikaamileh?

PT Trabalha frente ao ecrã de um computador? Durante todo o dia?

K Eske ou travay devan yon ekran konpitè ? Pendan tout jounin an ?

EL Εργάζεστε μπροστά από οθόνη υπολογιστή; Για ολόκληρη την ημέρα;
ergAzeste brostA apO othOnee eepologeestEE? geea olOkleeree teen eemEra?

HI क्या आप कंप्यूटर स्क्रीन के सामने कार्य करते हैं? पूरे दिन?
Kya aap computer screen ke saamne kaarya karte hain? poore din?

Do you have a mouth / neck problem? Which problem in particular?

ES   ¿Tiene algún problema en la boca / el cuello? ¿Qué problema es?

ZH   你有没有口腔 / 颈部问题？是什么问题呢？
nǐ yǒu méi yǒu kǒu qiāng / jǐng bù wèn tí? shì shén me wèn tí ne?

FR   Avez-vous un problème dans la bouche / le cou? Quel problème, en particulier?

DE   Haben Sie Probleme mit Ihrem Mund / Hals? Welche?

VI   Quý vị có vấn đề ở cổ / miệng không? Cụ thể, đó là vấn đề gì?

IT   Ha problemi alla bocca / al collo? Specificamente che problema?

KO   입 / 목에 문제가 있습니까? 구체적으로 어떤 문제입니까?
Ip / mo-ge mun-je-ga it-seum-ni-kka? Gu-che-jeo-geu-ro eo-tteon mun-je-im-ni-kka?

RU   Вас беспокоит рот / шея? Что именно?
Vas bespokoit rot / sheya? Chto imenno?

PL   Czy ma Pan(i) kłopoty z ustami / szyją? Jakiego konkretnie rodzaju jest to kłopot?

AR   هل عندك مشكلة في الفم \ الرقبة؟ اية مشكلة بالتحديد؟
Hal "indak mushkilah fil-famm / ar-ruqbah? Ayyi mushkilah bit-tahdeed?

PT   Tem um problema na boca / no pescoço? Que problema em particular?

FK   Eske ou gen pwoblèm bouch / kou? Ki pwoblèm an patikilye ?

EL   Έχετε πρόβλημα στο στόμα / λαιμό; Ποιο πρόβλημα συγκεκριμένα;
Ehete prOvleema sto stOma / lemO? peeo prOvleema seegegkreemEna?

HI   क्या आपके मुंह / गले में परेशानी है? विशे ॰ रूप से क्या परेशानी है? ...
Kya aapke moonh / gale mein pareshaani hai? Vishesh roop se kya pareshaani hai?

voice changes / dry mouth / sore throat

S cambios de la voz / boca seca / garganta irritada

H 声音变化 / 口干 / 喉咙痛
shēng yīn biàn huà / kǒu gān / hóu lóng tòng

R changement de la voix / bouche sèche / mal de gorge

DE Stimmveränderungen / trockener Mund / Halsschmerzen

VI đổi giọng / khô miệng / đau họng

IT cambiamento di voce / bocca secca / mal di gola

O 목소리 달라짐 / 목이 텁텁함 / 목안이 아픔
mok-sori dal-la-jim / mo-gi teop-teop-ham / mo-ga-ni a-peum

RU изменение голоса / сухость во рту / больное горло
izmenenie golosa / sukhost' vo rtu / bol'noe gorlo

PL zmiany głosu / suchość w ustach / ból gardła

AR التغيرات في الصوت \ الجفاف في الفم \ إلتهاب الحلقوم
At-taghyeeraat fis-sout / al-jafaaf fil-famm / iltihaab al-hulqoom

PT alterações da voz / boca seca / dor de garganta

FK chanjman vwa / bouch ou sèk / mal goj

EL αλλαγές στη φωνή / ξηροστομία / πονόλαιμος
alaGEs stee fonEE / xeerostomEEa / ponOlemos

HI आवाज़ बदलना / मुँह सूखना / गला दुखना ...
aawaz badalna / moonh sookhna / galaa dukhna

hoarseness / swallowing problems / changes in taste sensation

ES ronquera / problemas para tragar / cambio del sentido del gusto

ZH 声音沙哑 / 吞咽困难 / 吃饭味道变化
shēng yīn shā yǎ / tūn yàn kùn nán / chī fàn wèi dào biàn huà

FR raucité / problèmes de déglutition / changements dans la perception du goût

DE Heiserkeit / Schluckbeschwerden / Geschmacksveränderungen

VI khàn giọng / các vấn đề về nuốt / thay đổi về khẩu vị

IT raucedine / problemi a deglutire / modifica della sensazione del gusto

KO 목소리가 쉼 / 삼키는 데 불편 / 미각에 변화가 생김
mok-so-ri-ga swim / sam-ki-neun de bul-pyeon / mi-ga-ge byeon-hwa-ga saeng-gim

RU хрипота / нарушения глотания / нарушения вкуса
khripota / narusheniya glotaniya / narusheniya vkusa

PL chrypka / trudności w przełykaniu / zmiany w smaku

AR البحة \ الصعوبات في الابتلاع \ تغيرات في إحساس التذوق
Al-bahhah / as-su"oubaat fil-ibtilaa' / taghyeeraat fi ehsaas at-tadhawwuq

PT rouquidão / problemas de deglutição ou dificuldade em engolir / alterações no sentido do gosto

FK anwe / pwoblèm vale / chanjman nan sansasyon gou yon bagay

EL βραχνάδα / προβλήματα κατά την κατάποση / αλλαγές στην αίσθηση της γεύσης
vrahnAda / provlEEmata katA teen katApose / alagEs steen Estheesee tees gEfsees

HI कर्कशता / निगलने में परेशानी / स्वाद संवेदना में बदलाव ...
karkarshta / nigalne mein pareshaani / swaad samvednaa mein badlaav

increased salivation / tooth aches

ES salivación excesiva / dolor de dientes / muelas

ZH 口水增多 / 牙痛
kǒu shuǐ zēng duō / yá tòng

FR salivation augmentée / douleurs dentaires

DE vermehrter Speichelfluss / Zahnschmerzen

VI tiết ra nhiều nước miếng hơn / đau răng

IT aumento della salivazione / dolori ai denti

KO 타액(침) 증가 / 치통
ta-aek(chim) jeung-ga / chi-tong

RU повышенное слюноотделение / зубная боль
povyshennoe slyunootdelenie / zubnaya bol'

PL spotęgowanie ślinienia / ból zębów

AR التزايد في سيلان اللعاب \ الآلام في الأسنان
At-tazaayud fi saylaan al-lu"aab / al-'aalaam fil-asnaan

PT aumento da salivação / dores de dentes

FK fè plis saliv / dan fèmal

EL αυξημένη ποσότητα σίελου / πονόδοντος
afxeemEnee posOteeta sEEelu / ponOdondos

HI लार में वृद्धि / दांत में दर्द ...
laar me vridhi / daant mein dard

bleeding gums / canker sores / swollen lymph nodes

ES sangrado de encías / úlceras bucales (aftas) / ganglios inflamados

ZH 牙龈出血／口疮／淋巴结肿大
Yá yín chū xiě / kǒu chuāng / lín bā jié zhǒng dà

FR gencives qui saignent / ulcère douloureux / noeuds lymphatiques gonflés

DE Zahnfleischbluten / Geschwüre / dicke Lymphknoten

VI nướu răng chảy máu / viêm loét miệng / sưng hạch

IT gengive sanguinanti / afte / linfonodi gonfi

KO 잇몸에서 피가 나옴 / 구강궤양 / 부은 림프절
in-mo-me-seo pi-ga na-om / gu-gang-gwe-yang / bu-eun lim-peu-jeol

RU кровоточащие дёсны / афтозный стоматит / увеличение лимфатических узлов
krovotochashchie dyosny / aftoznyi stomatit / uvelichenie limfaticheskikh uzlov

PL krwawienie dziąseł / pleśniawki jamy ustnej / obrzmienie węzłów limfatycznych

AR نزيف الدم في اللثة \ القرحات \ التضخم في العقد اللمفاوية
Nazeef ad-damm fil-laththah \ al-qarhaat \ at-tadhakhkhum fil-"uqad al-limfaawiyyah

PT sangramento das gengivas / aftas na boca / nódulos linfáticos inchados

FK jansiv kap sinyen / blesi chank / glann anfle

EL αιμορραγία ούλων / στοματικό έκλωμα / διογκωμένοι λεμφαδένες
emoragEEa Ulon / stomateekO Ekloma / deeogomEnee lemfadEnes

HI मसूड़ों से खून बहना / नासूर / सूजे लिंफ नोड्स
masooDon se khoon behna / nasoor / sooze lymph nodes

Which tooth is hurting?

ES ¿Qué diente es el que le duele?

ZH 哪颗牙痛？
nǎ kē yá tòng?

FR Quelle dent fait mal?

DE Welcher Zahn tut weh?

VI Quý vị bị đau răng nào?

IT Quale dente Le duole?

KO 어떤 이가 아픕니까?
Eo-tteon i-ga a-peum-ni-kka?

RU Какой зуб болит?
Kakoi zub bolit?

PL Który ząb Pana / Panią boli?

AR اي سن من الأسنان توجعك؟
Ayyi sinn min al-asnaan touji"ak?

PT Que dente lhe dói?

FK Ki dan kap fè w mal?

EL Ποιο δόντι πονάει;
peeo dOdi ponAee?

HI कौन से दांत में परेशानी है?
Kaun se daant me pareshaani hai?

Do you have an ear problem? Which ear is affected?

ES ¿Tiene un problema en los oídos? ¿Qué oído es el afectado?

ZH 你耳朵有问题吗？是哪只耳朵？
nǐ ěr duǒ yǒu wèn tí ma? shì nǎ zhī ěr duǒ?

FR Avez-vous un problème d'oreille? Quelle oreille est atteinte?

DE Haben Sie Probleme mit den Ohren? Welches Ohr?

VI Quý vị có vấn đề gì về tai không? Tai nào bị bệnh?

IT Ha problemi ad un orecchio? A quale orecchio?

KO 귀에 문제가 있습니까? 어떤 귀에 문제가 있습니까?
Gwi-e mun-je-ga it-seum-ni-kka? Eo-tteon gwi-e mun-je-ga it-seum-ni-kka?

RU Вас беспокоят уши? Какое ухо болит?
Vas bespokoyat ushi? Kakoe ukho bolit?

PL Czy ma Pan(i) kłopoty z uszami? Którego ucha to dotyczy?

AR هل تعاني \ تعانين من مشكلة في الأذن؟ اي من الأذنين مصاب؟
Hal tu"aani / tu"aaneen min mushkilah fil-udhn? Ayyi min al-udhneyn musaab?

PT Tem um problema no ouvido? Que ouvido está afectado?

FK Eske ou gen pwoblèm nan zorèy? Nan ki zorèy?

EL Έχετε προβλήματα αυτιού; Ποιο αυτί επηρεάστηκε;
Ehete provlEEmata afteeU? peeo aftEE epeereAsteeke?

HI क्या आपके कान में परेशानी है? कौन–सा कान प्रभावित है? ...
Kya aapke kaan mein pareshaani hai? Kaun-sa kaan praBhavit hai?

ear pain / itching / ringing in the ears / ear noises

S dolor / picazón / zumbido de oídos / ruidos en el oído

H 耳朵痛 / 痒 / 嗡嗡声 / 耳鸣
ěr duǒ tòng / yǎng / wēng wēng shēng / ěr míng

R douleur auriculaire / démangeaisons / sifflement dans les oreilles / bruits

E Ohrenschmerzen / Juckreiz / Ohrensausen / Ohrgeräusche

VI đau tai / ngứa tai / ù tai / tiếng ồn trong tai

T dolore alle orecchie / prurito / ronzio nelle orecchie / rumori nelle orecchie

O 귀가 아픔 / 가려움 / 귀울림(이명) / 귀 잡음
gwi-ga a-peum / ga-ryeo-um / gwi-ul-lim(im-yeong) / gwi ja-beum

U ушная боль / зуд / звон в ушах / шум в ушах
ushnaya bol' / zud / zvon v ushakh / shum v ushakh

PL ból ucha / swędzenie / dzwonienie w uszach / dźwięki w uszach

AR الألم في الأذن \ الحك \ صوت الرنين في الأذنين \ الضوضاء في الأذنين
Al-alam fil-udhn / al-hakk / sout ar-raneen fil-udhneyn / adh-dhoudhaa' fil-udhneyn

PT Dor no ouvido / comichão / zumbido nos ouvidos / ruídos nos ouvidos

FK doulè nan zorèy / zorèy ou ap sonin / bouwi nan zorèy

EL πόνος αυτιού / κνησμός / βούισμα στα αυτιά / θόρυβοι στα αυτιά
pOnos afeeU / kneesmOs / vUeesma sta afteeA / thOreevee sta afteeA

HI कान में दर्द / खारिश / कान गूंजना / कान बजना ...
Kaan mein dard / khaarish / kaan goonjna / kaan bajnaa

hearing problems / dizziness / vomiting / liquid coming out of the ear

ES problemas para oír / vértigos / vómito / secreción de líquido por el oído

ZH 听觉问题 / 眩晕 / 呕吐 / 耳朵向外流液
tīng jué wèn tí / xuàn yūn / ǒu tù / ěr duǒ xiàng wài liú yè

FR problèmes d'audition / vertiges / vomissement / liquide qui s'écoule de l'oreille

DE Hörprobleme / Schwindel / Erbrechen / Flüssigkeit aus dem Ohr

VI các vấn đề về thính giác / chóng mặt / ói mửa / chất dịch lỏng chảy ra từ tai

IT problemi all'udito / capogiri / vomito / liquido che fuoriesce dall'orecchio

KO 청력 문제 / 현기증 / 구토 / 귀에서 액체가 나옴
cheon-ryeok mun-je / hyeon-gi-jeung / gu-to / gwi-e-seo aek-che-ga na-om

RU нарушения слуха / головокружение / рвота / выделение жидкости из уха
narusheniya slukha / golovokruzhenie / rvota / vydelenie zhidkosti iz ukha

PL problemy ze słyszeniem / zawroty głowy / wymioty / sączenie się płynu z ucha

AR المشاكل فى السمع \ الدوخة \ القيء \ إفراز سائل من الأذن
Al-mashaakil fis-sama" / ad-doukhah / al-qay' / ifraaz saa'il min al-udhn

PT problemas da audição / tonturas / vómitos / líquido a sair do ouvido

FK pwoblèm tande / vetij / vomisman / likid kap soti nan zorèy

EL προβλήματα ακοής / ζάλη / εμετός / υγρό να εξέρχεται από το αυτί
provlEEmata akoEEs / zAlee / emetOs / eegrO na exErhete apO to aftEE

HI सुनने में परेशानी / चक्कर आना / उलटी आना / कान से तरल बहना
sunne mein pareshaani / chakkar aana / ulti aana / kaan se taral behna

Can you hear me?

ES ¿Me oye bien?

ZH 你能听到我说话吗？
nǐ néng tīng dào wǒ shuō huà ma?

FR M'entendez-vous?

DE Können Sie mich hören?

VI Quý vị có thể nghe thấy tôi nói không?

IT Mi sente?

KO 제 말이 들립니까?
Je ma-ri deul-lim-ni-kka?

RU Вы меня слышите?
Vy menya slyshite?

PL Czy Pan(i) mnie słyszy?

AR هل تستطيع \ تستطيعين أن تسمعني \ تسمعيني؟
Hal tastatee" / tastatee"een an tasma"ni / tasma"eeni?

PT Pode ouvir-me?

FK Eske ou ka tande m?

EL Με ακούτε;
me akUte?

HI क्या आप मुझे सुन सकते हैं?
Kya aap mujhe sun sakte hain?

Is there a foreign body in your ear?

ES ¿Se le metió alguna cosa en el oído?

ZH 你耳朵里有什么异物吗？
nǐ ěr duǒ lǐ yǒu shén me yì wù ma?

FR Y a-t-il un corps étranger dans votre oreille?

DE Haben Sie einen Fremdkörper in Ihrem Ohr?

VI Có dị vật trong tai quý vị không?

IT C'è un corpo estraneo nel Suo orecchio?

KO 귀에 이물질이 있습니까?
Gwi-e i-mul-ji-ri it-seum-ni-kka?

RU У вас в ухе есть инородное тело?
U vas v ukhe est' inorodnoe telo?

PL Czy ma Pan(i) w uchu obce ciało?

AR هل هناك جسم غريب في أذنك؟
Hal hunaaka jism ghareeb fi udhnak?

PT Há um corpo estranho dentro do seu ouvido?

FK Eske gen yon ko etranje nan zorèy ou?

EL Υπάρχει ξένο αντικείμενο στο αυτί σας;
eepArhee xEno adeekEEmeno sto aftEE sas?

HI क्या आपके कान में कोई बाहरी तत्व है?
Kya aapke kaan mein koi bahari tatva hai?

Do you have a nasal problem? Which problem in particular?

ES ¿Tiene algún problema en la nariz? ¿Qué problema en especial?

ZH 你鼻子有问题吗？是什么问题？
nǐ bí zi yǒu wèn tí ma? shì shén me wèn tí?

FR Avez-vous un problème nasal? Quel problème, en particulier?

DE Haben Sie Probleme mit der Nase? Welche?

VI Quý vị có vấn đề về mũi không? Cụ thể, đó là bệnh gì?

IT Ha un problema al naso? Specificamente che problema?

KO 코에 문제가 있습니까? 구체적으로 어떤 문제 입니까?
Ko-e mun-je-ga it-seum-ni-kka? Gu-che-jeo-geu-ro eo-tteon mun-je im-ni-kka?

RU Вас беспокоит нос? Что именно?
Vas bespokoit nos? Chto imenno?

PL Czy ma Pan(i) jakieś kłopoty z nosem? Co to za kłopoty?

AR هل عندك مشكلة أنفية؟ اية مشكلة بالتحديد؟
Hal "indak mushkilah anfiyyah? Ayyi mushkilah bit-tahdeed

PT Tem um problema nasal? Que problemas em particular?

FK Eske ou gen pwoblèm nan nin? Ki pwoblèm an patikilye ?

EL Έχετε ρινικό πρόβλημα; Ποιο πρόβλημα συγκεκριμένα;
Ehete reeneekO prOvleema? peeo prOvleema seegekreemEna?

HI क्या आपके नाक में परेशानी है? विशेष रूप से कौन–सी परेशानी? ...
Kya aapke naak mein pareshaani hai? Vishesh roop se kaun-si pareshaani?

runny nose / nose bleeding / hay fever / pain

ES secreción constante / hemorragia nasal / fiebre del heno / dolor

ZH 流鼻涕 / 鼻出血 / 对花草过敏 / 痛
liú bí tì / bí chū xiě / duì huā cǎo guò mǐn / tòng

FR le nez qui coule / saignement / rhume des foins / douleur

DE Nasenausfluss / Nasenbluten / Heuschnupfen / Schmerzen

VI chảy nước mũi / chảy máu cam / bệnh sốt vào mùa hè / đau

IT naso che cola / naso che sanguina / febbre da fieno / dolore

KO 콧물이 나옴 / 코피 / 건초열 / 통증
kon-mu-ri na-om / ko-pi / geon-cho-yeol / tong-jeung

RU насморк / носовое кровотечение / сенная лихорадка / боль
nasmork / nosovoe krovotechenie / sennaya likhoradka / bol'

PL katar / krwawienie z nosa / katar sienny / ból

AR النزيف بالأنف \ نزيف الدم من الأنف \ حمى القش \ الألم
An-nazeef bil-anf / nazeef ad-damm min al-anf / hummaa al-qashsh / al-alam

PT corrimento no nariz / sangue do nariz / febre dos fenos / dor

FK nin koule / nin kap sinyin / lagrip lasezon / doulè

EL ρινόρροια / αιμορραγία από τη μύτη / αλλεργική ρινίτιδα / πόνος
reenOreea / emoragEEa apO tee mEEtee / alergeekEE reenEEteeda / pOnos

HI नाक बहना / नाक से खून बहना / परागज बुखार / दर्द
Naak behna / naak se khoon behna / paragaj bukhaar / dard

Is there a foreign body in your nose?

ES ¿Se le metió alguna cosa en la nariz?

ZH 你鼻子里有什么异物吗？
nǐ bí zi lǐ yǒu shén me yì wù ma?

FR Y a-t-il un corps étranger dans votre nez?

DE Haben Sie einen Fremdkörper in Ihrer Nase?

VI Trong mũi quý vị có dị vật không?

IT C'è un corpo estraneo nel Suo naso?

KO 코에 이물질이 있습니까?
Ko-e i-mul-ji-ri it-seum-ni-kka?

RU У вас в носу есть инородное тело?
U vas v nosu est' inorodnoe telo?

PL Czy ma Pan(i) w nosie jakieś obce ciało?

AR هل هناك جسم غريب موجود في أنفك؟
Hal hunaak jism ghareeb maujoud fi anfak?

PT Há um corpo estranho dentro do seu nariz?

FK Eske gen yon ko etranje nan nin w?

EL Υπάρχει ξένο αντικείμενο στη μύτη σας;
eepArhee xEno adeekEEmeno stee mEEtee sas?

HI क्या आपकी नाक में कोई बाहरी तत्व है?
Kya aapki naak me koi bahri tatva hai?

Have you noticed any changes in your sense of smell?

ES	¿Ha notado algún cambio en el sentido del olfato?
ZH	你感觉到嗅觉有什么变化吗？ nǐ gǎn jué dào xiù jué yǒu shén me biàn huà ma?
FR	Avez-vous remarqué un changement dans votre sens de l'odorat?
DE	Haben Sie Veränderungen des Geruchssinns?
VI	Quý vị có nhận thấy thay đổi gì về khứu giác không?
IT	Ha notato cambiamenti nel suo odorato?
KO	후각에 어떤 변화를 느끼셨습니까? Hu-ga-ge eo-tteon byeon-hwa-reul neu-kki-syeot-seum-ni-kka?
RU	Заметили ли вы у себя какие-нибудь изменения обоняния? Zametili li vy u sebia kakie-nibud' izmeneniya obonyaniya?
PL	Czy zauważył(a) Pan(i) u siebie jakieś zmiany jeśli chodzi o węch?
AR	هل لاحظت اية تغيرات في حاسة شمك؟ Hal laahadht ayyi taghyeeraat fi haasa shammak?
PT	Notou algumas alterações no seu sentido do gosto?
FK	Eske ou remake okinn chanjman nan jan nin w santi yon bagay?
EL	Παρατηρήσατε οποιαδήποτε αλλαγή στην αίσθηση της όσφρησής σας; parateerEEsate opeeadEEpote alagEE steen Estheesee tees OsfreesEEs sas?
HI	क्या आपने अपनी सूंघने की इंद्रिय में कोई बदलाव नोट किया है? Kay aapne apni sughne ki indriya mein koi badlaav note kiya hai?

Did this result from an accident?

ES ¿Fue a causa de algún accidente?

ZH 是因为意外事故造成的吗？
shì yīn wéi yì wài shì gù zào chéng de ma?

FR Cela fait-il suite à un accident?

DE War es ein Unfall?

VI Nguyên nhân có phải do tai nạn không?

IT È stato la conseguenza di un incidente?

KO 이것은 사고의 결과 입니까?
I-geo-seun sa-go-ui gyeol-gwa im-ni-kka?

RU Это произошло в результате травмы?
Eto proizoshlo v rezul'tate travmy?

PL Czy to było spowodowane wypadkiem?

AR هل حدث هذا نتيجة حادث؟
Hal hadath hadhaa nateejah haadith?

PT Isto foi consequência de um acidente?

FK Eske se rezilta yon aksidan?

EL Προέκυψε αυτό από ατύχημα;
proEkeepse aftO apO atEEheema?

HI क्या यह किसी दुर्घटना का परिणाम है?
Kya yeh kisi durghatna ka pariNaam hai?

10 Lung, Heart, Vessels

Do you experience pain while breathing / breathing difficulties?

ES ¿Tiene dolor al respirar / dificultad para respirar?

ZH 你呼吸时有没有感到痛 / 呼吸困难？
nǐ hū xī shí yǒu méi yǒu gǎn dào tòng / hū xī kùn nán?

FR Avez-vous mal lorsque vous respirez / avez-vous des difficultés à respirer?

DE Haben Sie Schmerzen beim Atmen / Atembeschwerden?

VI Quý vị có bị đau khi thở / khó thở không?

IT Prova dolore quando respira / ha difficoltà a respirare?

KO 숨을 쉴 때 통증을 느끼십니까 / 호흡 곤란?
Sum-eul swil ttae tong-jeung-eul neu-kki-sim-ni-kka / Ho-heup gollan?

RU Вы испытываете боль во время дыхания / затруднения дыхания?
Vy ispytyvaete bol' vo vremya dykhaniya / zatrudneniya dykhaniya?

PL Czy czuje Pan(i) ból podczas oddychania / czy ma Pan(i) trudności w oddychaniu?

AR هل تتعرض \ تتعرضين للألم عند التنفس \ الصعوبات في التنفس؟
Hal tit"arradh / tit'arradheen lil-alam "ind at-tanaffus / as-su"oubaat fit-tanaffus?

PT Sente dor enquanto respira / tem dificuldades respiratórias?

FK Eske ou gen doulè lè ou ap respire / difikilte respire ?

EL Νιώθετε πόνο όταν αναπνέετε / αναπνευστικές δυσκολίες;
neeOthete pOno Otan anapnEete / anapnefsteekEs deeskolEEes?

HI क्या आपने सांस लेने के दौरान दर्द / सांस लेने में परेशानी का अनुभव किया? ...
Kya aapne saans lene ke dauraan dard / saans lene mein pareshaani ka anubhav kiya?

constantly / during physical exertion / when lying flat

ES   constantemente / al hacer un esfuerzo / al estar acostado

ZH   持续性的 / 活动时 / 平躺的时候
chí xù xìng de / huó dòng shí / píng tǎng de shí hòu

FR   constamment / au cours d'un exercice physique / lorsque vous êtes couché(e) à plat

DE   ununterbrochen / bei Anstrengung / bei flachem Liegen

VI   luôn luôn / khi vận động mạnh / khi nằm thẳng người

IT   costantemente / quando faccio sforzi fisici / quando sono disteso / a

KO   항상 / 지나치게 육체 운동을 할 때 / 반드시 누울 때
hang-sang / ji-na-chin yuk-che un-dong-eul hal ttae / ban-deu-si nu-ul ttae

RU   постоянно / во время физического напряжения / лежа на спине
postoyanno / vo vremya fizicheskogo napryazheniya / lezha na spine

PL   stale / w czasie fizycznego wysiłku / leżąc na wznak

AR   بشكل دائم \ أثناء المشقة الجسمائية \ عند الإنبطاح
Bi-shekl daa'im / athnaa' al-mashaqqat il-jismaaniyyah / "ind al-inbitaah

PT   constantemente / durante o esforço físico / enquanto deitado(a)

FK   tout tan / pandan yon aktivite fizik / lè ou kouche plat sou do

EL   συνεχώς / κατά τη σωματική άσκηση / όταν είμαι ξαπλωμένος / η
seenehOs / katA tee somateekEE Askeesee / Otan EEme xaplomEnos / ee

HI   निरंतर / शारीरिक परिश्रम के दौरान / सी ६ो लेटते समय
Niranter / shaaririk pariShram ke dauraan / seedhe leTte samay

during inhalation / exhalation / at night / when climbing stairs

ES al inhalar / al exhalar / por la noche / al subir escaleras

ZH 吸气时 / 呼气时 / 夜间 / 上楼梯时
xī qì shí / hū qì shí / yè jiān / shàng lóu tī shí

FR au cours de l'inspiration / l'expiration / la nuit / en montant les escaliers

DE bei Ein- / Ausatmen / nachts / beim Treppensteigen

VI khi hít vào / thở ra / vào ban đêm / khi trèo cầu thang

IT Quando inspiro / espiro / la notte / quando salgo le scale

KO 숨을 들이 마실 때 / 숨을 내쉴 때 / 밤에 / 계단을 오를 때
sum-eul deu-ri ma-sil ttae / sum-eul nae-swil ttae / ba-me / gye-da-neul o-reul ttae

RU во время вдоха / выдоха / ночью / при подъёме по лестнице
vo vremya vdokha / vydokha / noch'yu / pri pod"yome po lestnitse

PL przy wdechu / wydechu / w nocy / przy wchodzeniu po schodach

AR عند الإستنشاق \ عند التنفس \ في الليل \ عند الصعود على السلم
"ind al-istinshaaq / "ind at-tanaffus / fil-leyl / "ind as-su"oud "ala as-sullam

PT durante a inalação / exalação / à noite / ao subir escadas

FK pandan ou app ran souf / lage souf ou / lan nwit / lè ou ap monte eskalye

EL κατά την εισπνοή / εκπνοή / τη νύχτα / όταν αναβαίνω σκάλες
katA teen eespnoEE / ekpnoEE / tee nEEhta / Otan anevEno skAles

HI सांस अंदर खींचते समय / निकालते हुए / रात को / सीढ़ियों पर चढ़ते समय
Sans ander kheenchte samay / nikaalte hue / raat ko / siDhiyon par chaDhte samay

Do you hear a whistling breathing sound / are you hoarse?

ES	¿Se oyen silbidos cuando respira / tiene ronquera?
ZH	你有没有听到哨声当你呼吸时 / 你的声音嘶哑吗？ nǐ yǒu méi yǒu tīng dào shào shēng dāng nǐ hū xī shí / nǐ de shēng yīn sī yǎ ma?
FR	Entendez-vous un sifflement lorsque vous respirez / êtes-vous enroué(e)?
DE	Haben Sie ein pfeifendes Atemgeräusch / sind Sie heiser?
VI	Quý vị có nghe thấy tiếng rít trong khi thở không / quý vị có bị khàn giọng không?
IT	Sente un fischio quando respira / soffre di raucedine?
KO	휘파람 소리같은 숨소리가 들립니까? / 목소리가 쇠셨습니까? Hwi-pa-ram so-ri-ga-teun sum-so-ri-ga deul-lim-ni-kka / mok-so-ri-ga soe-syeot-seum-ni-kka?
RU	Вы слышите свистящее дыхание / вы хрипите? Vy slyshite svistyashchee dykhanie / vy khripite?
PL	Czy słyszy Pan(i) gwizd oddechu / czy ma Pan(i) chrypę?
AR	هل تسمع \ تسمعين صوت صفير عند التنفس \ هل انت مبحوح \ مبحوحة؟ Hal tisma" / tisma"een sout safeer "ind at-tanaffus / hal inta / inti mabhooh / mabhoohah?
PT	Ouve um som sibilante enquanto respira / está rouco(a)?
FK	Eske ou tande yon sifleman lè ou ap resoire / vwa ou anwe?
EL	Ακούτε αναπνευστικό σφύριγμα / έχετε βραχνάδα; akUte anapnefsteekO sfEEreegma / Ehete vrahnAda?
HI	क्या आपकी सांस में सीटी की आवाज सुनाई देती है / क्या आपकी आवाज फटी हुई है? Kya aapki saans mein citi ki aawaz sunaai deti hai / kya aapki aawaaz faTi hui hai?

Did this occur suddenly?

ES ¿Esto empezó de repente?

ZH 这是突然发生的吗？
zhè shì tū rán fā shēng de ma?

FR Cela s'est-il produit subitement?

DE Hat es plötzlich begonnen?

VI Hiện tượng này có xảy ra đột ngột không?

IT Ciò è avvenuto improvvisamente?

KO 이것은 갑자기 생긴 일입니까?
I-geo-seun gap-ja-gi saeng-gin i-rim-ni-kka?

RU Это появилось внезапно?
Eto poyavilos' vnezapno?

PL Czy to się stało nagle?

AR هل حدث هذا فجأة؟
Hal hadath hadha faj'atan?

PT Isto ocorre de repente?

FK Eske sa a fèt sibitman?

EL Συμβαίνει αυτό ξαφνικά;
seemvEnee aftO xafneekA?

HI क्या यह अचानक हुआ था?
Kya yeh achaanak hua tha?

Have you experienced this before? When?

ES ¿Ya lo había tenido antes? ¿Cuándo?

ZH 你以前有过这种情况吗？什么时候？
nǐ yǐ qián yǒu guò zhè zhǒng qíng kuàng ma? shén me shí hòu?

FR Avez-vous déjà eu cela auparavant? Quand?

DE Ist das früher schon einmal passiert, wann?

VI Quý vị đã bao giờ gặp hiện tượng này chưa? Khi nào?

IT Le è già capitato prima? Quando?

KO 이전에도 이런 일을 경험한 적이 있습니까? 언제?
I-jeon-e-do i-reon i-reul gyeong-heom-han jeo-gi it-seum-ni-kka? Eon-je?

RU Было ли такое раньше? Когда?
Bylo li takoe ran'she? Kogda?

PL Czy doświadczał(a) Pan(i) tego już wcześniej? Kiedy?

AR هل تعرضت لهذا من قبل؟ متى؟
Hal ta"arradht li-hadha min qabl? Mattaa?

PT Já alguma vez sentiu isto? Quando?

FK Eske ou te janm gen sa avan? Kil è ?

EL Το έχετε βιώσει αυτό πριν; Πότε;
to Ehete veeOsee aftO preen? pOte?

HI क्या आपने पहले इसका अनुभव किया था? कब?
Kya aapne pehle iska anubhav kiya tha? Kab?

Did you inhale anything unusual?

ES	¿Inhaló algún objeto extraño?
ZH	你有没有吸入过不正常的东西？ nǐ yǒu méi yǒu xī rù guò bù zhèng cháng de dōng xī?
FR	Avez-vous inhalé quelque chose d'inhabituel?
DE	Haben Sie etwas Ungewöhnliches eingeatmet?
VI	Quý vị có hít phải vật gì bất thường không?
IT	Ha inalato qualcosa di insolito?
KO	보통 흡입하지 않는 것을 흡입하셨습니까? Bo-tong heu-bi-pa-ji an-neun geo-seul heu-bi-pa-syeot-seum-ni-kka?
RU	Вы вдохнули что-нибудь необычное? Vy vdokhnuli chto-nibud' neobychnoe?
PL	Czy wdychał(a) Pan(i) coś niezwyczajnego?
AR	هل إستنشقت أيّ شئ غير عادي؟ Hal istanshaqt ay shey' gheyr "aadi?
PT	Inalou algo de invulgar?
FK	Eske ou respire yon bagay ki pa nomal?
EL	Εισπνεύσατε κάτι ασυνήθιστο; eespnEfsate kAtee aseenEEtheesto?
HI	क्या आपने सांस के साथ कुछ असामान्य खींच लिया? Kya aapne saans ke saath kuchh asaamanya kheench liya?

Do you have pain in the area of the ribs / chest pain?

ES ¿Siente dolor en la zona de las costillas / dolor de pecho?

ZH 你有没有感到过肋骨下痛 / 胸痛？
nǐ yǒu méi yǒu gǎn dào guò lèi gǔ xià tòng / xiōng tòng?

FR Ressentez-vous de la douleur dans la région des côtes / avez-vous mal dans le thorax?

DE Haben Sie Schmerzen in Ihren Rippen / Brustschmerzen?

VI Quý vị có bị đau ở vùng xương sườn / tức ngực không?

IT Prova dolore nell'area delle costole / dolore al petto?

KO 갈비 부분에 통증 / 가슴에 통증이 있으십니까?
Gal-bi bu-bun-e tong-jeung / ga-seu-me tong-jeung-i i-seu-sim-ni-kka?

RU У вас есть боль в области ребер / боль в груди?
U vas est' bol' v oblasti reber / bol' v grudi?

PL Czy odczuwa Pan(i) ból w okolicy żeber / ból w klatce piersiowej?

AR هل لك ألم في منطقة الأضلاع / ألم في صدر؟
Hal lak alam fi mantiqat il-adhlaa" / alam fis-sadr?

PT Tem dores na zona das costelas / dores no peito?

FK Eske ou gen doulè bo kot ou / doulè nan pwatrin ou ?

EL Έχετε πόνο στην περιοχή των πλευρών / θωρακικό πόνο;
Ehete pOno steen pereeohEE ton plevrOn / thorakeekO pOno?

HI क्या आपको पसली / सीने में दर्द है?
Kya aapko pasli / seene me dard hai?

How long did the pain last?

ES	¿Cuánto tiempo le duró el dolor?
ZH	痛了多久了？ tòng le duō jiǔ le?
FR	Depuis quand avez-vous mal?
DE	Wie lange hat er angehalten?
VI	Tình trạng đau này kéo dài bao lâu?
IT	Quanto è durato il dolore?
KO	통증이 얼마나 계속 되었습니까? Tong-jeung-i eol-ma-na gye-sok doe-eot-seum-ni-kka?
RU	Как долго длилась боль? Kak dolgo dlilas' bol'?
PL	Jak długo ten ból trwał?
AR	كم مدة دام الألم؟ Kam muddah daam al-alam?
PT	Quanto tempo durou a dor?
FK	Pandan konbyen tan ou te gen doulè a?
EL	Πόσο κράτησε ο πόνος; pOso krAteese o pOnos?
HI	दर्द कितने समय तक रहा? Dard kitne samay tak raha?

Do you still feel the pain?

ES ¿Todavía siente ese dolor?

ZH 现在还痛吗？
xiàn zài hái tòng ma?

FR Avez-vous encore mal?

DE Spüren Sie den Schmerz immer noch?

VI Quý vị có còn thấy đau nữa không?

IT Sente ancora dolore?

KO 아직도 통증이 있습니까?
A-jik-do tong-jeung-i it-seum-ni-kka?

RU Вы все ещё испытываете боль?
Vy vse eshchyo ispytyvaete bol'?

PL Czy dalej czuje Pan(i) ten ból?

AR هل ما زلت تشعر\ تشعرين بالألم؟
Hal maa zilt tish"ur / tish"ureen bil-'alam?

PT Ainda sente a dor?

FK Eske ou santi doulè a toujou?

EL Νιώθετε ακόμη τον πόνο;
neeOthete akOmee ton pOno?

HI क्या आप अब भी दर्द महसूस कर रहे हैं?
Kya aap abhi bhi dard mehsoos kar rahe hain?

Where does it hurt?

ES	¿Dónde le duele?
ZH	那个地方痛？ něi gè dì fāng tòng?
FR	Où avez-vous mal?
DE	Wo schmerzt es
VI	Quý vị đau ở chỗ nào?
IT	Dove Le fa male?
KO	어디가 아프십니까? Eo-di-ga a-peu-sim-ni-kka?
RU	Где именно болит? Gde imenno bolit?
PL	Gdzie Pana (Panią) boli?
AR	أين الألم بالتحديد؟ Ayn al-alam bit-tahdeed?
PT	Onde é que dói?
FK	Ki kote li fè w mal?
EL	Πού πονάτε; pu ponAte?
HI	यह कहां चोट करता है? Yeh kahaan chot karta hai?

When did you start feeling the pain? ... Minutes, ... hours, ... days

¿Cuándo empezó a sentir el dolor? ... Minutos, ... horas, ... días

你从什么时候开始感到痛的？... 几分钟，... 几小时，... 几天
nǐ cóng shén me shí hòu kāi shǐ gǎn dào tòng de? ... jǐ fēn zhōng, ... jǐ xiǎo shí, ... jǐ tiān

Quand a commencé la douleur? ... minutes, ... heures, ... jours

Wann hat es angefangen? ... Minuten, ... Stunden, ... Tage

Quý vị bắt đầu thấy đau khi nào? ... Phút, ... giờ, ... ngày

Quando ha iniziato a provare dolore? ... minuti, ... ore, ... giorni

언제 통증을 느끼기 시작하셨습니까? ... 분, ... 시간, ... 일 전
Eon-je tong-jeung-eul neu-kki-gi si-jak-ha-syeot-seum-ni-kka? ... bun, ... si-gan, ... il jeon

Когда вы стали чувствовать боль? ... минут, ... часов, ... дней
Kogda vy stali chuvstvovat' bol'? ... minut, ... chasov, ... dney

Kiedy zaczął(a) Pan(i) odczuwać ból? ... Minut, ... godzin, ... dni

متى بدأت أن تشعر \ تشعري بالألم؟ ... دقيقة ... ساعة ... يوم
Mattaa bada't an tash"ur / tash"uree bil-alam? ... daqeeqah ... saa"ah ... youm

Quando é que começou a sentir a dor? ... minutos, ... horas, ... dias

Ki lè ou komanse santi doulè a ? ... Minit ... hètan ... jou

Πότε αρχίσατε να νιώθετε τον πόνο; ... λεπτά, ... ώρες, ... ημέρες
pOte arhEEsate na neeOthete ton pOno? ... leptA, ... Ores, ... eemEres

आपको दर्द महसूस होना कब शुरू हुआ था? ... मिनट, ... घंटे, ... दिन
Aapko dard mehsoos hona kab shuru hua tha? ... minute, ... ghante, ... din

When do you feel the pain?

ES	¿En que momento siente el dolor?
ZH	什么时候痛？ shén me shí hòu tòng?
FR	Quand avez-vous ressenti la douleur?
DE	Wann spüren Sie den Schmerz?
VI	Quý vị thấy đau khi nào?
IT	Quando sente dolore?
KO	언제 통증을 느끼십니까? Eon-je tong-jeung-eul neu-kki-sim-ni-kka?
RU	Когда вы чувствуете боль? Kogda vy chuvstvuete bol'?
PL	Kiedy odczuwa Pan(i) ten ból?
AR	متى تشعر \ تشعرين بالألم؟ Mattaa tish"ur / tish"ureen bil-alam?
PT	Quando é que sente a dor?
FK	Ki lè ou santi doulè a ?
EL	Πότε νιώθετε τον πόνο; pOte neeOthete ton pOno?
HI	आपको दर्द कब महसूस हुआ? ... Aapko dard kab mehsoos hua?

constantly, during exertion / at night / during the day

S
constantemente, al hacer un esfuerzo / por la noche / en el día

H
持续性的，活动时 / 夜间 / 白天
chí xù xìng de, huó dòng shí / yè jiān / bái tiān

R
constamment / au cours d'un exercice / la nuit / pendant la journée

E
ununterbrochen, bei Anstrengung / nachts / tagsüber

VI
lúc nào cũng thấy đau, khi vận động mạnh / vào ban đêm / ban ngày

IT
costantemente / quando faccio sforzi / la notte / durante il giorno

O
항상, 몸을 많이 움직일 때 / 밤에 / 낮에
hang-sang, mo-meul ma-ni um-ji-gil ttae / ba-me / na-je

RU
постоянно, во время нагрузок / ночью / днём
postoyanno, vo vremya nagruzok / noch'yu / dnyom

PL
cały czas, podczas wysiłku fizycznego / w nocy / w ciągu dnia

AR
بشكل دائم، عند المشقة او العمل الشاق \ في الليل \ أثناء اليوم
Bi-shekl daa'im, "ind al-mashaqqah au al-"amal ash-shaaq / fil-leyl / athnaa' al-youm

PT
Constantemente, durante o esforço físico / à noite / o dia

FK
tout tan, pandan egzesis / lan nwit / pandan la jounin

EL
συνεχώς, κατά την άσκηση / τη νύχτα / κατά τη διάρκεια της ημέρας
seenehOs, katA teen Askeesee / tee nEEhta / katA tee deeArkeea tees eemEras

HI
लगातार, परिश्रम के दौरान / रात को / दिन में
lagaatar, pariShram ke dauraan / raat ko / din me

When you breathe, do you notice a change in the intensity of the pain?

ES Cuando respira, ¿siente que el dolor cambia de intensidad?

ZH 当你呼吸时，疼痛有没有变化？
dāng nǐ hū xī shí, téng tòng yǒu méi yǒu biàn huà?

FR Lorsque vous respirez, percevez-vous un changement dans l'intensité de la douleur?

DE Verändert sich der Schmerz, wenn Sie atmen?

VI Khi thở, quý vị có thấy sự thay đổi về mức độ đau không?

IT Quando respira nota un cambiamento nell'intensità del dolore?

KO 숨을 쉴 때, 통증의 정도가 달라지는 것을 느끼십니까?
Su-meul swil ttae, tong-jeung-ui jeong-do-ga dal-la-ji-neun geo-seul neu-kki-sim-ni-kka?

RU Вы замечаете изменение интенсивности боли во время дыхания?
Vy zamechaete izmenenie intensivnosti boli vo vremya dykhaniya?

PL Czy podczas oddychania zauważa Pan(i) zmianę w nasileniu bólu?

AR هل تلاحظ / تلاحظين عند التنفس تغيراً في شدة الألم؟
Hal tulaahidh / tulaahidheen "ind at-tanaffus taghyeeran fi shiddat il-alam?

PT Quando respira, nota alguma alteração na intensidade da dor?

FK Lè w ap respire, eske ou remake yon chanjman nan intansite doulè a?

EL Όταν αναπνέετε, παρατηρείτε αλλαγή στην ένταση του πόνου;
Otan anapnEete, parateerEEte alagEE steen Edasee tu pOnu?

HI जब आप सांस लेते हैं, क्या आपने दर्द की तीव्रता में बदलाव नोट किया?
Jab aap saans lete hain, Kya aapne dard ki teevrta mein badlaav note kiya?

Does the pain radiate in a particular direction? Please specify.

.S ¿Se irradia el dolor en determinada dirección? Por favor especifique

H 这个痛向哪里放射吗？具体说一下
zhè gè tòng xiàng nǎ lǐ fàng shè ma? jù tǐ shuō yī xià

R La douleur irradie-t-elle dans une direction particulière? veuillez spécifier

E Strahlt der Schmerz aus? Wohin?

VI Tình trạng đau có lan tỏa theo một hướng cụ thể nào đó không? Xin trình bày rõ

IT Il dolore si irradia in una direzione particolare? La prego di specificare

KO 통증이 일정한 방향으로 뻗어 나갑니까? 구체적으로 밝히십시오
Tong-jeung-i il-jeong-han bang-hyang-eu-ro ppeo-deo na-gam-ni-kka? Gu-che-jeo-geu-ro bal-ki-sip-si-o

RU Боль отражается в каком-то определенном направлении? Пожалуйста, уточните.
Bol' otrazhaetsya v kakom-to opredelennom napravlenii? Pozhaluysta, utochnite.

PL Czy ból rozchodzi się w jakimś konkretnym kierunku? Proszę bliżej określić

AR هل ينتشر الألم باتجاه معين؟ الرجاء تحديد جهة إنتشار الألم.
Hal yantashir al-alam bi-ittijaah mu''ayyan? Ar-rajaa' tahdeed jihhat intishaar al-alam

PT A dor irradia numa direcção especial? Por favor, especifique.

FK Eske doulè a al nan yon direksyon an patikilye? Tanpri spesifye

EL Διαχέεται ο πόνος προς κάποια συγκεκριμένη κατεύθυνση; Παρακαλώ καθορίστε.
deeahEete o pOnos pros kApeea seegekreemEnee katEftheensee? parakalO kathorEEste

HI क्या दर्द किसी निश्चित दिशा की ओर बढता है? कृपया स्पष्ट करें ...
Kya dard kisi nishchit disha ki or baDhta hai? Kripya spaST karein

along the left / right arm / towards the back / the shoulder

ES	por el brazo izquierdo / derecho / hacia la espalda / el hombro
ZH	沿着左 / 右臂 / 向背部 / 向肩部 yán zhe zuǒ / yòu bì / xiàng bèi bù / xiàng jiān bù
FR	le long du bras gauche / droit / vers le dos / l'épaule
DE	den linken / rechten Arm entlang / in den Rücken / die Schulter
VI	dọc theo cánh tay trái / phải / về phía lưng / vai
IT	lungo il braccio sinistro / destro / verso la schiena / la spalla
KO	왼 / 오른 팔을 따라 / 등 / 어깨 쪽으로 oen / o-reun pa-reul tta-ra / deung / eo-kkae jjo-geu-ro
RU	в левую / правую руку / в спину / в плечо v levuyu / pravuyu ruku / v spinu / v plecho
PL	wzdłuż lewej ręki / prawej ręki / w plecy / do ramienia
AR	على طول الذراع الأيسر \ الأيمن \ نحو الظهر \ الكتف "alaa tool adh-dhiraa al-aysar / al-ayman / nahu adh-dhuhr / al-katf
PT	ao longo do braço esquerdo / braço direito / em direcção às costas / ao ombro
FK	nan bra goch / swat / nan zon pa deye / zepol
EL	προς το αριστερό / δεξί άνω άκρο / προς την πλάτη / τον ώμο pros to areesterO / dexEE Ano Akro / pros teen plAtee / ton Omo
HI	दाईं / बाईं भुजा के साथ / कमर की तरफ / क ६ ौ में ... daanyi / baanyi bhuja ke saath / kamar ki taraf / kandhe mein

towards the back of the neck / the jaw / towards the stomach

S
H hacia la nuca / la mandíbula / el estómago

R 向脖子后面 / 向颚部 / 向腹部
xiàng bó zi hòu miàn / xiàng è bù / xiàng fù bù
E
T vers la nuque / vers la mâchoire / vers l'estomac
I
T in den Nacken / den Kiefer / zum Magen hin
O
U về phía sau cổ / hàm / về phía bao tử
R
verso la nuca / la mandíbola / lo stomaco

L 목 뒤 쪽으로 / 턱 쪽으로 / 배 쪽으로
mok dwi jjo-geu-ro / teok jjo-geu-ro / bae jjo-geu-ro

T в заднюю область шеи / в челюсть / в живот
K v zadnyuyu oblast' shei / v chelyust' / v zhivot
I
نحو خلف الرقبة \ الفكّ \ نحو المعدة
Nahu khalf ar-ruqubah / al-fakk / nahu al-ma"idah

em direcção à parte de trás do pescoço / ao maxilar / em direcção ao estômago

nan zon deye kou / machwa / nan zon vant

προς το πίσω μέρος του λαιμού / τη γνάθο / προς το στομάχι
pros to pEEso mEros tu lemU / tee gnAtho / pros to stomAhee

गर्दन के पिछली ओर / जबड़ा / पेट की ओर
Gardan ki piChli or / jabDa / pet ki or

Have you noticed the following changes on yourself?

ES	¿Ha tenido alguno de los siguientes síntomas?
ZH	你有没有发现自己有以下的变化？ nǐ yǒu méi yǒu fā xiàn zì jǐ yǒu yǐ xià de biàn huà?
FR	Avez-vous remarqué par vous-même, les changements suivants?
DE	Haben Sie folgende Veränderungen bei sich bemerkt?
VI	Quý vị có nhận thấy các thay đổi sau đây trong người không?
IT	Ha notato in Lei i seguenti cambiamenti?
KO	다음의 변화가 스스로에 생긴 것을 느끼셨습니까? Da-eu-mui byeon-hwa-ga seu-seu-ro-e saeng-gin geo-seul seu-kki-syeot-seum-ni-kka?
RU	Вы заметили у себя следующие изменения? Vy zametili u sebya sleduyushchie izmeneniya?
PL	Czy zauważył Pan(i) u siebie następujące zmiany?
AR	هل لاحظت التغيرات التالية على نفسك؟ Hal laahadht at-taghyeeraat it-taaliyah "alaa nafsak?
PT	Notou, em si, algumas das seguintes alterações?
FK	Eske ou remake chanjman swivan yo lakay ou?
EL	Παρατηρήσατε τις ακόλουθες αλλαγές στον εαυτό σας; parateerEEsate tees akOluthes alagEs ston eaftO sas?
HI	क्या आपने स्वयं में निम्नलिखित परिवर्तन नोट किए? ... Kya aapne swayam mein nimnlikhit parivartan note kiye?

Nausea / sweating / unconsciousness / fever

ES Náusea / sudoración / inconsciencia / fiebre

ZH 恶心 / 多汗 / 昏迷 / 发烧
ě xīn / duō hàn / hūn mí / fā shāo

FR Nausée / transpiration / inconscience / fièvre

DE Übelkeit / Schwitzen / Ohnmacht / Fieber

VI Buồn nôn / đổ mồ hôi / bất tỉnh / sốt

IT Nausea / sudorazione / perdita dei sensi / febbre

KO 구토증 / 땀흘리기 / 의식 잃음 / 열
gu-to-jeung / ttam-heul-li-gi / ui-sik i-reum / yeol

RU Тошнота / потливость / потеря сознания / повышение температуры
Toshnota / potlivost' / poterya soznaniya / povyshenie temperatury

PL Nudności / poty / utratę przytomności / gorączkę

AR الغثيان \ التعرّق \ فقدان الوعي \ الحمّى
Al-ghithyaan / at-ta"arruq / fuqdaan al-wa'ei / al-hummaa

PT Náusea / sudação / perda de sentidos / febre

FK Noze / swe / pedi konesans / lafyev

EL ναυτία / εφίδρωση / απώλεια αισθήσεων / πυρετός
naftEEa / efEdrosee / apOleea esthEEseon / peeretOs

HI मतली / पसीना / मूर्छित अवस्था / बुखार
Matli / pasina / moorChit awastha / bukhaar

Was your ribcage impacted by something / have you hurt yourself in other ways?

ES ¿Recibió algún golpe en el tórax / se lastimó de alguna otra forma?

ZH 你的胸廓有没有受到挤压 / 你有没有受过伤？
nǐ de xiōng kuò yǒu méi yǒu shòu dào jǐ yā / nǐ yǒu méi yǒu shòu guò shāng？

FR Votre cage thoracique a-t-elle été heurtée par quelque chose? Vous êtes-vous cogné à quelque chose?

DE Haben Sie Ihren Brustkorb gestoßen / sich anders verletzt?

VI Xương sườn của quý vị có bị một vật nào đó va chạm vào không / quý vị có tự làm hại mình bằng cách khác không?

IT La sua cassa toracica è stata colpita da qualcosa / si è fatto / a male in altri modi?

KO 흉곽을 무엇인가에 부딪히셨습니까 / 다른 방식으로 다치셨습니까?
Hyung-gwa-geul mu-eo-sin-ga-e bu-dit-chi-syeot-seum-ni-kka / da-reun bang-si-geu-ro da-chi-syeot-seum-ni-kka?

RU Была ли у вас травма грудной клетки / травмировали ли вы себя другим образом?
Byla li u vas travma grudnoy kletki / travmirovali li vy sebya drugim obrazom?

PL Czy doznał(a) Pan(i) uderzenia czymś w klatkę piersiową / czy zrobił(a) Pan(i) sobie krzywdę w jakiś inny sposób?

AR هل اصيب قفص أضلاعك بشيءٍ ١ هل تأذيت بأشكال أخرى؟
Hal useeb qafs adhlaa"ak bi-shey' / hal ta'adhdheyt bi-ashkaal ukhraa?

PT Sofreu algum impacto nas suas costelas com algo/magoou-se de qualquer outra forma?

FK Eske gen yon bagay ki frape kot ou / eske ou andomaje tet nan ninpòt ki fason ?

EL Συγκρούστηκε κάτι με το θωρακικό κλωβό σας / τραυματιστήκατε με οποιονδήποτε άλλο τρόπο;
seegrUsteeke kAtee me to thorakeekO klovO sas / travmateestEEkate me opeeondEEpote Alo trOpo?

HI क्या आपकी पसली का ढांचा किसी चीज से प्रभावित हुआ / आपने स्वयं को किसी अन्य तरीके से नुकसान पहुंचाया?
Kya aapki pasli ka Dhancha kisi cheez se prabhavit hua / aapne swayam ko kisi anya tareeke se nuksaan pahunchaya?

Have you already been diagnosed with heart / coronary heart disease?

ES ¿Le han diagnosticado enfermedad cardíaca / de las coronarias?

ZH 医生说你有心脏病 / 冠心病吗？
yī shēng shuō nǐ yǒu xīn zàng bìng / guàn xīn bìng ma?

FR Vous a-t-on déjà diagnostiqué une maladie du cœur ou des artères coronaires?

DE Ist bei Ihnen bereits eine Herz-(Gefäß)erkrankung festgestellt worden?

VI Có phải gần đây quý vị đã được chẩn đoán là mắc bệnh tim / bệnh vành tim không?

IT Le è già stata diagnosticata una malattia cardiaca / malattia cardiaca coronarica?

KO 이미 심장 / 관상 동맥성 심장 질환 진단을 받으셨습니까？
I-mi sim-jang / gwan-sang dong-maek-seong sim-jang jil-hwan jin-da-neul ba-deu-syeot-seum-ni-kka?

RU Вам ставили диагноз заболевания сердца / ишемической болезни сердца?
Vam stavili diagnoz zabolevaniya serdtsa / ishemicheskoy bolezni serdtsa?

PL Czy zdiagnozowano już u Pana(i) chorobę serca / wieńcową chorobę serca?

AR هل سبق أن تم تشخيص مرض القلب / مرض قلب تاجي عندك؟
Hal sabaq an tamm tashkhees maradh al-qalb / maradh qalb taaji "indak?

PT Já foi diagnosticado(a) com uma cardiopatia / cardiopatia coronária?

FK Eske yo te fè diagnostic ke ou gen maladi kè / kowonè?

EL Σας έχει ήδη γίνει διάγνωση καρδιακής / στεφανιαίας νόσου;
sas Ehei EEdee gEEnee deeAgnosee kardeeakEEs / stefaneeEas nOsu?

HI क्या पहले ही आपके हृदय / वलयकार हृदय बीमारी की पहचान हो गई थी?
Kya pahle hi aapke hirdey / valaykaar hirdey beemari ki pehchaan ho gayi thi?

congenital heart defect / coronary heart disease / high blood pressure

ES defecto cardíaco congénito / cardiopatía coronaria / hipertensión

ZH 先天性心脏病 / 冠心病 / 高血压
xiān tiān xìng xīn zàng bìng / guàn xīn bìng / gāo xuè yā

FR malformation cardiaque congénitale / maladie du coeur / pression sanguine élevée

DE angeborener Herzfehler / koronare Herzkrankheit / Bluthochdruck

VI loạn nhịp tim bẩm sinh / bệnh vành tim / huyết áp cao

IT difetto cardiaco congenito / malattia cardiaca coronarica / pressione alta

KO 선천성 심장 결함 / 관상 동맥성 심장 질환 / 고혈압
seon-cheon-seong sim-jang gyeol-ham / gwan-sang dong-maek-seong sim-jang jil-hwan / go-hyeo-rap

RU врожденный порок сердца / ишемическая болезнь сердца / повышенное кровяное давление
vrozhdennyi porok serdtsa / ishemicheskaya bolezn' serdtsa / povyshennoe krovyanoe davlenie

PL wrodzoną wadę serca / wieńcową chorobę serca / nadciśnienie

AR عيب قلب ميرائي \ مرض قلب تاجي \ ضغط دمّ عالٍ
"eyb qalb meeraathi / maradh qalb taaji / dhaght damm "aali

PT defeito cardíaco congénito / cardiopatia coronária / hipertensão ou tensão arterial alta

FK tar kè konjenital / maladi kè / tansyon

EL εκ γενετής καρδιακή ανωμαλία / στεφανιαία νόσος / υψηλή αρτηριακή πίεση
ek genetEEs kardeeakEE anomalEEa / stefaneeEa nOsos / eespeelEE arteereeakEE pEEesee

HI जन्मजात हृदय कमी / वलयकार हृदय बीमारी / उच्च रक्तचाप ...
janmjaat hirdey kami / valeykaar hirdey beemari / uchch raktchaap

arterial occlusive disease / pacemaker / artificial heart valve

ES enfermedad oclusiva arterial / marcapasos / válvula cardíaca artificial

ZH 动脉栓塞 / 起搏器 / 人工心脏瓣膜
dòng mài shuān sāi / qǐ bó qì / rén gōng xīn zàng bàn mó

FR maladie artérielle occlusive / pacemaker / valve cardiaque artificielle

DE arterielle Verschlusskrankheit / Schrittmacher / künstliche Herzklappe

VI bệnh nghẽn động mạch vành / máy điều hòa nhịp tim / van tim nhân tạo

IT malattia occlusiva arteriosa / pacemaker / valvola cardiaca artificiale

KO 동맥 폐쇄 질환 / 인공 심박 조율기 / 인공 심장판막
dong-maek pye-swae jil-hwan / in-gong sim-bak jo-yul-gi / in-gong sim-jang-pan-mak

RU облитерация артерий / кардиостимулятор / искусственный клапан сердца
obliteratsiya arteriy / kardiostimulyator / iskusstvennyi klapan serdtsa

PL zarostową chorobę tętnic / rozrusznik serca / sztuczną zastawkę serca

AR مرض شرياني إنسدادي \ منظّم قلب \ صمام قلب إصطناعي
Maradh shiryaani insidaadi / munadhdhim qalb / sammam qalb istinaa"ei

PT doença oclusiva arterial / pacemaker / válvula cardíaca artificial

FK maladi oklusif arteryak / stimulate kadyak (aparey nan kè) / valv kè atifisyel

EL νόσος αρτηριακής απόφραξης / βηματοδότης / τεχνητή βαλβίδα καρδίας
nOsos arteereeakEes apOfraxees / veematodOtees / tehneetE valvEEda kardeeAs

HI ६ मनीय रो ६ गी बीमारी / पेसमेकर / कृत्रिम हृदय वाल्व
Dhamniye rodhi beemari / pacemaker / kratrim hirdey valve

Did / do you have a feeling of constriction in the chest?

ES ¿Sintió / siente una opresión en el pecho?

ZH 现在／过去你有没有感到胸部发紧？
xiàn zài / guò qù nǐ yǒu méi yǒu gǎn dào xiōng bù fā jǐn?

FR Avez-vous ressenti / ressentez-vous une sensation de constriction dans le thorax?

DE Hatten / haben Sie ein Engegefühl im Brustkorb?

VI Quý vị có / đã cảm thấy đau thắt ở vùng ngực không?

IT Ha avuto / ha una sensazione di oppressione al petto?

KO 가슴이 조이는 느낌이 드십니까?
Ga-seu-mi jo-i-neun neu-kki-mi deu-sim-ni-kka?

RU Испытывали / испытываете ли вы чувство стеснения в груди?
Ispytyvali / ispytyvaete li vy chuvstvo stesneniya v grudi?

PL Czy odczuwa Pan(i) ucisk w klatce piersiowej?

AR هل عندك \ كان عندك شعوراً بالتقيد في الصدر؟
Hal "indak / kaan "indak shu"oor bit-taqyeed fis-sadr?

PT Sente / sentiu uma sensação de constrição no peito?

FK Eske ou janm santi / ou santi pwatrin ou sere?

EL Είχατε / Έχετε αίσθημα σύσφιξης στο στήθος;
EEhate / Ehete Estheema sEEsfeexees sto stEEthos?

HI क्या आप हृदय में संकुचनशिलता महसूस करते हैं / थे?
Kya aap hirdey mein sankuchanshilta mehsoos karte hain / the?

Did this cause anxiety in you?

ES ¿Le produjo angustia esa sensación?

ZH 这些让你焦虑吗？
zhè xiē ràng nǐ jiāo lǜ ma?

FR Cela vous donne-t-il de l'anxiété?

DE Hatten Sie Angst?

VI Tình trạng này có khiến quý vị cảm thấy lo lắng không?

IT Ciò Le ha provocato ansia?

KO 이것 때문에 불안하십니까?
I-geot ttae-mu-ne bu-ran-ha-sim-ni-kka?

RU Это вызывало у вас чувство страха?
Eto vyzyvalo u vas chuvstvo strakha?

PL Czy to powoduje u Pana(i) lęk?

AR هل أثار هذا فيك القلق؟
Hal athaar hadha feek al-qalaq?

PT Isto causou-lhe ansiedade?

FK Eske sa lakòz ke ou angwas (panike)?

EL Σας προκάλεσε αυτό άγχος;
sas prokAlese aftO Aghos?

HI क्या इस कारण आपको चिंता हुई?
Kya is kaaraN aapko chinta hui?

Have you noticed anything unusual in your heart beat?

ES ¿Ha notado algo extraño en el latido del corazón?

ZH 你有没有感到心跳有什么异常？
    nǐ yǒu méi yǒu gǎn dào xīn tiào yǒu shén me yì cháng?

FR Avez-vous remarqué quelque chose d'inhabituel dans le battement de votre coeur?

DE Ist Ihnen an Ihrem Herzschlag etwas Ungewöhnliches aufgefallen?

VI Quý vị có nhận thấy điều gì bất thường trong nhịp tim của mình không?

IT Ha notato nulla di insolito nel Suo battito cardiaco?

KO 심장 박동에 이상을 느끼신 적이 있습니까?
    Sim-jang bak-dong-e i-sang-eul neu-kki-sin jeo-gi it-seum-ni-kka?

RU Заметили ли вы какие-либо отклонения в сердцебиении?
    Zametili li vy kakie-libo otkloneniya v serdtsebienii?

PL Czy zauważył Pan(i) coś dziwnego w biciu swojego serca?

AR هل لاحظت أيّ شيء غير عادي في نبض قلبك؟
    Hal laahadht ay shey' gheyr "aadi fi nabdh qalbak?

PT Notou algo de invulgar nos seus batimentos cardíacos?

FK Eske ou remake okinn bagay ki pa nomal nan jan kè w ap bat?

EL Παρατηρήσατε κάτι ασυνήθιστο στον καρδιακό σας ρυθμό;
    parateerEEsate kAtee aseenEEtheesto ston kardeeakO sas reethmO?

HI क्या आपने अपनी हृदय गति में कुछ असामान्य नोट किया? ...
    Kya aapne apni hirdey gati mein kuCh A-saamanya note kiya?

accelerated / irregular heartbeat / heartbeat sensation

ES	ritmo acelerado / irregular / siente los latidos
ZH	加快的 / 心跳异常 / 心慌 jiā kuài de / xīn tiào yì cháng / xīn huāng
FR	accélération / battement irrégulier / sensation du battement
DE	vermehrtes / unregelmäßiges Herzschlagen / fühlbares Herzklopfen
VI	nhịp tim nhanh hơn / bất thường / tim đập mạnh
IT	battito accelerato / irregolare / sensazione di battito cardiaco
KO	더 빨리 뛰는 / 불규칙한 심장 박동 / 심장 박동이 느껴짐 deo ppal-li ttwi-neun / bul-gyu-chik-han sim-jang bak-dong / sim-jang bak-dong-i-neu-kkyeo-jim
RU	учащенное / нерегулярное сокращение сердца / ощущение пульсации сердца uchashchennoe / neregulyarnoe sokrashchenie serdtsa / oshchushchenie pul'satsii serdtsa
PL	przyspieszone / nieregularne bicie serca / odczuwanie bicia serca
AR	نبض قلب مسرع \ نبض قلب غير نظامي \ إحساس نبض قلب Nabdh qalb musarra" / nabdh qalb gheyr nidhaami / ihsaas nabdh qalb
PT	batimentos cardíacos acelerados / irregulares / sensação de batimentos cardíacos
FK	bat vit / batman kè iregilye / sansasyon batman kè
EL	επιταχυμένος / ακανόνιστος καρδιακός παλμός / αίσθημα καρδιακού παλμού epeetaheemEnos / akanOneestos kardeeakOs palmOs / Estheema kardeeakU palmU
HI	तेज / अनियमित हृदय गति / हृदय गति संवेदना Tez / A-niyamit hirdey gati / hirdey gati samvedna

Do you often have to go to the toilet at night for urination? How often?

ES ¿Va muy seguido al baño a orinar en la noche? ¿Con qué frecuencia?

ZH 你是否经常晚上起来小便？一晚有几次？
nǐ shì fǒu jīng cháng wǎn shàng qǐ lái xiǎo biàn? yī wǎn yǒu jǐ cì?

FR Avez-vous souvent été à la toilette la nuit pour uriner? Combien de fois?

DE Müssen Sie nachts oft auf die Toilette zum Wasserlassen? Wie oft?

VI Quý vị có thường đi tiểu tiện vào ban đêm không? Bao lâu một lần?

IT Deve andare spesso al bagno la notte per urinare? Quanto spesso?

KO 밤에 소변을 보러 가는 일이 잦습니까? 얼마나 자주?
Ba-me so-byeo-neul bo-reo ga-neun i-ri jat-seum-ni-kka? Eol-ma-na ja-ju?

RU Часто ли вам ночью приходится ходить в туалет мочиться? Как часто?
Chasto li vam noch'yu prikhoditsya khodit' v tualet mochit'sya? Kak chasto?

PL Czy Pan(i) często wstawać w nocy w celu oddania moczu? Jak często?

AR هل يجب عليك كثرة إستعمال المرحاض في الليل للتبوّل؟ كم مرة؟
Hal yajib "alayk kathrah isti"maal al-mirhaadh fil-leyl lit-tabawwul? Kam marrah?

PT Durante a noite, vai muitas vezes à casa de banho para urinar? Quantas vezes?

FK Eske ou ale souvan nan twalet pandan lan nwit pou al pipi? Konbyen fwa?

EL Πρέπει να πηγαίνετε συχνά στην τουαλέτα τη νύχτα για ούρηση; Πόσο συχνά;
prEpee na peegEnete seehnA steen tualEta tee nEEhta geea Ureesee? pOso seehnA?

HI क्या आपको रात में पेशाब के लिए कई बार जाना पड़ता है? कितनी बार?
Kya aapko raat mein peshaab ke liye kayi baar jana paDta hai? Kitni baar?

Do you sometimes have swollen legs? In which situations?

ES ¿A veces se le hinchan las piernas? ¿En qué situaciones?

ZH 你有时候腿肿吗？在什么情况下出现的？
nǐ yǒu shí hòu tuǐ zhǒng ma? zài shén me qíng kuàng xià chū xiàn de?

FR Avez-vous parfois les pieds gonflés? Dans quelles circonstances?

DE Haben Sie manchmal geschwollene Beine? Wann?

VI Thỉnh thoảng, chân quý vị có bị sưng không? Trong những trường hợp nào?

IT A volte Le si gonfiano le gambe? In quali situazioni?

KO 다리가 붓는 적이 가끔 있습니까? 어떤 때에?
Da-ri-ga bun-neun jeo-gi ga-kkeum it-seum-ni-kka? Eo-tteon ttae?

RU У вас иногда отекают ноги? В каких случаях?
U vas inogda otekayut nogi? V kakikh sluchayakh?

PL Czy często puchną Panu(i) nogi? W jakich sytuacjach?

AR هل تعاني / تعانين احناناً من انتفاخ الرجلين؟ في اي ظروف؟
Hal tu"aani / tu"aaneen ahyaanah min intifaakh ar-rijleyn? Fi ayyi dhuroof?

PT Às vezes, tem as pernas inchadas? Em que situações?

HK Eske janb ou kon anfle ? Nan ki situasyon ?

EL Έχετε μερικές φορές πρησμένα κάτω άκρα; Σε ποιες περιπτώσεις;
Ehete mereekEs forEs preesmEna kAto Akra? se peeEs pereeptOsees?

HI क्या आपकी टांगें कभी-कभी सूज जाती हैं? किस स्थिति में?...
Kya aapki taangein kabhi-kabhi sooz jaati hain? Kis sthiti mein?

always / in the evening

ES	siempre / por la noche
ZH	经常的 / 在晚上 jīng cháng de / zài wǎn shàng
FR	toujours / le soir
DE	immer / am Abend
VI	luôn luôn / vào buổi tối
IT	sempre / la sera
KO	항상 / 저녁에 hang-sang / jeo-nyeo-ge
RU	всегда / вечером vsegda / vecherom
PL	stale / wieczorem
AR	دائماً \ في المساء Daa'iman / fil-masaa'
PT	sempre / à noite
FK	tout tan / nan aswe
EL	πάντα / το απόγευμα pAnda / to apOgevma
HI	हमेशा / शाम में Hamesha / shaam me

Do you have strongly visible veins? Do you have varicose veins?

ES ¿Tiene las venas muy abultadas? ¿Tiene várices?

ZH 你有能明显看见的静脉吗？你有静脉曲张吗？
nǐ yǒu néng míng xiǎn kàn jiàn de jìng mài ma? nǐ yǒu jìng mài qū zhāng ma?

FR Avez-vous des veines fortement apparentes? avez-vous des varices?

DE Treten Ihre Venen stark hervor? Haben Sie Krampfadern?

VI Quý vị có nhìn thấy rõ các tĩnh mạch không? Quý vị có bị giãn tĩnh mạch không?

IT Ha vene molto visibili? Ha vene varicose?

KO 아주 두드러진 정맥이 있으십니까? 정맥류 정맥이 있으십니까?
A-ju dudeu-reo-jin jeong-mae-gi i-seu-sim-ni-kka? Jeong-maeng-nyu jeong-mae-gi i-seu-sim-ni-kka?

RU Есть ли у вас отчетливо видимые вены? Есть ли у вас варикозно расширенные вены?
Est' li u vas otchetlivo vidimye veny? Est' li u vas varikozno rasshirennye veny?

PL Czy ma Pan(i) silnie uwidocznione żyły? Czy ma Pan(i) żylaki?

AR هل عروقك ظاهرة بشكل واضح جداً؟ هل عندك عروق دوالية؟
Hal "urooqak dhaahirah bi-shekl waashidh jiddan? Hal "indak "urooq dawwaaliyyah?

PT Tem veias muito visíveis? Tem varizes?

FK Eske ven ou parèt anpil? Eske ou gen ven varikez

EL Έχετε πολύ ορατές φλέβες; Έχετε κιρσούς φλεβών;
Ehete polEE oratEs flEves? Ehete keersUs flevOn?

HI क्या आपकी नसें बहुत अधिक दिखाई देती हैं? क्या आपकी नसें सूजी हुई हैं?
Kya aapki nasein bahut adhik dikhaayi deti hain? Kya aapki nasein suji hui hain?

Have you ever experienced heart problems / a heart attack / a stroke?

ES ¿Ha tenido problemas del corazón / ataque cardíaco / embolia?

ZH 你有没有过心脏病发作 / 心脏梗塞 / 中风？
nǐ yǒu méi yǒu guò xīn zàng bìng fā zuò / xīn zàng gěng sāi / zhòng fēng?

FR Avez-vous déjà eu des problèmes cardiaques? une attaque cardiaque / une apoplexie?

DE Hatten Sie jemals Herzprobleme / einen Herzanfall / Schlaganfall?

VI Quý vị đã bao giờ gặp các vấn đề về tim / nhồi máu cơ tim / đột quỵ chưa?

IT Ha mai avuto problemi al cuore / un attacco cardiaco / un ictus?

KO 심장에 문제가 있은 / 심장 마비가 있은 / 뇌졸중이 있은 적이 있습니까?
Sim-jang-e mun-je-ga i-seun / sim-jang ma-bi-ga i-seun / noe-jol-jeung-i i-seun jeo-gi it-seum-ni-kka?

RU У вас когда-нибудь были проблемы с сердцем / инфаркт / инсульт?
U vas kogda-nibud' byli problemy s serdtsem / infarkt / insul't?

PL Czy miał(a) Pan(i) kiedykolwiek problemy z sercem / zawał serca / udar?

AR هل سبق أن عانيت من مشاكل قلبية \ نوبة قلبية \ جلطة دماغية؟
Hal sabaq an "aanayt min mashaakil qalbiyyah / noubah qalbiyyah / jultah dimaaghiyah?

PT Alguma vez teve problemas cardíacos / um ataque de coração / um acidente vascular cerebral?

FK Eske ou te jam, gen pwoblèm kè / yon kriz kadyak / yon estwok ?

EL Έχετε βιώσει ποτέ καρδιακά προβλήματα / καρδιακή προσβολή / εγκεφαλικό επεισόδιο;
Ehete veeOsee potE kardeeakA provlEEmata / kardeeakEE prosvolEE / egefaleekO epeesOdeeo?

HI क्या आपको कभी हृदय की समस्या / दिल का दौरा / आघात हुआ है ?
Kya aapko kabhi hirdey ki samasya / dil ka daura / aaghat hua hai?

How high is your blood pressure? Normal / high / low

ES ¿Cómo anda de la presión arterial? Normal / alta / baja

ZH 你的血压有多高？正常 / 偏高 / 偏低
nǐ de xuè yā yǒu duō gāo? zhèng cháng / piān gāo / piān dī /

FR Quelle est votre pression sanguine? Normale / élevée / basse

DE Wie ist Ihr Blutdruck? normal / hoch / niedrig

VI Huyết áp của quý vị cao tới mức nào? Bình thường / cao / thấp

IT Quale è la sua pressione? Normale / alta / bassa

KO 혈압이 어떻습니까? 정상 / 높다 / 낮다
Hyeo-ra-bi eo-tteo-sseum-ni-kka? Jeong-sang / nop-da / nat-da

RU Какое у вас артериальное давление? Нормальное / высокое / низкое
Kakoe u vas arterial'noe davlenie? Normal'noe / vysokoe / nizkoe

PL Jakie ma Pan(i) ciśnienie? Normalne / wysokie / nieskie

AR ما هو ارتفاع ضغط دمّك؟ عادي \ مرتفع \ واطي
Maa huwa irtifaa dhaght dammak? "Aadi \ murtafi" / waati'

PT Como é a sua tensão arterial? Normal / alta / baixa

FK Kijan tansyon w ye? Nomal / wo / ba

EL Πώς είναι η αρτηριακή πίεση σας; Κανονική / Υψηλή / Χαμηλή
pOs EEne e arteereeakE pEEesEE sas? kanoneekEE / eepseelEE / hameelEE

HI आपका रक्तचाप कितना उच्च है? सामान्य / उच्च / निम्न
Apka raktchaap kitna uchch hai? saamanya / uchch / nimn

Are you taking any heart medication? Please specify.

ES	¿Toma ahora medicamentos para el corazón? ¿De qué tipo?
ZH	你在使用什么心脏病药物吗？是什么药 nǐ zài shǐ yòng shén me xīn zàng bìng yào wù ma? shì shén me yào
FR	Prenez-vous un médicament pour le coeur? Lequel?
DE	Nehmen Sie Herzmedikamente? Welche?
VI	Quý vị có đang dùng loại thuốc điều trị bệnh tim nào không? Xin trình bày rõ
IT	Sta prendendo farmaci per il cuore? Prego specificare
KO	심장 약 드시는 게 있으십니까? 구체적으로 밝혀주십시오 Sim-jang yak deu-si-neun ge i-seu-sim-ni-kka? Gu-che-jeo-geu-ro bal-kyeo-ju-sip-si-o
RU	Вы принимаете какие-нибудь сердечные лекарства? Пожалуйста, уточните Vy prinimaete kakie-nibud' serdechnye lekarstva? Pozhaluysta, utochnite
PL	Czy przyjmuje Pan(i) leki na serce? Proszę szerzej określić.
AR	هل تأخذ \ تأخذين أي دواء للقلب؟ الرجاء بيانه. Hal ta'khudh / ta'khudheen ayy dawaa lil-qalb? Ar-rajaa' bayaanoh
PT	Está a tomar algum medicamento para o coração? Por favor, especifique.
FK	Eske ou ap pran okinn medikaman pou kè? Tanpri spesifye
EL	Λαμβάνετε φάρμακα για την καρδιά; Παρακαλώ καθορίστε. lamvAnete fArmaka geea teen kardeeA? parakalO kathorEEste
HI	क्या आप हृदय की कोई दवा ले रहे हैं? कृपया स्पष्ट करें ... Kya aap hirdey ki koi davaa le rahe hain? Kripya spaSt karein

nitroglycerine / digitalis / diuretics

S nitroglicerina / digital / diuréticos

H 硝酸甘油 / 洋地黄 / 利尿药
xiāo suān gān yóu / yáng dì huáng / lì niào yào

R nitroglycérine / digitaline / diurétique

E Nitroglyzerin / Digitalis / Diuretika

I nitroglycerine / lá mao địa hoàng / thuốc lợi tiểu

I nitroglicerina / digitaleina / diuretici

O 니트로글리세린 / 디기탈리스 / 이뇨제
ni-teu-ro-geul-li-se-rin / di-gi-tal-li-seu / i-nyo-je

U нитроглицерин / дигиталис / мочегонные
nitroglitserin / digitalis / mochegonnye

L nitroglicerynę / naparstnicę / leki moczopędne

R نتروجليسرين \ ديجيتاليس \ مدّرات بول
Nitroglycerine / digitalis / mudarriraat baul

T nitroglicerina / digitalina / diuréticos

K nitwoglyserin / digitalis / duretik

L νιτρογλυκερίνη / δακτυλίτιδα / διουρητικά
neetrogleekerEEnee / dakteelEEteeda / deeureetikA

नाइट्रोग्लिसरीन / नागफनी का रस / मूत्रवर्धक ...
nitroglycerine / naahphani ka ras / mootravardhak

tablets against high blood pressure / which are placed under the tongue

ES	pastillas contra la hipertensión / las que se ponen debajo de la lengua
ZH	抗高血压药片 / 放到舌头下面的那一种 kàng gāo xuè yā yào piàn / fàng dào shé tóu xià miàn de nà yī zhǒng
FR	des comprimés contre l'hypertension / des comprimés placés sous la langue
DE	Tabletten gegen hohen Blutdruck / die man unter die Zunge legt
VI	thuốc viên điều trị chứng cao huyết áp / các loại thuốc ngậm dưới lưỡi
IT	compresse contro la pressione alta / che si mettono sotto la lingua
KO	고혈압 내리는 약 / 혀 밑에 넣는 약 go-hyeo-rap nae-ri-neun yak / hyeo mi-te neon-neun yak
RU	таблетки от высокого давления / подъязычные таблетки tabletki ot vysokogo davleniya / pod"yazychnye tabletki
PL	tabletki obniżające ciśnienie / które wprowadza się pod język
AR	أقراص مضادة لضغط الدمّ العالي \ التي توضع تحت اللسان Aqraas mudhaadah li-dhaght ad-damm al-"aali / alati toodha" taht il-lisaan
PT	comprimidos contra a tensão arterial alta / quais são colocados debaixo da língua
FK	gren pou tansyon / ke yo plase anba lang
EL	δισκία κατά της υπέρτασης / που τοποθετούνται κάτω από τη γλώσσα deeskEEa katA tees eepErtasees / pu topothetUde kAto apO tee glOsa
HI	उच्च रक्तचाप के विरुद्ध गोलियां /जो जीभ के नीचे रखी जाती हैं Uchch raktchaap ke virudh goliyan / jo jeebh ke neeche rakkhi jati hain

Do you cough / have a common cold? For how long?

S ¿Tiene tos / está resfriado? ¿Desde hace cuánto?

H 你咳嗽吗 / 患感冒吗？多久了？
nǐ ké sòu ma / huàn gǎn mào ma? duō jiǔ le?

R Toussez-vous / avez-vous un rhume banal? / depuis quand?

E Haben Sie Husten / Schnupfen / eine Erkältung? Wie lange schon?

T Quý vị có bị ho / cảm lạnh thông thường không? Trong bao lâu?

I Tossisce / ha il raffreddore? Da quanto tempo?

O 기침하십니까 / 일반 감기가 있으십니까? 얼마나 오래 됐습니까?
Gi-chim-ha-sim-ni-kka / il-ban gam-gi-ga i-seu-sim-ni-kka? Eol-ma-na o-rae
dwaet-seum-ni-kka?

U У вас есть кашель / простуда? Как долго?
U vas est' kashel / prostuda? Kak dolgo?

L Czy ma Pan(i) kaszel / jest przeziębiony(a)? Od jak dawna?

R هل عندك سعال \ هل عندك زكام عادي؟ كم مدة كان عندك إياه؟
Hal "indak su"aal / hal "indak zukkaam "aadi? Kam muddah kaan "indak iyyah?

T Tem tosse / está constipado(a)? Há quanto tempo?

K Eske ou ap touse / gen la grip ? Pandan konbyen tan ?

L Βήχετε / Έχετε κοινό κρυολόγημα; Για πόσο καιρό;
vEEhete / Ehete keenO kreeolOgeema? Geea pOso kerO?

HI क्या आपको खांसी / सामान्य जुकाम है? कब से?
Kya aapko Khaansi / saamanya jukaam hai? Kab se?

Do you (often) have a cold?

ES ¿Está usted resfriado (muy seguido)?

ZH 你咳嗽带痰吗？
nĭ ké sòu dài tán ma?

FR Avez-vous (souvent) des rhumes?

DE Sind Sie (oft) erkältet?

VI Quý vị có bị ho ra đờm không (chất nhầy)?

IT Ha (spesso) il raffreddore?

KO 기침할 때 침 (점액)이 나옵니까?
Gi-chim-hal ttae chim (jeom-aek) i na-om-ni-kka?

RU У вас есть (часто бывает) простуда?
U vas est' (chasto byvaet) prostuda?

PL Czy często jest Pan(i) przeziębiony(a)?

AR هل تصاب / تصابين (كثيراً) بالزكام؟
Hal tusaab / tusaabeen (kathiiran) biz-zukaam?

PT Constipa-se (com frequência)?

FK Eske ou touse kracha (bil)?

EL Έχετε (συχνά) κρυολόγημα;
Ehete (seehnA) kreeolOgeema?

HI क्या आपकी खांसी में बलगम आ रहा है (कफदार)?
Kya aapki khaansi mein balgam aa raha hai (cuffdar)?

Are you coughing out sputum (mucous)?

ES ¿Tose mucosidad (esputo)?

ZH 带血丝的 / 有血块 / 有脓 / 粘的
dài xiě sī de / yǒu xuè kuài / yǒu nóng / nián de

FR Avez-vous émis des crachats (muqueux) en toussant?

DE Husten Sie Schleim ab?

VI kèm theo các vết máu / các cục máu khô / có mủ / có chất nhầy

IT Espettora quando tossisce (muco)?

KO 피가 섞여 / 굳은 피가 덩어리져서 / 화농성의 / 점액성의
pi-ga seok-kyeo / gu-deun pi-ga deong-eo-ri-jyeo-seo / hwa-nong-seong-ui / jeom-aek-seong-ui

RU Вы отхаркиваете мокроту (слизь)?
Vy otkharkivaete mokrotu (sliz')?

PL Czy odksztusza Pan(i) flegmę (śluz)?

AR هل يخرج البلغم عند السعال؟
Hal yakhruj al-balgham "ind as-su"aal?

PT Está a tossir com expectoração (mucosidade)?

FK ki gen san / boul san / purulan (pus) / larim

EL Βήχετε πτύελα (βλέννη);
vEEhete ptEEela (vlEnee)?

HI खून की जांच से / रक्त के ठोस गुमड़े पड़ जाना / पीव वाला / चिपचिपा
Khoon ki jaanch se / rakt ke Thos gumDe pad jaana / peev vala / chipchipa

with traces of blood / lumps of solidified blood / purulent / viscous

ES	con rastros de sangre / coágulos / pus / pegajosa
ZH	低粘性的 / 黄色的 / 绿色的 / 棕色的 / 白色的 dī nián xìng de / huáng sè de / lǜ sè de / zōng sè de / bái sè de
FR	avec des traces de sang / avec des fragments de sang coagulé / purulents / visqueux
DE	mit Blutspuren / Blutklumpen / eitrig / dickflüssig
VI	ít nhầy / vàng / xanh / nâu / trắng
IT	con tracce di sangue / grumi di sangue solidificato / purulento / viscoso
KO	점액성이 낮은 / 노란 / 녹색의 / 갈색의 / 하얀 jeom-aek-seong-i na-jeun / no-ran / nok-saeg-ui / gal-sae-gui / ha-yan
RU	со следами крови / сгустками затвердевшей крови / гнойную / вязкую so sledami krovi / sgustkami zatverdevshey krovi / gnoynuyu / vyazkuyu
PL	ze śladowymi ilościami krwi / z grudkami skrzepłej krwi / ropną / lepką
AR	فيه آثار الدمّ \ فيه كتل الدمّ المتجمد / شكله قيحي / شكله لزج Feehe aathaar ad-damm / feehe kutal ad-damm al-mutajammid / shakloh qayhee / shakloh lazij
PT	com vestígios de sangue / pedaços de sangue coagulado / purulenta / viscosa
FK	pa anpil larim / jaun / vet / mawon / blan
EL	με ίχνη αίματος / σβόλους στερεοποιημένου αίματος / πυώδη / ιξώδες me EEhnee Ematos / svOlus stereopee-eemEnu Ematos / peeOdee / eexOdes
HI	कम चिपचिपापन / पीला / हरा / भूरा / सफेद Kam chipchipapan / peela / haraa / Bhuraa / safed

of low viscosity / yellow / green / brown / white

ES de poca viscosidad / amarillo / verde / marrón (café) / blanco

ZH 你 / 你的家人有没有得过结核？
nǐ / nǐ de jiā rén yǒu méi yǒu dé guò jiē hé?

FR de faible viscosité / jaunes / verts / bruns / blancs

DE dünnflüssig / gelb / grün / braun / weiß

VI Quý vị / thành viên trong gia đình quý vị đã bao giờ mắc bệnh lao chưa?

IT a bassa viscosità / giallo / verde / marrone / bianco

KO 본인이나 가족 일원 중에 결핵이 있은 사람이 있습니까?
Bo-ni-n-i-na ga-jok ir-won jung-e gyeol-hae-gi it-seun sa-ra-mi it-seum-ni-kka?

RU маловязкую / желтую / зеленую / коричневую / белую
malovyazkuyu / zheltuyu / zelenuyu / korichnevuyu / beluyu

PL o niskiej kleistości / żółtą / zieloną / brązową / białą

AR لزوجته منخفضة \ لونه أصفر \ لونه أخضر \ لونه أسمر \ لونه أبيض
Luzoojteh munkhafidhah / lonoh asfar / lonoh akhdhar / lonoh asmar / lonoh abyadh

PT de viscosidade baixa / amarelada / esverdeada / acastanhada / esbranquiçada

FK Eske ou menm / yon moun nan fanmi out e janm gen tibekiloz?

EL χαμηλού ιξῶδους / κίτρινο / πράσινο / καφέ / λευκό
hameelU eexOdus / kEEtreeno / prAseeno / kafE / lefkO

HI क्या आपको / आपके परिवार के किसी सदस्य को कभी क्षय रोग हुआ था?
Kya aapko / aapke parivar ke kisi sadasya ko kabhi kShay rog hua tha?

Have you / has a family member ever had tuberculosis?

ES	¿Ha tenido tuberculosis usted / un miembro de la familia?
ZH	你呼吸时喘气吗？ nǐ hū xī shí chuǎn qì ma?
FR	Avez-vous un membre de votre famille qui a / qui a eu la tuberculose?
DE	Haben Sie / ein Familienmitglied Tuberkulose gehabt?
VI	Quý vị có thở khò khè khi thở không?
IT	Lei / un Suo familiare ha mai avuto la tubercolosi?
KO	숨을 쉴 때 쌕쌕 소리가 납니까? Su-meul swil ttae ssae-kssaek so-ri-ga nam-ni-kka?
RU	У вас / у члена вашей семьи был туберкулёз? U vas / u chlena vashey sem'i byl tuberkulyoz?
PL	Czy Pan(i) lub ktoś z rodziny chorował kiedykolwiek na gruźlicę?
AR	هل سبق لك او لأحد أفراد عائلتك الإصابة بمرض السلّ؟ Hal sabaq lak au li-ahad afraad "aa'ilatak al-isaabah bi-maradh as-sull?
PT	Você já teve / ou algum familiar seu já teve tuberculose?
FK	Eske ou gen bwi sifleman lè ou ap respire ?
EL	Είχατε εσείς / είχε κάποιο οικογενειακό μέλος ποτέ φυματίωση; EEhate esEEs / EEhe kApeeo eekogeneeakO mElos potE feematEEosee?
HI	क्या आपको सांस लेते हुए घरघराहट होती है? Kya aapko saans lete hue ghargharahat hoti hai?

Do you wheeze when breathing?

ES ¿Cuando respira se oyen silbidos?

ZH 你抽烟吗？一天抽多少？抽了几年了？
nǐ chōu yān ma? yī tiān chōu duō shǎo? chōu le jǐ nián le?

FR Sifflez-vous en respirant?

DE Atmen Sie keuchend?

VI Quý vị có hút thuốc không? Bao nhiêu điếu mỗi ngày? Quý vị đã hút thuốc trong bao nhiêu năm?

IT Rantola quando respira?

KO 담배 피우십니까? 하루에 얼마나? 몇 년 동안?
Dam-bae pi-u-sim-ni-kka? Ha-ru-e eol-ma-na? Myeot nyeon dong-an?

RU У вас свистящее дыхание?
U vas svistyashchee dykhanie?

PL Czy ma Pan(i) świszczący oddech?

AR هل تئز \ تزين أثناء التنفس؟
Hal ta'izz / ta'izeen athnaa' at-tanaffus?

PT Tem pieira quando respira?

FK Eske ou fimin? Konbyen ou fimin pa jou? Pandan konbyen ane ?

EL Σφυρίζετε όταν αναπνέετε;
sfeerEEzete Otan anapnEete?

HI क्या आप धूम्रपान करते हैं? दिन में कितनी बार? कितने वर्षों से?
Kya aap Dhumrapaan karte hain? Din me kitni baar? Kitne varShon se?

Do you smoke? How much per day? For how many years?

ES ¿Fuma usted? ¿Cuántos cigarrillos al día? ¿Por cuántos años?

ZH 你对什么东西过敏吗？
nǐ duì shén me dōng xī guò mǐn ma?

FR Fumez-vous? Combien par jour? depuis combien d'années?

DE Rauchen Sie? Wie viel am Tag? Wie viele Jahre schon?

VI Quý vị có bị dị ứng với vật gì không?

IT Fuma? Quanto al giorno? Da quanti anni?

KO 알레르기가 있으십니까?
Al-le-reu-gi-ga i-seu-sim-ni-kka?

RU Вы курите? Сколько в день? Сколько лет?
Vy kurite? Skol'ko v den'? Skol'ko let?

PL Czy pali Pan(i) papierosy ? Ile dziennie? Od ilu lat?

AR هل تدخّن \ تدخنين؟ كم سيجارة باليوم؟ ولكم سنة؟
Hal tudakhkhin / tudakhkhineen? Kam seejaarah bil-youm? Wa li-kam sanah?

PT Fuma? Quanto fuma por dia? Há quantos anos?

FK Eske ou fè alèji a okinn bagay?

EL Καπνίζετε; Πόσο την ημέρα; Για πόσα χρόνια;
kapnEEzete? pOso teen eemEra? geea pOsa hrOneea?

HI क्या आपको किसी चीज से एलर्जी है? ... क्यूक्यूएूए
Kya aapko kisi cheez se allergy hai?

Are you allergic to something?

ES ¿Es usted alérgico a algo?

ZH 你有哮喘吗？
nǐ yǒu xiào chuǎn ma?

FR Etes-vous allergique à quelque chose?

DE Sind Sie gegen irgendetwas allergisch?

VI Quý vị có bị bệnh suyễn không?

IT È allergico / a a qualcosa?

KO 천식이 있으십니까?
Cheon-si-gi i-seu-sim-ni-kka?

RU У вас есть аллергия к чему-либо?
U vas est' allergiya k chemu-libo?

PL Czy jest Pan(i) na cokolwiek uczulony(a)?

AR هل عندك حساسية لشيء؟
Hal "indak hassaasiyyah li-shey'?

PT É alérgico(a) a algum coisa?

FK Eske ou soufri opresyon?

EL Είστε αλλεργικοί σε κάτι;
EEste alergeekEE se kAtee?

HI क्या आपको अस्थमा है?
Kya aapko asthma hai?

Do you have asthma?

ES ¿Es usted asmático?

ZH 你（经常）感冒吗？
nǐ (jīng cháng) gǎn mào ma?

FR Avez-vous de l'asthme?

DE Haben Sie Asthma?

VI Quý vị có (thường) bị cảm lạnh không?

IT Soffre di asma?

KO 감기가 (자주) 있으십니까?
Gam-gi-ga (ja-ju) i-seu-sim-ni-kka?

RU У вас есть астма?
U vas est' astma?

PL Czy ma Pan(i) astmę?

AR هل تعاني \ تعانين من الربو؟
Hal tu"aani / tu"aaneen min ar-rabou?

PT Tem asma?

FK Eske ou gen lagrip souvan?

EL Έχετε άσθμα;
Ehete Asthma?

HI क्या आपको (अक्सर) जुकाम हो जाता है?
Kya aapko (aksar) jukaam ho jata hai?

1 Gastroenterology

Do you feel upper abdominal pain? At which times?

ES ¿Le duele en la parte de arriba del abdomen? ¿A qué horas?

CH 你有没有感觉上腹部痛？什么时间痛？
nǐ yǒu méi yǒu gǎn jué shàng fù bù tòng? shén me shí jiān tòng?

FR Avez-vous ressenti de la douleur dans l'abdomen supérieur? A quels moments?

GE Haben Sie Schmerzen im Oberbauch? Wann?

VI Quý vị có cảm thấy đau ở vùng bụng trên không? Vào những lúc nào?

IT Ha dolori alla parte alta dell'addome? Quando?

KO 윗 배가 아프십니까? 어떤 때 아프십니까?
Wit bae-ga a-peu-sim-ni-kka? Eo-tteon ttae a-peu-sim-ni-kka?

RU Испытываете ли вы боли в верхней части живота? В какое время?
Ispytyvaete li vy boli v verkhney chasti zhivota? V kakoe vremya?

PL Czy odczuwa Pan(i) ból w górnej części brzucha? Kiedy?

AR هل تشعر\ تشعرين بالألم في البطن؟ في أية اوقات؟
Hal tash"ur / tash"ureen bil-alam fil-batn? Fi ayyati auqaat?

PT Sente dores na região abdominal superior? Em que momentos?

HK Eske ou santi tranche? Ki lè ?

GL Νιώθετε πόνο στην άνω περιοχή της κοιλιάς; Ποιες ώρες;
neeOthete pOno steen Ano pereeoHee tees keeleeAs; peeEs Ores?

HI क्या आपको पेट के ऊपरी भाग में दर्द महसूस होता है? किस समय? ...
Kya aapko pet ke upari bhaag mein dard mehsoos hota hai? Kis samay?

after meals / alcohol consumption / on empty stomach / after eating fatty foods

ES	después de comer / al beber alcohol / con el estómago vacío / después de alimentos grasosos

ZH 饭后 / 酒后 / 空腹时 / 吃了油腻食品之后
fàn hòu / jiǔ hòu / kōng fù shí / chī le yóu nì shí pǐn zhī hòu

FR Après les repas / de la consommation d'alcool / à jeun / après un repas gras

DE nach dem Essen / Alkoholgenuss / bei leerem Magen / nach fettigem Essen

VI sau khi ăn / uống rượu / khi đói bụng / sau khi ăn đồ ăn có nhiều chất béo

IT dopo i pasti / consumo di alcol / a stomaco vuoto / dopo aver mangiato cibi grassi

KO 식사 후 / 음주 / 공복에 / 고지방 음식 먹은 후
siksa hu / eum-ju / gong-bo-ge / go-ji-bang eum-sik meo-geun hu

RU после еды / употребления алкоголя / на пустой желудок / после приема жирной пищи
posle edy / upotrebleniya alkogolya / na pustoy zheludok / posle priema zhirnoy pishchi

PL po posiłkach / po alkoholu / na czczo / po jedzeniu tłustych potraw

AR بعد تناول الغذاء \ بعد إستهلاك الكحول \ عند خلاء المعدة \ بعد تناول الأغذية الغنية بالدهن
Ba"d tanaawul al-ghadhaa' / ba'd istihlaak al-kuhool / "ind khalaa al-ma"idah / ba"d tanaawul al-aghdhiyyah al-ghaniyyah bid-dihn

PT depois das refeições / do consumo de álcool / com o estômago vazio / depois de ter comido comidas gordas

FK Apre ou fin manje / bouwè tafya / vant vid / apre ou fin manje ki gen anpil gres

EL μετά από γεύματα / κατανάλωση αλκοόλ / με άδειο στομάχι / μετά από κατανάλωση λιπαρών τροφίμων
metA apO gEvmata / katanAlosee alkoOl / me Adeeo stomAhee / metA apO katanAlosee leeparOn trofEEmon

HI खाना खाने के बाद / शराब पीने / खाली पेट / वसायुक्त भोजन खाने के बाद
Khaana khaane ke baad / shraab peene / khaali pet / vasaayukt bhojan khaane ke baad

Do you have swallowing problems / heartburn / cramps / bloating?

¿Tiene dificultad para deglutir / acidez / cólicos / inflamación abdominal?

你有没有吞咽困难 / 感觉烧心 / 绞痛 / 胀痛？
nǐ yǒu méi yǒu tūn yàn kùn nán / gǎn jué shāo xīn / jiǎo tòng / zhàng tòng?

Avez-vous des problèmes de déglutition? Des brûlures d'estomac / des crampes / des lourdeurs?

Leiden Sie unter Schluckstörungen / Sodbrennen / Krämpfen / Blähungen?

Quý vị có các vấn đề về nuốt / ợ nóng / chứng vọp bẻ / sưng phồng không?

Ha difficoltà ad inghiottire / bruciori allo stomaco / crampi / gonfiore?

삼키는 데 문제가 / 가슴쓰림이 / 급격한 복통이 / 더부룩함이 있습니까?
Sam-ki-neun de mun-je-ga / ga-seum-sseu-ri-mi / geup-gyeo-kan bok-tong-i / deo-bu-ruk-ha-mi it-seum-ni-kka?

У вас есть нарушения глотания / изжога / спазмы / вздутие живота?
U vas est' narusheniya glotaniya / izzhoga / spazmy / vzdutie zhivota?

Czy ma Pan(i) problemy z połykaniem / zgagą / kurczami / wzdęciami?

هل تعاني \ تعانين من مشاكل في الإبتلاع \ الحموضة المعوية \ التشنجات \ النفخ؟
Hal tu"aani / tu"aaneen min mashaakil fil-ibtilaa" / al-humoodhah al-mi"awiyyah / at-tashannujaat / an-nafkh?

Tem problemas de deglutição / azia / cólicas / sensação de enfartamento?

Eske ou gen pwoblèm pou vale / lestomak si / kramp / santi ou gonflé (gaz) ?

Έχετε προβλήματα όταν καταπίνετε / καούρα / κράμπες / τυμπανισμό;
Ehete provlEEmata Otan katapEEnete / kaUra / krAbes / teebaneesmO?

क्या आपको निगलने में परेशानी / कलेजा–जलना / ऐंठन / सूजन है?
Kya aapko nigalne mein pareshaani / kaleja-jalna / ainThan / suzan hai?

Do you take any stomach medications? Which ones in particular?

ES ¿Toma medicamentos para el estómago? ¿Cuáles en particular?

ZH 你在吃治胃病的药吗？ 什么药呢？
nǐ zài chī zhì wèi bìng de yào ma? shén me yào ne?

FR Prenez-vous des médicaments pour l'estomac? Lesquels, en particulier?

DE Nehmen Sie Medikamente für Ihren Magen ein? Welche?

VI Quý vị có dùng thuốc chữa bệnh bao tử không? Cụ thể, đó là những loại thuốc nào?

IT Prende medicine per lo stomaco? Specificamente quali?

KO 위장약 드시는 게 있습니까? 구체적으로 어떤 약을 드십니까?
Wi-jang-yag deu-si-neun ge it-seum-ni-kka? Gu-che-jeo-geu-ro eo-tteon ya-geul deu-sim-ni-kka?

RU Вы принимаете какие-нибудь желудочные лекарства? Какие именно?
Vy prinimaete kakie-nibud' zheludochnye lekarstva? Kakie imenno?

PL Czy przyjmuje Pan(i) leki na żołądek? Jakie konkretnie?

AR هل تأخذ \ تأخذين أية أدوية للمعدة؟ اية أدوية بالتحديد؟
Hal ta'khudh / ta'khudheen ayyi adwiyyah lil-ma"idah? Ayyi adwiyyah bit-tahdeed?

PT Toma medicamentos para o estômago? Quais são os medicamentos específicos?

FK Eske ou pran okinn medikaman pou vant ou? Ki les an patikilye?

EL Παίρνετε οποιαδήποτε φάρμακα για το στομάχι; Ποια συγκεκριμένα;
pErnete opeeadEEpote fArmaka geea to stomAhee? peea seegekreemEna?

HI क्या आप कोई पेट की दवा ले रहे हैं? विशेष रूप से कौन-सी?
Kya aap koi pet ki davaa le rahe hain? Vishesh roop se kaun-si?

Do you feel nauseated / did you vomit?

ES ¿Tiene ascos (náuseas) / ha tenido vómito?

ZH 你是否感到恶心 / 呕吐过吗？
nǐ shì fǒu gǎn dào ě xīn / ǒu tù guò ma?

FR Vous sentez-vous nauséeux (-euse) / avez-vous vomi?

DE Haben Sie Brechreiz / erbrochen?

VI Quý vị có cảm thấy buồn nôn / quý vị có bị ói mửa không?

IT Prova nausea / ha vomitato?

KO 구토증을 느끼십니까 / 토하셨습니까?
Gu-to-jeung-eul neu-kki-sim-ni-kka? / to-ha-syeot-seum-ni-kka?

RU Вас тошнит / была ли рвота?
Vas toshnit / byla li rvota?

PL Czy odczuwa Pan(i) nudności / czy Pan(i) wymiotował(a)?

AR هل تشعر\ تشعرين بالتقزز \ هل تقيأت؟
Hal tash"ur / tash"ureen bit-taqazzuz / hal taqayya't?

PT Sente náuseas / vomitou?

FK Eske ou gen nozè / eske ou vomi?

EL Νιώθετε ναυτία / Κάνατε εμετό;
neeOthete naftEEa / kAnate emetO?

HI क्या आप मतली महसूस कर रहे / क्या आपने उल्टी की?
Kya aap matli mehsoos kar rahe hain / Kya aapne ulti ki?

bloody / bitter / coffee-grounds-like / stomach content

ES sanguinolento / amargo / como asientos de café / contenido estomacal

ZH 带血的 / 苦味的 / 咖啡色的 / 吃进去的东西
dài xiě de / kǔ wèi de / kā fēi sè de / chī jìn qù de dōng xī

FR du sang / quelque chose d'amer / quelque chose ressemblant à du marc de café / le contenu de l'estomac

DE blutig / bitter / kaffeesatzartig / Mageninhalt

VI chất ói mửa có máu / đắng / giống như cà phê xay

IT con tracce di sangue / amaro / come caffè macinato / contenuto dello stomaco

KO 피가 섞인 / 쓴 / 커피 가루같은 / 위 내용물
pi-ga seo-kkin / sseun / keo-pi ga-ru-ga-teun / wi nae-yong-mul

RU кровавая / горькая / цвета кофейной гущи / содержимым желудка
krovavaya / gor'kaya / tsveta kofeinoy gushchi / soderzhimym zheludka

PL krwawa / gorzka / podobna do mielonej kawy / zawartość żołądka

AR دامي \ مرّ \ مثل بن القهوة \ محتويات المعدة
Daami / murr / mithl bunn al-qahwah / muhtawayaat al-ma"idah

PT com sangue / sabor amargo / com o aspecto de borras de café / conteúdo do estômago

FK gen san / anme / kouwè gren kafe / sa ki nan vant

EL αιματώδης / πικρός / σαν κόκκοι καφέ / περιεχόμενο στομαχιού
ematOdees / peekrOs / san kOkee kafE / peree-ehOmeno stomaheeU

HI रक्तयुक्त / कड़ुवा / कॉफी–आ ६ ।ार जैसी / पेट के तत्व
raktyukt / kaDuya / coffee-aadhar jaisi / pet ke tatv

Do you have diarrhea?

ES ¿Ha tenido diarrea?

CH 你腹泻吗？
nǐ fù xiè ma?

FR Avez-vous de la diarrhée?

DE Haben Sie Durchfall?

VI Quý vị có bị tiêu chảy không?

IT Ha la diarrea?

KO 설사하십니까?
Seol-sa-ha-sim-ni-kka?

RU У вас есть понос?
U vas est' ponos?

PL Czy ma Pan(i) biegunkę?

AR هل عندك إسهال؟
Hal "indak is'haal?

PT Tem diarreia?

FK Eske ou gen dyare?

EL Έχετε διάρροια;
Ehete deeAreea?

HI क्या आपको अतिसार है? ...
Kya aapko atisaar hai?

bloody / viscous / black / watery

ES	sanguinolenta / viscosa / negra / acuosa
ZH	带血的 / 粘性的 / 黑色的 / 水样的 dài xiě de / nián xìng de / hēi sè de / shuǐ yàng de
FR	sanguinolente / visqueuse / noire / aqueuse
DE	blutig / dickflüssig / schwarz / wässrig
VI	ra kèm máu / sền sệt / có màu đen / lỏng
IT	con tracce di sangue / viscosa / nera / acquosa
KO	피가 섞인 / 점액성의 / 검은 / 묽은 pi-ga seo-kkin / jeo-maek-seong-ui / geo-meun / mul-geun
RU	кровавый / слизистый / черный / водянистый krovavyi / slizistyi / chernyi / vodyanistyi
PL	krwawą / lepką / czarną / wodnistą
AR	دامى \ لزج \ أسود \ مائى، سائل Daami / lazij / aswad / maa'ee, saa'il
PT	sanguinolenta / viscosa / preta / aquosa
FK	gen san / viske / mwa / likid
EL	αιματώδης / ιξώδης / μαύρη / υδαρή ematOdees / eexOdees / mAvree / eedarEE
HI	रक्तयुक्त / चिपचिपा / काला / पानीयुक्त Raktyukt / chipchipa / kala / paniyukt

How often does it occur? ... times daily / ... times a week

ES ¿Con qué frecuencia ocurre? ... veces al día / ... veces a la semana

ZH 多久一次？ ... 一天有几次 / ... 一星期有几次？
duō jiǔ yī cì? ... yī tiān yǒu jǐ cì / ... yī xīng qī yǒu jǐ cì?

FR Combien de fois cela s'est-il produit? ... fois par jour / ... fois par semaine

DE Wie oft? ... mal täglich / ... mal wöchentlich

VI Hiện tượng này xảy ra thường xuyên như thế nào? ... lần hàng ngày / ... lần một tuần

IT Quanto spesso succede? ... volte al giorno / ... volte alla settimana

KO 얼마나 자주 있습니까? 매일 ... 번 / 매주 ... 번
Eol-ma-na ja-ju i-sseum-ni-kka? Mae-il ... beon / mae-ju ... beon

RU Как часто это происходит? ... раз в день / ... раз в неделю
Kak chasto eto proiskhodit? ... raz v den' / ... raz v nedelyu

PL Jak często to ona występuje? ... razy dziennie / ... razy w tygodniu

AR كم مرة يحدث عندك؟ __ مرة باليوم \ __ مرة بالأسبوع
Kam marrah yahduth "indak? ___ times per day / ___ times per week

PT Com que frequência é que isso ocorre? ... vezes por dia / ... vezes por semana

FK Pandan konbyen fwa sa rive? ... . Fwa pa jou / ... fwa pa semèn

EL Πόσο συχνά συμβαίνει; ... φορές την ημέρα / ... φορές την εβδομάδα
pOso seehnA seemvEnee? ... forEs teen eemEra / ... forEs teen evdomAda

HI यह कितनी बार होता है? ... बार प्रतिदिन / ... बार प्रति सप्ताह
Yeh kitni bar hota hai? ... bar pratidin / ... bar prati saptaah

Do you also experience diarrhea at night?

ES	¿Tiene diarrea también en la noche?
ZH	你夜里也拉肚子吗？ nǐ yè lǐ yě lā dù zi ma?
FR	Avez-vous la diarrhée la nuit?
DE	Haben Sie auch in der Nacht Durchfall?
VI	Ngoài ra, quý vị quý vị có bị tiêu chảy vào ban đêm không?
IT	Ha la diarrea anche la notte?
KO	밤에도 설사를 하십니까? Ba-me-do seol-sa-reul ha-sim-ni-kka?
RU	У вас также бывает понос по ночам? U vas takzhe byvaet ponos po nocham?
PL	Czy miewa Pan(i) także biegunkę w nocy?
AR	هل تعاني \ تعانين من الإسهال بالليل أيضاً؟ Hal tu"aani / tu"aaneen min al-is'haal bil-leyl aydhan?
PT	Também tem diarreia durante a noite?
FK	Eske ou kon gen dyare lan nwit?
EL	Παθαίνετε επίσης διάρροια τη νύχτα; pathEnete epEEsees diAreea tee nEEhta?
HI	क्या आपने रात में भी अतिसार अनुभव किया है? Kya aapne raat mein bhi atisaar anubhav kiya hai?

Do you suffer from constipation?

ES ¿Padece estreñimiento?

ZH 你有便秘吗？
nǐ yǒu biàn mì ma?

FR Souffrez-vous de constipation?

DE Haben Sie Verstopfung?

VI Quý vị có bị táo bón không?

IT Soffre di stipsi?

KO 변비가 있으십니까?
Byeon-bi-ga i-seu-sim-ni-kka?

RU Вы страдаете запорами?
Vy stradaete zaporami?

PL Czy cierpi Pan(i) na zaparcie?

AR هل تعاني \ تعانين من الإمساك؟
Hal tu"aani / tu"aaneen min al-imsaak?

PT Sofre de prisão de ventre?

FK Eske ou soufri ak konstipasyon?

EL Πάσχετε από δυσκοιλιότητα;
pAshete apO deeskeeleeOteeta?

HI क्या आप कब्ज से पीड़ित हैं?
Kya aap kabz se pidit hain?

When was your last bowel movement?

ES	¿Cuánto hace que evacuó por última vez?
ZH	你最后一次大便是什么时候？ nǐ zuì hòu yī cì dà biàn shì shén me shí hòu?
FR	Quand avez-vous été à la selle pour la dernière fois?
DE	Wann hatten Sie das letzte Mal Stuhlgang?
VI	Quý vị đi cầu lần gần đây nhất là khi nào?
IT	Quando è stata l'ultima volta che è andato / a di corpo?
KO	마지막으로 대변을 보신 게 언제 입니까? Ma-ji-ma-geu-ro dae-byeo-neul bo-sin ge eon-je im-ni-kka?
RU	Когда вы последний раз испражнялись? Kogda vy posledniy raz isprazhnyalis'?
PL	Kiedy miał(a) Pan(i) ostatnie wypróżnienie?
AR	متى جاءك الغائط آخر مرة؟ Mattaa jaa'ak al-ghaa'it aakhiri marrah?
PT	Quando foi a sua última evacuação intestinal?
FK	Ki denye fwa ou al nan twalet?
EL	Πότε ενεργηθήκατε για τελευταία φορά; pOte energeethEEkate geea teleftEa forA?
HI	अंतिम बार आपकी आंत में गति कब हुई थी? Antim bar aapki aant me gati kab hui thi?

Do you take laxatives?

ES ¿Toma laxantes?

ZH 你在吃通大便的药吗？
nǐ zài chī tōng dà biàn de yào ma?

FR Prenez-vous des laxatifs?

DE Nehmen Sie Abführmittel?

VI Quý vị có dùng thuốc nhuận tràng không?

IT Prende lassativi?

KO 하제를 드십니까?
Ha-je-reul deu-sim-ni-kka?

RU Вы принимаете слабительные?
Vy prinimaete slabitel'nye?

PL Czy przyjmuje Pan(i) środki przeczyszczające?

AR هل تستعمل \ تستعملين المسهلات؟
Hal tasta"mil / tasta"mileen al-mus'hilaat?

PT Toma laxativos?

FK Eske ou pran laksatif?

EL Παίρνετε καθαρτικά;
pErnete katharteekA?

HI क्या आप दस्तावर लेते हैं?
Kya aap dastavar lete hain?

Have you noticed any stool changes?

ES ¿Ha notado cambios en el excremento?

ZH 你的大便有什么变化吗？
nǐ de dà biàn yǒu shén me biàn huà ma?

FR Avez-vous mal quand vous allez à la selle?

DE Hat sich Ihr Stuhl verändert?

VI Quý vị có nhận thấy thay đổi gì trong phân không?

IT Ha notato un cambiamento nelle feci?

KO 대변이 달라진 것이 있습니까?
Dae-byeo-ni dal-la-jin geo-si it-seum-ni-kka?

RU Заметили ли вы какие-нибудь изменения в кале?
Zametili li vy kakie-nibud' izmeneniya v kale?

PL Czy zauważył(a) Pan(i) jakieś zmiany w swoim stolcu?

AR هل لاحظت تغيرات في الغائط؟
Hal laahadht taghyeeraat fil-ghaa'it?

PT Notou alguma alteração nas fezes?

FK Eske ou remake okinn chanjman nan watè w?

EL Παρατηρήσατε αλλαγές στα κόπρανά σας;
parateerEEsate alagEs sta kOpranA sas?

HI क्या आपने अपने मल में कोई भी बदलाव महसूस किया है? ...
Kya aapne apne mal mein koi bhi badlaav mehsoos kiya hai?

brighter / darker / bloody / more watery / harder / changing appearance

ES más brillante / oscuro / con sangre / acuoso / duro / cambia de aspecto

ZH 颜色变浅 / 变黑 / 带血 / 变稀 / 变硬 / 形状改变
yán sè biàn qiǎn / biàn hēi / dài xiě / biàn xī / biàn yìng / xíng zhuàng gǎi biàn

FR plus claires / plus sombres / sanguinolentes / aqueuses / plus dures / d'aspect changeant

DE heller / dunkler / blutig / flüssiger / härter / wechselt häufig

VI có màu sáng hơn / sẫm hơn / có máu / lỏng hơn / rắn hơn / thay đổi về khuôn dạng

IT più chiare / più scure / con tracce di sangue / più acquose / più dure / l'aspetto cambia

KO 더 밝은 색 / 더 어두운 색 / 피가 섞인 / 더 묽은 / 더 굳은 / 외형 변화
deo bal-geun saek / deo eo-du-un saek / pi-ga so-kkin / deo mul-geun / deo gu-deun / oe-hyeong byeon-hwa

RU светлее / темнее / кровавый / более водянистый / плотнее / другой на вид
svetleye / temneye / krovavyy / boleye vodyanistyi / plotneye / drugoy na vid

PL jaśniejszy / ciemniejszy / krwawy / bardziej wodnisty / zmieniony wygląd

AR أفتح \ أدكن \ دامي \ اكثر سائلاً \ اجمد \ متغير او متنوع الشكل
Aftah / adkan / daami / akthar saa'ilan / ajmad / mutaghayyir au mutanawwi" ash-shakl

PT mais claras / mais escuras / com sangue / mais aquosas / mais duras / mudando de aparência

FK pli vif / pli fonse / gen san / pli likid / pli di / aparans li chanjè

EL φωτεινότερα / σκουρότερα / αιματώδη / πιο υδαρά / πιο σκληρά / εμφάνιση που αλλάζει
foteenOtera / skurOtera / ematOdee / peeo eedarA / peeo skleerA / emfAneesee pu alAzee

HI अधिक चमकदार / गहरी / रक्तयुक्त / अधिक पानीयुक्त / सख्त / बदली शक्ल
Adhik chamakdar / gehri / raktyukt / adhik paniyukt / saKht / badli Shakl

Have you noticed a change in the smell of your stool?

ES	¿Ha notado algún cambio en el olor del excremento?
ZH	大便的气味有什么变化吗？ dà biàn de qì wèi yǒu shén me biàn huà ma?
FR	Avez-vous remarqué un changement d'odeur dans les selles?
DE	Ist Ihr Stuhl im Geruch verändert?
VI	Quý vị có thấy thay đổi gì về mùi phân không?
IT	Ha notato un cambiamento nell'odore delle Sue feci?
KO	대변 냄새가 달라진 게 있습니까? Dae-byeon naem-sae-ga dal-la-jin ge it-seum-ni-kka?
RU	Заметили ли вы изменение запаха кала? Zametili li vy izmenenie zapakha kala?
PL	Czy zauważył(a) Pan(i) zmianę w zapachu swego stolca?
AR	هل لاحظت تغيراً في رائحة غائطك؟ Hal laahadht taghyeeran fi raa'ihati ghaa'itak?
PT	Notou uma alteração no cheiro das suas fezes?
FK	Eske ou remake gen yon chanjman nan odè watè w?
EL	Παρατηρήσατε αλλαγή στην οσμή των κοπράνων σας; parateerEEsate alagEE steen osmEE ton koprAnon sas?
HI	क्या आपने अपने मल की गंध में कोई बदलाव नोट किया है? Kya aapne apne mal ki gandh mein koi badlaav note kiya hai?

Do you have pain during bowel movements?

ES ¿Siente dolor al evacuar?

ZH 大便时痛吗？
dà biàn shí tòng ma?

FR Avez-vous mal au cours des mouvements intestinaux?

DE Haben Sie Schmerzen beim Stuhlgang?

VI Quý vị có bị đau khi đi ngoài không?

IT Prova dolore quando va di corpo?

KO 대변보실 때 통증이 있습니까?
Dae-byeon-bo-sil ttae tong-jeung-i it-seum-ni-kka?

RU Испытываете ли вы боль во время дефекации?
Ispytyvaete li vy bol' vo vremya defekatsii?

PL Czy odczuwa Pan(i) ból podczas wypróżniania?

AR هل تعاني \ تعانين من الألم عند التغوط؟
Hal tu"aani / tu"aaneen min al-alam "ind at-taghawwut?

PT Sente dor durante as evacuações intestinais?

FK Eske ou gen doulè lè ou al nan watè?

EL Νιώθετε πόνο κατά τον εντερικό περισταλτισμό;
neeOthete pOno katA ton edereekO pereestalteesmO?

HI क्या आपको आंत में गति होने पर दर्द होता है?
Kya aapko aant mein gati hone par dard hota hai?

Have you gained / lost weight?

ES   ¿Ha subido / bajado de peso?

ZH   你的体重有没有增加／减少？
nǐ de tǐ zhòng yǒu méi yǒu zēng jiā / jiǎn shǎo?

FR   Avez-vous gagné / perdu du poids?

DE   Haben Sie an Gewicht zugenommen / verloren?

VI   Quý vị có bị tăng / giảm cân không?

IT   È aumentato / a / diminuito / a / di peso?

KO   체중이 늘었습니까 / 줄었습니까?
Che-jung-i neu-reot-seum-ni-kka / ju-reot-seum-ni-kka?

RU   Вы поправились / похудели?
Vy popravilis' / pokhudeli?

PL   Czy stracił(a) / zyskał(a) Pan(i) na wadze?

AR   هل زاد \ قل وزنك؟
Hal zaad / qalla waznak?

PT   Aumentou / perdeu peso?

FK   Eske ou gwosi / megri?

EL   Πήρατε / Χάσατε βάρος;
pEErate / hAsate vAros?

HI   क्या आपका वजन बढ़ा / घटा है?
Kya aapka vajan badha / Ghata hai?

Do you have hemorrhoids / jaundice / yellow discoloration of the white of your eye?

S ¿Tiene hemorroides / ictericia / tono amarillento de lo blanco de los ojos?

H 你有没有痔疮 / 黄疸 / 眼睑变黄？
nĭ yŏu méi yŏu zhì chuāng / huáng dăn / yăn jiăn biàn huáng?

R Avez-vous des hémorrhoïdes / de la jaunisse / une coloration jaune du blanc de vos yeux

E Haben Sie Hämorrhoiden / Gelbsucht / gelbes Augenweiß?

T Quý vị có bị bệnh trĩ / vàng da / lòng trắng mắt chuyển sang màu vàng không?

T Ha le emorroidi / l'ittero / macchie gialle nel bianco dell'occhio?

O 치질 / 황달 / 눈 흰자위가 노란 색으로 변함이 있습니까?
chi-jil / hwang-dal / nun huin-ja-wi-ga no-ran sae-geu-ro byeon-ha-mi it-seum-ni-kka?

U У вас есть геморрой / желтуха / желтушность белков глаз?
U vas est' gemorroi / zheltukha / zheltushnost' belkov glaz?

L Czy ma Pan(i) hemoroidy / żółtaczkę / żółte zabarwienie białej części oka?

R هل عندك بواسير \ اليرقان \ تغيير لون أصفر في الجزء الأبيض من عينك؟
Hal "indak bawaseer / al-yarqaan / taghyeer laun asfar fi al-jiz' il-abyadh min "aynak?

T Tem hemorróides / icterícia / descoloração amarela da córnea dos seus olhos?

K Eske ou gen emowoyid / la jonis / pati blan zye w gen koulè jaun?

L Έχετε αιμορροΐδες / ίκτερο / κίτρινο αποχρωματισμό του λευκού των ματιών σας;
Ehete emoroEEdes / EEktero / kEEtreeno apohromateesmO tu lefkU ton mateeOn sas?

I क्या आपको बवासीर / पीलिया / आपकी आंख का सफेद भाग पीला पड़ जाता है?
Kya aapko bavaaseer / peeliya / aapki aankh ka safed bhaag peela paDh jata hai?

Have you noticed a change in the color of your urine? ... darker

ES ¿Ha notado cambios en el color de la orina? ... más oscura

ZH 小便颜色有什么变化吗？ ... 颜色变深
xiǎo biàn yán sè yǒu shén me biàn huà ma? yán sè biàn shēn

FR Avez-vous remarqué un changement dans la couleur de vos urines? Plus foncées?

DE Hat sich die Farbe Ihres Urins verändert? ... dunkler

VI Quý vị có nhận thấy thay đổi trong màu nước tiểu không? ... sẫm hơn

IT Ha notato un cambiamento nel colore delle Sue urine? ... più scure

KO 소변 색이 달라진 것이 있습니까? ... 더 어두운
So-byeon sae-gi dal-la-jin geo-si it-seum-ni-kka? ... deo eo-du-un?

RU Заметили ли вы изменение цвета мочи? ... темнее
Zametili li vy izmenenie tsveta mochi? ... temneye

PL Czy zauważył(a) Pan(i) zmianę w barwie swego moczu? ... ciemniejszy

AR هل لاحظت تغيراً في لون بولك؟ ... ادكن؟
Hal laahadht taghyeeran fi laun baulak? ... adkan?

PT Notou alguma alteração na cor da sua urina? ... mais escura

FK Eske ou remake yon chanjman nan koulè pipi w? ... pli fonse

EL Παρατηρήσατε αλλαγή στο χρώμα των ούρων σας; ... πιο σκούρα
parateerEEsate alagEE sto hrOma ton Uron sas? ... peeo skUra

HI क्या आपने अपने मूत्र के रंग में कोई बदलाव नोट किया है? ... गहरा
Kya aapne apne mootra ke rang mein koi badlaav note kiya hai? ... gehra

Where do you have pain / where did the pain begin?

¿Donde le duele / dónde comenzó el dolor?

你现在那里痛 / 刚开始什么地方痛？
nǐ xiàn zài nà li tòng / gāng kāi shǐ shén me dì fāng tòng?

Où avez-vous mal / où la douleur a-t-elle commencé?

Wo haben Sie Schmerzen / Wo fing der Schmerz an?

Quý bị bị đau ở đâu / bắt đầu thấy đau từ khi nào?

Dove ha dolore / dove è iniziato il dolore?

어디에 통증이 있습니까 / 어디서 통증이 시작되었습니까?
Eo-di-e tong-jeung-i it-seum-ni-kka / eo-di-seo tong-jeung-i si-jak-doe-eot-seum-
ni-kka?

Где у вас болит / где эта боль появилась?
Gde u vas bolit / gde eta bol' poyavilas'?

Gdzie odczuwa Pan(i) ból / kiedy ten ból się zaczął

أين تشعر \ تشعرين بالألم؟ \ أين بدأ الألم؟
Ayna tash"ur / tash"ureen bil-alam? / Min ayna bada' al-alam?

Onde sente a dor / onde é que a dor começou?

Ki bo ou gen doulè a / ki bo doulè a komanse ?

Πού έχετε τον πόνο / Πού ξεκίνησε ο πόνος;
pu Ehete ton pOno / pu xekEEneese o pOnos?

आपको कहां दर्द हो रहा है / दर्द कहां से शुरु हुआ था?
Aapko kahaan dard ho raha hai / dard kahaan se shuru hua tha?

What alleviates the pain?

ES	¿Con qué se alivia el dolor?
ZH	什么能使疼痛减轻？ shén me néng shǐ téng tòng jiǎn qīng?
FR	Qu'est-ce qui soulage la douleur?
DE	Wird der Schmerz durch irgendetwas gelindert?
VI	Cách gì giúp làm giảm cơn đau?
IT	Cosa allevia il dolore?
KO	어떻게 하면 통증이 완화됩니까? Eo-tteo-ke ha-myeon tong-jeung-i wan-hwa-doem-ni-kka?
RU	Что облегчает эту боль? Chto oblegchaet etu bol'?
PL	Co łagodzi ten ból?
AR	ما هو الذي يخفف الألم؟ Ma huwa aladhi yukhaffif al-alam?
PT	O que alivia a dor?
FK	Kisa ki soulajè doulè a?
EL	Τι ανακουφίζει τον πόνο; tee anakufEEzee ton pOno?
HI	कौन दर्द से राहत पहुंचाता है? ... Kaun dard se rahat pahuchata hai?

eating / drinking / positional change / heat / cold / rest / medications (specify!)

al comer / beber / cambiar de posición / con el calor / frío / reposo / con medicamentos (¡especifíque!)

当吃东西时 / 喝东西 / 体位变化 / 热 / 冷 / 休息 / 药物（具体说明）
dāng chī dōng xī shí / hē dōng xī / tǐ wèi biàn huà / rè / lěng / xiū xi / yào wù (jù tǐ shuō míng)

manger / boire / changer de position / le chaud / le froid / le repos / des médicaments (spécifiez lesquels)

Essen / Trinken / Positionswechsel / Wärme / Kälte / Ruhe / Medikamente (welche?)

ăn / uống / thay đổi tư thế / nóng / lạnh / nghỉ ngơi / dùng thuốc (trình bày rõ!)

mangiare / bere / cambiare posizione / il calore / il freddo / il riposo / medicine (specificare!)

먹기 / 마시기 / 자세를 바꿈 / 따뜻하게 함 / 차갑게 함 / 휴식 / 약 (약 이름을 명시하시오)
meok-gi / ma-si-gi / ja-se-reul ba-kkum / tta-tteu-ta-ge ham / cha-gap-ge ham / hyu-sik / yak (yak i-reu-meul myeong-si-ha-si-o)

приём пищи / жидкости / изменение положения тела / тепло / холод / покой / лекарства (уточните!)
priyom pischi / zhidkosti / izmenenie polozheniya tela / teplo / kholod / pokoy / lekarstva (utochnite!)

jedzenie / picie / zmiana pozycji / gorąco / zimno / odpoczynek / leki (proszę bliżej opisać)

تناول الغذاء \ الشرب \ تغيير موقف الجسم \ الحرارة \ البرد \ الراحة \ الأدوية (بيانها بالتحديد!)
Tanaawul al-ghadhaa' / ash-sharb / taghyeer mauqif al-jism / al-haraarah / al-bard / ar-raahah / al-adwiyah (bayaanihaa bit-tahdeed!)

comer / beber / mudança de posição / calor / frio / descanso / medicamentos (especificar quais!)

lè ou manje / bouwè / chanje pozisyon / chalè / fredi / repoze w / medikaman (spesifye)

φαγητό / ποτό / αλλαγή στάσης / θερμότητα / κρύο / ξεκούραση / φάρμακα (καθορίστε!)
fageetO / potO / alagEE stAsees / thermOteeta / krEEo / xekUrasee / fArmaka (kathoreeste!)

खाना / पीना / स्थितिक बदलाव / गर्मी / सर्दी / आराम / दवा (विनिर्दि ष्ट!)
Khana / peena / stithik badlaav / garmi / sardi / aaram / davaa (vinirdisht!)

Have you ever had an ulcer?

ES ¿Ha tenido úlcera?

ZH 以前有过溃疡吗？
yǐ qián yǒu guò kuì yáng ma?

FR Avez-vous jamais eu un ulcère?

DE Hatten Sie ein Geschwür?

VI Quý vị có bao giờ bị lở loét không?

IT Ha mai avuto un'ulcera?

KO 위궤양이 있은 적이 있습니까?
Wi-gwe-yang-i i-seun jeo-gi it-seum-ni-kka?

RU Была ли у вас когда-нибудь язва?
Byla li u vas kogda-nibud' yazva?

PL Czy kiedykolwiek miał(a) Pan(i) wrzody?

AR هل سبق لك أن عانيت من قرحة؟
Hal sabaqa lak an "aanayt min qarhah?

PT Alguma vez teve uma úlcera?

FK Eske ou te janm gen yon ilsè?

EL Είχατε ποτέ έλκος;
EEhate potE Elkos?

HI क्या आपको कभी नासूर हुआ है?
Kya aapko kabhi nasoor hua hai?

2 Endocrinology

Have you noticed any changes in yourself?

ES ¿Ha notado cambios en usted?

ZH 你感觉自己身体最近有什么变化吗.？
nǐ gǎn jué zì jǐ shēn tǐ zuì jìn yǒu shén me biàn huà ma?

FR Avez-vous remarqué l'un ou l'autre changement en vous?

DE Haben Sie Veränderungen an sich bemerkt?

VI Quý vị có nhận thấy thay đổi nào trong người không?

IT Ha notato in Lei cambiamenti?

KO 본인한테 변화가 일어난 것을 느끼셨습니까?
Bo-nin-han-te byeon-hwa-ga i-reo-nan geo-seul neu-kki-syeot-seum-ni-kka?

RU Заметили ли вы у себя какие-нибудь изменения?
Zametili li vy u sebya kakie-nibud' izmeneniya?

PL Czy zauważył Pan(i) u siebie jakiekolwiek zmiany?

AR هل لاحظت بعض التغيرات فى نفسك؟
"hal laahadht ba"dh at-taghyeeraat fi nafsak?"

PT Notou algumas alterações em si?

FK Eske ou remake okinn chanjman nan ou menm?

EL Παρατηρήσατε οποιεσδήποτε αλλαγές στον εαυτό σας;
parateerEEsate opee-esdEEpote alagEs ston eaftO sas?

HI क्या आपने अपने अंदर कुछ बदलाव देखे? ......
Kyaa aapne apne andar kuchh badlaav dekhe?

dizziness attacks / hunger / weight changes / shivering / thirst

ES	mareos / cambios en el hambre / el peso / temblores / sed
ZH	一阵阵头晕 / 饥饿 / 体重变化 / 哆嗦 / 口渴 yī zhèn zhèn tóu yūn / jī è / tǐ zhòng biàn huà / duō suo / kǒu kě
FR	attaques de vertiges / faim / changement de poids / tremblement / soif
DE	Schwindelanfälle / Hunger / Gewichtsveränderungen / Zittern / Durst
VI	những cơn chóng mặt / đói / thay đổi về cân nặng / rét run / khát
IT	attacchi di capogiri / fame / cambiamento di peso / brividi / sete
KO	현기증 발병 / 배고품 / 체중 변화 / 떨림 / 목마름 hyeon-gi-jeung bal-byeong / bae-go-peum / che-jung byeon-hwa / tteol-lim / mong-ma-reum
RU	приступы головокружения / чувство голода / изменения веса / дрожь / жажда pristupy golovokruzheniya / chuvstvo goloda / izmeneniya vesa / drozh' / zhazhda
PL	zawroty głowy / głód / zmiany w wadze / dreszcze / pragnienie
AR	حملات من الدوخة \ الجوع \ تغيرات في الوزن \ الإرتجاف \ العطش Hamlaat minadd-dowkhah / al-joo"a / at-taghyeeraat fil-wazn / al-irtijaaf / al-"atash
PT	ataques de vertigens / fome / mudanças de peso / calafrios / sede
FK	atak ventij / grangou / chanjman nan pwa oufrison / swaf
EL	προσβολές ζάλης / πείνα / αλλαγές βάρους / ρίγος / δίψα prosvolEs zAlees / pEEna / allagEs vArus / rEEgos / dEEpsa
HI	चक्कर आना /भूख /वज़न में बदलाव /कँपना /प्यास लगना..... chakkar aana / bhookh / vazan mein badlaav / kaampna / pyaas lagnaa

frequent urination / fungal infection / sweating / visual problems

ES orina frecuente / infección por hongos / sudores / problemas visuales

ZH 尿频 / 真菌感染 / 出汗 / 视力障碍
niào pín / zhēn jūn gǎn rǎn / chū hàn / shì lì zhàng ài

FR miction fréquente / infection par des champignons / transpiration / troubles visuels

DE häufiges Wasserlassen / Pilzinfektion / Schwitzen / Sehprobleme

VI thường xuyên đi tiểu / viêm nhiễm nấm / đổ mồ hôi / các vấn đề về thị lực

IT minzione frequente / infezioni fungine / sudorazione / problemi alla vista

KO 잦은 배뇨 / 진균(곰팡이) 감염 / 땀 흘림 / 시각 장애
ja jeun bae-nyo / gom-pang-i gam-yeom / ttam-heul-lim / si-gak jang-ae

RU частое мочеиспускание / грибковая инфекция / потливость / нарушения зрения
chastoe mocheispuskanie / gribkovaya infektsiya / potlivost' / narusheniya zreniya

PL Częste oddawanie moczu / zakażenie grzybiczne / poty / problemy ze wzrokiem

AR التبول المتكرر \ الإلتهابات الفطرية \ التعرق \ مشاكل في البصر
At-tabawwul al-mutakarrir / al- iltihaabaat al-futriyah / at-ta"arruq / mahsaakil fil-bassar

PT micção frequente / infecção micótica / sudorese / problemas visuais

FK pipi anpil / infeksyon fongis / swe anpil / pwoblè vizyon

EL συχνουρία / μυκητιασική λοίμωξη / εφίδρωση / προβλήματα όρασης
seehnurEEa / meekeeteeaseekEE IEEmoxee / efEEdrosee / provIEEmata Orasees

HI लगातार मूत्र करना / फन्गल संक्रमण / पसीना आना / दृष्टि संबंधी तकलीफें......
lagaataar mootra karma / fungal sankramaN / pasiiana aanaa / drishti sambandhi
takliifen

kidney problems (dialysis) / numbness in feet / erectile dysfunction

ES trastorno (diálisis) renal / insensibilidad en los pies / disfunción eréctil

ZH 肾脏疾病（透析）/ 脚麻木 / 阴颈勃起困难
shèn zàng jí bìng (tòu xī) jiǎo má mù / yīn jìng bó qǐ kùn nán

FR problèmes rénaux (dialyse) / engourdissement des pieds / dysfonction érectile

DE Nierenprobleme (Dialyse) / Taubheitsgefühl der Füße / Impotenz

VI các vấn đề về thận (thẩm tách) / tê liệt bàn chân / hiện tượng cương cứng bất thường

IT problemi renali (dialisi) / intorpidimento dei piedi / disfunzioni erettili

KO 신장 장애 (투석) / 발 저림 / 발기 기능이상
sin-jang jang-ae (tu-seok) / bal jeo-rim / bal-gi gi-neung-i-sang

RU заболевания почек (диализа) / онемение стоп / эректильная дисфункция
zabolevaniya pochek (dializ) / onemenie stop / erektil'naya disfunktsiya

PL problemy z nerkami (dializa) / cierpnięcie stóp / zaburzenia erekcji

AR مشاكل في الكلى (في عملية غسل الكلى) \ احساس الخدران في الأقدام / العجز الإنتصابي
Mashaakil fil-kilaa (fi "amaliyah ghuslil-kilaa) / ihsaas al-khudraan fil-aqdaam / al-"ajz ul-intisaabi

PT problemas dos rins (diálise) / entorpecimento dos pés / disfunção eréctil

FK pwoblèm nan ren (dialys) / pa gen sensasyon nan pye / paka bande

EL προβλήματα με τους νεφρούς (αιμοκάθαρση) / μούδιασμα στα πόδια / στυτική δυσλειτουργία
provlEEmata me tus nefrUs (emokAtharsee) / mUdeeasma sta pOdeea / seeteekEE deesleeturgEEa

HI गुर्दे की तकलीफ़ें (डायलेसिस) / पैरों में सुन्नता / लिंग दुषिक्रिया......
gurde ki takleefein (dialysis) / pairon mein sunnta / ling dushikriya

intolerance to heat or low temperatures / goiter / bulging eyes

ES intolerancia al calor o a las bajas temperaturas / bocio / ojos saltones

ZH 怕热或怕冷 / 甲状腺肿 / 眼球外突
pà rè huò pà lěng / jiǎ zhuàng xiàn zhōng / yǎn qiú wài tū

FR intolérance à la chaleur, aux basses températures / goitre / gonflement des yeux

DE Intoleranz Hitze oder Kälte / Kropf / hervortretende Augen

VI không chịu được nhiệt độ cao hoặc thấp / bướu cổ / mắt bị lồi

IT intolleranza al calore o alle basse temperature / gozzo / occhi sporgenti

KO 고온 혹은 저온을 못참음 / 갑상성종 / 튀어나온 눈
go-on ho-geun jeo-on-eul mot-cham-eum / gap-sang-seong-jong / twi-eo-na-on nun

RU непереносимость жары или холода / зоб / пучеглазие
neperenosimost' zhary ili kholoda / zob / pucheglazie

PL nietolerowanie wysokiej lub niskiej temperatury / wole / wypukłe oczy

AR عدم تحمل درجات عالية او واطئة من الحرارة \ مرض الدراق \ تنوء العيون
"adam tahammul darajaat "aaliyah aw waati'ahmin al-haraarah / maradh ad-duraaq / nutoo' al-"uyoon

PT intolerância ao calor ou temperaturas baixas / bócio / olhos salientes

FK pake tolere chalè oswa fredi / maladi gwo kou (gwat) / zye ekszorbite

EL δυσανεξία σε υψηλές ή χαμηλές θερμοκρασίες / βρογχοκήλη / εξόφθαλμος
deesanexEEa se eepseelEs ee hameelEs thermokrasEEes / vroghokEElee / exOfthalmos

HI गर्मी या कम तापमान के प्रति असहिष्णुता / गलगल / आँखों में सूजन.....
garmi yak am taapmaan ke prati asahishNuta / galgal / aankhon mein soojan

abnormal hair growth / male breast development

ES crecimiento anormal del pelo corporal / de los pechos

ZH 毛发异常生长／男性乳房发育
máo fà yì cháng shēng zhǎng / nán xìng rǔ fáng fā yù

FR croissance anormale des poils / développement des seins chez l'homme

DE abnormer Haarwuchs / Brustentwicklung beim Mann

VI lông tóc mọc bất thường / sự phát triển tuyến vú ở đàn ông

IT crescita pilifera anormale / sviluppo del seno nei soggetti maschili

KO 체모 이상 발달 / 남성 유방 발달
che-mo i-sang bal-dal / nam-seong yu-bang bal-dal

RU патологический рост волос / увеличение молочных желез у мужчин
patologicheskiy rost volos / uvelichenie molochnykh zhelez u muzhchin

PL nienormalny porost włosów / rozwój piersi u mężczyzny

AR نمو غير طبيعي في الشعر / تطور الصدر عند الذكور
Numoow gheyr tabee'ei fish-sha"r / tatawwur as-sadr "indadh-dhukoor

PT crescimento piloso anormal / desenvolvimento da mama no homem

FK cheve w pouse nan yon fason ki pa normal / gason devlope pwatrin

EL μη φυσιολογική τριχοφυία / ανάπτυξη μαστού στους άνδρες
mee feeseeologeekEE treehofeeEEa / anApteexee mastU stus Andres

HI बालों का असाधारण विकास / मर्द की छाती का विकास
baalon ka asaadhaaraN vikaas / mard ki chhaati ka vikaas

Do you have hyperthyroidism / hypothyroidism?

ES ¿Tiene hipertiroidismo / hipotiroidismo?

ZH 你有甲状腺亢进 / 甲状腺低下吗？
nǐ yǒu jiǎ zhuàng xiàn kàng jìn / jiǎ zhuàng xiàn dī xià ma?

FR Avez-vous souffert d'hyperthyroïdie / d'hypothyroïdie?

DE Haben Sie eine Schilddrüsen Über/unterfunktion?

VI Quý vị có mắc chứng cường tuyến giáp / thiếu năng tuyến giáp không?

IT È affetto / a da ipertiroidismo / ipotiroidismo?

KO 갑상선 기능 항진증 / 갑상선 기능 저하증이 있으십니까?
Gap-sang-seon gi-neung hang-jin-jeung / gap-sang-seon gi-neung jeo-ha-jeung-
i is-eu-sim-ni-kka?

RU Есть ли у вас гипертиреоз / гипотиреоз?
Est' li u vas gipertireoz / gipotireoz?

PL Czy ma Pan(i) nadczynność tarczycy / niedoczynność tarczycy?

AR هل تعاني \ تعانين من فرط او نقص الدراق؟
Hal tu"aani \ tu"aaneen min fart au naqs ad-duraaq?

PT Tem hipertireoidismo / hipotireoidismo?

FK Eske ou gen ipetiwoyid / ipotiwoyid?

EL Έχετε υπερθυροειδισμό / υποθυροειδισμό;
Ehete eepertheeroeedeesm0 / eepotheeroeedeesm0?

HI क्या आपको थाइराॅयड की अतिक्रियता / अल्पक्रियता है ?
Kya aapko thyroid ki atikriyataa / alpakriyataa hai?

Have you recently been sick / unconscious?

ES ¿Recientemente se ha mareado / desmayado?

ZH 你最近有没有生病 / 昏迷？
nǐ zuì jìn yǒu méi yǒu shēng bìng / hūn mí?

FR Avez-vous été malade récemment / inconscient(e)?

DE Waren Sie in letzter Zeit krank / bewusstlos?

VI Gần đây quý vị có bị đau bệnh / bất tỉnh không?

IT Recentemente è stato / a male / ha perso i sensi?

KO 최근에 아픈 / 의식을 잃은 적이 있습니까?
Choe-geun-e a-peun / ui-sig-eul i-reun jeog-i it-seum-ni-kka?

RU Недавно вы были больны / теряли сознание?
Nedavno vy byli bol'ny / teryali soznanie?

PL Czy ostatnio był(a) Pan(i) chory(a) / stracił(a) przytomność?

AR هل اصبت فى الوقت الأخير بمرض \ فقدان الوعى؟
Hal usibt fil-waqt al-akheer bi-maradh / fuqdaan al-wa"ei?

PT Recentemente esteve doente / perdeu os sentidos?

FK Eske ou te malad / pedi konesans resamman?

EL Ήσασταν πρόσφατα άρρωστοι / αναίσθητοι;
EEsastan prOsfata Arostee / anEstheetee?

HI क्या आप हाल में बीमार / बेहोश रहे हैं ?
Kya aap haal mein beemaar / behosh rahe hain?

Are you a diabetic? Since when?

ES ¿Tiene usted diabetes? ¿Desde cuándo?

ZH 你有糖尿病吗？从什么时候开始？
nǐ yǒu táng niào bìng ma? cóng shén me shí hòu kāi shǐ?

FR Avez-vous un diabète? depuis quand?

DE Sind Sie Diabetiker? Seit wann?

VI Quý vị có mắc bệnh tiểu đường không? Kể từ bao giờ?

IT È diabetico / a? Da quando?

KO 당뇨병이 있으십니까? 언제 부터 입니까?
Dang-nyo-byeong-i is-eu-sim-ni-kka? Eon-je bu-teo im-ni-kka?

RU Вы диабетик? С какого года?
Vy diabetik? S kakogo goda?

PL Czy choruje Pan(i) na cukrzycę? Od jak dawna?

AR هل تعانى \ تعانين من مرض السكر؟ منذ متى؟
Hal tu"aani / tu"aneen min maradh as-sukkar? / mundhu mattaa?

PT É diabético(a)? Desde quando?

FK Eske ou fè sik? Depi ki lè?

EL Είστε διαβητικοί; Από πότε;
EEste deeaveeteekEE? apO pOte?

HI क्या आपको मधुमेह है ? कबसे है ?
Kya aapko madhumeh hai? Kase hai?

Do you inject insulin? Type / how many units?

ES ¿Se inyecta insulina? ¿De que tipo / cuántas unidades?

ZH 你在打胰岛素吗？哪一种 / 多大剂量？
nǐ zài dá yí dǎo sù ma? nǎ yī zhǒng / duō dà jì liàng?

FR Vous injectez-vous de l'insuline? Quel type? Combien d'unités?

DE Spritzen Sie Insulin? Typ / wie viele Einheiten?

VI Quý vị có tiêm insulin không? Loại nào / bao nhiêu đơn vị?

IT Si inietta insulina? Che tipo / quante unità?

KO 인슐린 주사를 맞으십니까? 종류 / 몇 대나?
In-syul-lin ju-sa-reul ma-jeu-sim-ni-kka? Jong-nyu / Myeot dae-na?

RU Вы делаете уколы инсулина? Какой тип / сколько единиц?
Vy delaete ukoly insulina? Kakoy tip / skol'ko edinits?

PL Czy stosuje Pan(i) insulinę w zastrzykach? Jakiego rodzaju / ile jednostek?

AR هل تستعمل \ تستعملين حقن من الإنسولين؟
Hal tasta"mil / tasta"mileen huqan min al-insulin?

PT Injecta insulina? De que tipo e quantas unidades?

FK Eske ou pran piki insulin? Tip / ki dòz ?

EL Κάνετε ενέσεις ινσουλίνης; Τύπος / Πόσες μονάδες;
kAnete enEsees eensulEEnees? tEEpos / pOses monAdes?

HI क्या आप इन्सुलिन का इंजेक्शन लेते हैं ? किस प्रकार का /कितने यूनिट ?
Kya aap insulin ka injection lete hain? Kis prakaar ka / kitne unit?

Do you take antidiabetics? Types you use / how many?

S ¿Toma antidiabéticos? ¿De qué tipo / en qué cantidad?

H 你在用抗增生素吗？哪一种／多大剂量？
nǐ zài yòng kàng zēng shēng sù ma? nǎ yī zhòng / duō dà jì liàng?

R Prenez-vous des antidiabétiques? Quels types utilisez-vous? Combien?

E Nehmen Sie Antidiabetika? Welche / wie viele?

VI Quý vị có uống thuốc chữa tiểu đường không? Quý vị dùng loại nào / liều lượng bao nhiêu?

T Prende farmaci antidiabetici? Che tipi usa / quanti?

O 당뇨약을 드십니까? 사용하는 종류 / 몇 개?
Dang-nyo-ya-geul deu-sim-ni-kka? Sa-yong-ha-neun jong-nyu / Myeot gae?

RU Вы принимаете лекарство от диабета? Тип / доза лекарства?
Vy prinimaete lekarstvo ot diabeta? Tip / doza lekarstva?

PL Czy przyjmuje Pan(i) leki przeciwcukrzycowe? Jakiego rodzaju / ile?

AR هل تأخذ \ تأخذين مضادات لمرض السكر؟ الأنواع التي تستعملها \ تستعمليها \ كم منها؟
Hal ta'khudh / ta'khudheen mudhaataat li-maradh as-sukkar? Al-anwaa" alati tista"milha / tista"mileeha / kam minha?

PT Toma antidiabéticos? Tipos que toma / quantos?

K Eske ou pran antydyabetik? Kalite ou sevi a / konbyen?

EL Παίρνετε αντιδιαβητικά φάρμακα; Τύπτοι που χρησιμοποιείτε / Πόσα;
pErnete adeedeeaveeteekA fArmaka; tEEpee pu hreeseemopeeEEte / pOsa;

HI क्या आप मधुमेह प्रतिरोधी लेते हैं ? किस प्रकार के /कितने ?
Kya aap madhumeh pratirodhi lete hain? Kis prakaar ke / kitne?

Are you on a diabetic diet? How many bread units?

ES   ¿Lleva una dieta para diabéticos? ¿Cuántos panes come?

ZH   你在吃糖尿病餐吗？有几个面包单位？
nǐ zài chī táng niào bìng cān ma? yǒu jǐ ge miàn bāo dān wèi?

FR   Avez-vous un régime pour diabétique? Combien d'unités de pain?

DE   Halten Sie eine Diabetes-Diät? wie viele Broteinheiten?

VI   Quý vị có áp dụng chế độ ăn kiêng dành cho người mắc bệnh tiểu đường
không? Quý vị dùng bao nhiêu lượng bánh mì?

IT   Segue una dieta diabetica? Quante unità di pane?

KO   당뇨 식이법을 시행하십니까? 빵은 몇 개나?
Dang-nyo si-gi-beob-eul si-haeng-ha-sim-ni-kka? Ppang-eunMyeot gae-na?

RU   Вы соблюдаете диабетическую диету? Сколько съедаете кусков хлеба?
Vy soblyudaete diabeticheskuyu dietu? Skol'ko s"edaete kuskov khleba?

PL   Czy jest Pan(i) na diecie cukrzycowej? Ile jednostek chleba?

AR   هل انت على ريجيم خاص لمرض السكر؟ كم من الوحدات الخبزية؟
Hal inta (male) / inti (female) "alaa reezheem khaas li-maradh as-sukkar? Kam min
al-wihdaat al-khubziyah?

PT   Segue um regime alimentar para diabéticos? Quantas unidades de pão?

FK   Eske ou ap swiv rejim dyabetik? Ki vale pin?

EL   Ακολουθείτε δίαιτα για διαβητικούς; Πόσες μονάδες ψωμιού τρώτε;
akoluthEEte dEEeta geea deeaveeteekUs? pOses monAdes psomeeU trOte?

HI   क्या आप मधुमेह संबंधित खुराक पर हैं ? दिन में ब्रेड के कितने यूनिट ?
Kya aap madhumeh sambandhit khurak per hain? Din mein bread ke kitne unit?

When was your most recent insulin injection?

ES ¿Cuándo se aplicó la última inyección de insulina?

ZH 你最后一次打胰岛素是什么时候？
nǐ zuì hòu yī cì dǎ yí dǎo sù shì shén me shí hòu?

FR Quand avez-vous reçu votre injection d'insuline la plus récente?

DE Wann haben Sie zuletzt Insulin gespritzt?

VI Lần quý vị tiêm insulin gần đây nhất là khi nào?

IT Quando ha iniettato l'insulina l'ultima volta?

KO 가장 최근에 인슐린 주사 맞은 게 언제입니까?
Ga-jang choe-geun-e in-syul-lin ju-sa ma-jeun ge eon-je-im-ni-kka?

RU Когда был последний укол инсулина?
Kogda byl posledniy ukol insulina?

PL Kiedy brał(a) Pan(i) ostatni zastrzyk insuliny?

AR متى كان آخر مرة إستعملت حقنة من الإنسولين؟
Mattaa kaan aakhir marrah ista"malt huqnah min al-insulin?

PT Quando administrou a sua mais recente injecção de insulina?

FK Ki lè ou pran denye piki insilin ou ?

EL Πότε ήταν η πιο πρόσφατη ένεση ινσουλίνης;
pOte EEtan ee peeo prOsfatee Enesee eensulEEnees?

HI आपने हालमें इनसूलिन का इंजेक्शन कब लिया था ?
Aapne haalmein insulin ka injection kab liya tha?

When was your most recent meal?

ES	¿A qué hora comió la última vez?
ZH	你最后一次用餐是什么时候？ nǐ zuì hòu yī cì yòng cān shì shén me shí hòu?
FR	Quand avez-vous pris votre dernier repas?
DE	Wann haben Sie zuletzt gegessen?
VI	Lần dùng bữa gần đây nhất của quý vị là khi nào?
IT	Quando ha mangiato l'ultima volta?
KO	가장 최근에 언제 식사하셨습니까? Ga-jang choe-geun-e eon-je sik-sa-ha-syeot-seum-ni-kka?
RU	Когда вы последний раз ели? Kogda vy posledniy raz eli?
PL	Kiedy jadł(a) Pan(i) ostatni posiłek?
AR	ما هي آخر وجبة غذاء تناولتها؟ Maa hiya aakhir wajbah ghadhaa tanaawalt-haa?
PT	Quando tomou a sua refeição mais recente?
FK	A ki lè ou te manje denye fwa a?
EL	Πότε ήταν το πιο πρόσφατο γεύμα σας; pOte EEtan to peeo prOsfato gEvma sas?
HI	आपने हालमें कब खाना खाया था ? Aapne haalmein khaanaa kab khaayaa tha?

Does diabetes run in your family?

ES ¿Ha habido diabetes en su familia?

ZH 糖尿病是你家的遗传病吗？
tàng niào bìng shì nǐ jiā de yí chuán bìng ma?

FR Y-a-t-il du diabète dans votre famille?

DE Haben Sie Diabetes in der Familie?

VI Bệnh tiểu đường có di truyền trong gia đình quý vị không?

IT Il diabete presenta caratteri di ereditarietà nella sua famiglia?

KO 본인 가족에 당뇨병이 유전됩니까?
Bon-in ga-jo-ge dang-nyo-byeong-i yu-jeon-doem-ni-kka?

RU Кто-нибудь в вашей семье болел диабетом?
Kto-nibud' v vashey sem'e bolel diabetom?

PL Czy cukrzyca występuje w Pana(i) rodzinie?

AR هل يوجد مرض السكر عند أفراد آخرين من أهلك؟
Hal youjad maradh as-sukkar "ind afraad aakhareen min ahlak?

PT A diabetes existe na sua família?

FK Eske maladi sik la nan fanmi w?

EL Είναι ο διαβήτης κληρονομικός στην οικογένειά σας;
EEne o deeaveetees kleeronomeekOs steen eekogEneeA sas?

HI क्या आपके परिवार में मधुमेह का इतिहास है ?
Kya aapke parivaar mein madhumeh ka itihaas hai?

Are you receiving / have you received cortisone therapy?

ES	¿Lo están tratando / lo han tratado con cortisona?
ZH	你是否在用 / 曾经用过可的松？ nǐ shì fǒu zài yòng / céng jīng yòng guò kě de sōng?
FR	Recevez-vous / avez-vous reçu un traitement à la cortisone?
DE	Haben / hatten Sie eine Therapie mit Cortison?
VI	Quý vị có đang / đã được điều trị bằng cortisone không?
IT	Sta seguendo / ha seguito una terapia a base di cortisone?
KO	코티존 치료를 현재 받거나 받으신 적이 있습니까? Ko-ti-jon chi-ryo-reul hyeon-jae bat-geo-na ba-deu-sin jeo-gi it-seum-ni-kka?
RU	Лечитесь / лечились ли вы кортизоном? Lechites' / lechilis' li vy kortizonom?
PL	Czy przechodzi / przechodził(a) Pan(i) terapię kortyzonową?
AR	هل انت حالياً \ سبق لك أن تكون \ تكونين تحت العلاج بالكورتيزون؟ Hal inta / inti haaliyan sabaq lak an takoun / takouneen taht al-"ilaaj bil-cortizone?
PT	Está receber / já recebeu tratamento com cortisona?
FK	Eske ou ap resevwa / te janm resevwa terapi kotizon?
EL	Λαμβάνετε / Λάβατε θεραπεία με κορτιζόνη; lamvAnete / lAvate therapEEa me korteezOnee?
HI	क्या आप कॉर्टिज़ोन उपचार ले रहे हैं / कभी लिया था ? Kya aap cortisone upchaar le rahe hain / kabhi liya thaa?

Do you have high blood pressure / cholesterol?

ES ¿Tiene presión arterial alta / colesterol alto?

ZH 你有没有高血压 / 高血脂？
nǐ yǒu méi yǒu gāo xuè yā / gāo xiě zhī?

FR Avez-vous une pression sanguine élevée / du cholestérol?

DE Haben Sie hohe(n) Blutdruck / Cholesterinwerte?

VI Quý vị có bị huyết áp cao / cholesterol trong máu cao không?

IT Ha la pressione alta / il colesterolo alto?

KO 고혈압 / 고 콜레스테롤이 있으십니까?
Go-hyeo-rap / go kol-le-seu-te-ro-ri it-seu-sim-ni-kka?

RU У вас повышенное давление / холестерин?
U vas povyshennoe davlenie / kholesterin?

PL Czy ma Pan(i) nadciśnienie / wysoki cholesterol?

AR هل تعاني \ تعانين من ضغط دم \ مستوى كوليستيرول مرتفع؟
Hal tu"aani / tu"aaneen min dhaght damm / mustawaa cholesterol murtafi"?

PT Sofre de tensão alta / colesterol?

FK Eske ou souvri ak tansyon / kolestewòl ?

EL Έχετε υψηλή αρτηριακή πίεση / χοληστερίνη;
Ehete eepseelEE arteereeakEE pEEesee / holeesterEEnee?

HI क्या आपको उच्च रक्तचाप / कोलेस्टेरोल है ?
Kya aapko uchch raktachaap / cholesterol hai?

Do you have gestational diabetes?

ES ¿Tiene diabetes del embarazo?

ZH 你有妊辰性糖尿病吗？
nǐ yǒu rèn chén xìng táng niào bìng ma?

FR Avez-vous un diabète de grossesse?

DE Haben Sie Schwangerschaftsdiabetes?

VI Quý vị có mắc bệnh tiểu đường trong khi mang thai không?

IT Ha il diabete gestazionale?

KO 임신성 당뇨병이 있으십니까?
Im-sin-seong dang-nyo-byeong-i it-seu-sim-ni-kka?

RU У вас есть гестационный диабет?
U vas est' gestatsionnyi diabet?

PL Czy ma Pan(i) cukrzycę ciążową?

AR هل تعاني \ تعانين من مرض سكر حملي؟
Hal tu"aani / tu"aaneen min maradh sukkar hamli?

PT Sofre de diabetes gestacional?

FK Eske ou gen diabèt jestasyonèl ?

EL Έχετε διαβήτη κύησης;
Ehete deeavEEtee kEEeesees?

HI क्या आपको जेस्टेशनल मधुमेह है?
Kya aapko gestational madhumeh hai?

13 Genitourinary System

Do you have pain during urination?

ES ¿Siente dolor al orinar?

ZH 你小便时感到痛吗？
nǐ xiǎo biàn shí gǎn dào tòng ma?

FR Avez-vous mal en urinant?

DE Haben Sie Schmerzen beim Wasserlassen?

VI Quý vị có thấy đau khi tiểu tiện không?

IT Prova dolore durante l'urinazione?

KO 소변보실 때 통증이 있으십니까?
So-byeon-bo-sil ttae tong-jeung-i i-seu-sim-ni-kka?

RU Вам больно мочиться?
Vam bol'no mochit'sya?

PL Czy odczuwa Pan(i) ból podczas oddawania moczu?

AR هل تشعر \ تشعرين بالألم عند التبول؟
Hal tish"ur / tish"ureen bil-alam "ind at-tabawwul?

PT Sente dor durante a micção?

FK Eske ou gen doulè lè w ap pipi?

EL Έχετε πόνο κατά την ούρηση;
Ehete pOno katA teen Ureesee?

HI क्या आपको पेशाब के दौरान दर्द होता है?
Kya aapko peshaab ke dauraan dard hota hai?

Have you noticed a change in the color of your urine?

ES ¿Ha notado cambios en el color de la orina?

ZH 你小便的颜色有变化吗？
nǐ xiǎo biàn de yán sè yǒu biàn huà ma?

FR Avez-vous remarqué un changement dans la couleur de vos urines?

DE Hat sich die Farbe Ihres Urins verändert?

VI Quý vị có thấy màu nước tiểu thay đổi không?

IT Ha notato un cambiamento nel colore delle urine?

KO 소변 색깔에 변화가 생겼습니까?
So-byeon saek-kka-re byeon-hwa-ga saeng-gyeot-seum-ni-kka?

RU Вы заметили изменение цвета мочи?
Vy zametili izmenenie tsveta mochi?

PL Czy zauważył(a) Pan(i) zmianę w barwie swego moczu?

AR هل لاحظت تغيراً في لون بولك؟
Hal laahadht taghyeeran fi loun baulak?

PT Notou alguma alteração na cor da sua urina?

FK Eske ou remake pipi w chanje koulè?

EL Παρατηρήσατε αλλαγή στο χρώμα των ούρων σας;
parateerEEsate alagEE sto hrOma ton Uron sas?

HI क्या आपने अपने पेशाब के रंग में परिवर्तन नोट किया है? ...
Kya aapne apne peshaab ke rang mein parivartan note kiya hai?

bloody / dark / cloudy

S	con sangre / oscura / turbia
H	有血的 / 深色 / 混浊 yǒu xiě de / shēn sè / hn zhuó
R	souillées de sang / sombres / troubles
VI	blutig / dunkel / trüb
VI	có máu / sẫm màu / đục
T	tracce di sangue / scure / torbide
O	피가 섞인 / 어두운 / 탁한 pi-ga seo-kkin / eo-du-un / tak-han
RU	кровавая / темная / мутная krovavaya / temnaya / mutnaya
PL	krwisty / ciemny / mętny
AR	دام \ داكن \ متغيم اللون Daami / daakin / mutaghayyim al-loun
T	sanguinolenta / escura / turva
K	gen san / fonse / nuwaje
L	αιματώδη / σκούρα / θολά ematOdee / skUra / tholA
HI	रक्तयुक्त / गहरा / धुँधला Raktyukt / gehra / dhundhla

Have you noticed a change in the smell of your urine?

ES	¿Ha notado algún cambio en el olor de la orina?
ZH	你小便的气味有什么变化吗？ nĭ xiăo biàn de qì wèi yŏu shén mè biàn huà ma?
FR	Avez-vous noté un changement dans l'odeur de vos urines?
DE	Hat sich der Geruch Ihres Urins verändert?
VI	Quý vị có thấy mùi nước tiểu thay đổi không?
IT	Ha notato un cambiamento nell'odore delle urine?
KO	소변 냄새에 변화가 생겼습니까? So-byeon naem-sae-e byeon-hwa-ga saeng-gyeot-seum-ni-kka?
RU	Вы заметили изменение запаха мочи? Vy zametili izmenenie zapakha mochi?
PL	Czy zauważył(a) Pan(i) zmianę w zapachu swego moczu?
AR	هل لاحظت تغيراً في رائحة بولك؟ Hal laahadht taghyeeran fi reehat baulak?
PT	Notou alguma mudança no cheiro da sua urina?
FK	Eske ou remake yon chanjman nan sant pipi w?
EL	Παρατηρήσατε αλλαγή στην οσμή των ούρων σας; parateerEEsate alagEE steen osmEE ton Uron sas?
HI	क्या आपने अपने पेशाब की गंध में परिवर्तन नोट किया है? ... Kya aapne apne peshaab ki gandh mein parivartan note kiya hai?

Are you suffering from incontinence? Are you leaking urine?

¿Tiene incontinencia (no controla la orina)? ¿Tiene escapes de orina?

你有没有小便失禁？有没有不自主的滴尿？
nǐ yǒu méi yǒu xiǎo biàn shī jìn? yǒu méi yǒu bù zì zhǔ de dī niào?

Souffrez-vous d'incontinence urinaire? Perdez-vous vos urines?

Sind Sie inkontinent? Verlieren Sie Urin?

Quý vị có gặp tình trạng không kiềm chế được tiểu tiện không? Quý vị có bị són tiểu không?

È incontinente? Ha perdite di urina?

요실금이 있으십니까? 소변이 흘러나오는 문제가 있으십니까?
Yo-sil-geum-i i-seu-sim-ni-kka? So-byeo-ni heul-leo-na-o-neun mun-je-ga i-seu-sim-ni-kka?

Вы страдаете недержанием? Моча непроизвольно вытекает?
Vy stradaete nederzhaniem? Mocha neproizvol'no vytekaet?

Czy cierpi Pan(i) na nietrzymanie moczu? Czy mocz wycieka?

هل تعاني \ تعانين من السلس في التبول؟ هل يصب منك البول لا تستطيع \ تستطيعين السيطرة عليه؟
Hal tu"aani / tu"aaneen min as-salas fit-tabawwul? Hal yasibb minnak al-baul wa la tastatee" / tastatee"een as-saytarah "alaihi?

Sofre de incontinência? Sofre de perda involuntária de urina?

Eske w ap soufri inkontinans? Eske w ap koule pipi?

Πάσχετε από ακράτεια; Έχετε διαρροή ούρων;
pAshete apO akrAteea? Ehete deearoEE Uron?

क्या आप असंयमता से पीड़ित हैं? क्या आपका पेशाब निकलता रहता है? ...
Kya aap A-saiyamtaa se peeDit hain? Kya aapka peshaab nikalta rehta hai?

Do you have a frequent urge to urinate?

ES   ¿Siente frecuentemente el impulso de orinar?

ZH   你有没有尿频尿急？
nǐ yǒu méi yǒu niào pín niào jí?

FR   Avez-vous souvent un besoin urgent d'uriner?

DE   Haben Sie häufig einen Drang zum Wasserlassen?

VI   Quý vị có luôn cảm thấy mót tiểu không?

IT   Ha bisogno di urinare con frequenza?

KO   소변을 보고 싶은 생각이 자주 드십니까?
So-byeo-neul bo-go si-peun saeng-ga-gi ja-ju deu-sim-ni-kka?

RU   Часто ли вы испытываете позывы помочиться?
Chasto li vy ispytyvaete pozyvy pomochit'sya?

PL   Czy często odczuwa Pan(i) parcia na mocz?

AR   هل انت مضطر \ مضطرة كثيراً على التبول؟
Hal inta / inti mudhtarr / mudhtarrah katheeran "alaa at-tabawwul?

PT   Tem uma vontade premente de urinar, com frequência?

FK   Eske ou toujou anvi pipi?

EL   Έχετε συχνή ανάγκη να ουρείτε;
Ehete seehnEE anAgee na urEEte?

HI   क्या आप बार–बार पेशाब आता है? ...
Kya aapko baar-baar peshaab aata hai?

always / often / especially at night

S
todo el tiempo / a menudo / principalmente en la noche

H
不断的 / 经常的 / 特别是在晚上
bù duàn de / jīng cháng d / e tè bié shì zài wǎn shàng

R
toujours / souvent / spécialement la nuit

E
immer / oft / vor allem nachts

V
luôn luôn / thường xuyên / đặc biệt là vào buổi tối

I
sempre / spesso / specialmente la notte

T
항상 / 자주 / 특히 밤에
hang-sang / ja-ju / teuk-hi ba-me

O
всегда / часто / особенно ночью
vsegda / chasto / osobenno noch'yu

U
stale / często / szczególnie w nocy

'L
دائماً \ كثيراً \ بصفة خاصة بالليل
Daa'iman / katheeran / bi-siffah khaasah bil-leyl

.R
sempre / muitas vezes / especialmente à noite

T
tout tan / souvan / soutou lan nwit

K
πάντα / συχνά / ειδικά τη νύχτα
pAnda / seehnA / eedeekA tee nEEhta

L
हमेशा / अक्सर / विशेष रूप से रात में
hamesha / aksar / vishesh roop se raat mein

Do you have back pain / pain on your side?

ES ¿Tiene dolor de espalda / en un costado?

ZH 你有没有腰痛／腰侧痛？
nǐ yǒu méi yǒu yāo tòng / yāo cè tòng?

FR Avez-vous mal dans le dos / dans le côté?

DE Haben Sie Schmerzen in der Seite / im Rücken?

VI Quý vị có bị đau lưng / đau bên người không?

IT Ha dolori alla schiena / dolori laterali?

KO 등이 아프십니까 / 옆구리가 아프십니까?
Deung-i a-peu-sim-ni-kka / yeop-gu-ri-ga a-peu-sim-ni-kka?

RU У вас болит спина / бок?
U vas bolit spina / bok?

PL Czy odzuwa Pan(i) ból krzyża / w boku?

AR عندك ألم فى الظهر \ ألم فى ضلعك؟
"Indak alam fidh-dhuhr / alam fi dhil"ak?

PT Tem dores nas costas / dores de lado?

FK Eske ou gen doulè nan do w / doulè sou kote w?

EL Έχετε πόνο στην πλάτη / πόνο στα πλευρά;
Ehete pOno steen plAtee / pOno sta plevrA?

HI क्या आपको कमर में दर्द / साइड में दर्द होता है?
Kya aapko kamar me dard / side mein dard hota hai?

Have you had / do you have stones in your urine / kidney stones?

S ¿Ha tenido / tiene piedras (cálculos) en la orina / renales?

H 你现在 / 从前有没有得过尿结石 / 肾结石？
nǐ xiàn zài / cóng qián yǒu méi yǒu dé guò niào jié shí / shèn jié shí?

R Avez-vous eu / avez-vous des calculs dans vos urines / des calculs rénaux?

E Hatten / haben Sie Steine im Urin / in den Nieren?

I Quý vị đã bao giờ có / hiện có sỏi trong nước tiểu / sỏi thận không?

T Ha avuto / ha calcoli nelle urine / calcoli renali?

O 소변에 돌(결석)이 나온 적이 / 신장 결석이 있은 적이 있으십니까 / 있습니까??
So-byeo-ne dol(gyeol-seok)-i na-on jeog-i it-seum-ni-kka / sin-jang gyeol-seog-i i-seun jeog-i i-seu-sim-ni-kka?

U У вас были / есть камни в моче / в почках?
U vas byli / est' kamni v moche / v pochkakh?

L Czy miał(a) / ma Pan(i) kamienie w moczu / kamienie nerkowe?

R ؟هل سبق أن كان عندك \ هل عندك حصى في بولك \ حصى في الكلى
Hal sabaq an kaan "indak / hal "indak hassaa fi baulak / hassaa fil-kilaa?

T Já teve / tem pedras na urina / pedras nos rins?

K Eske ou te gen / ou genyen kalke (wòch) nan piti w / kalke (wòch) nan ren?

L Είχατε / Έχετε πέτρες στα ούρα / πέτρες στα νεφρά;
EEhate / Ehete pEtres sta Ura / pEtres sta nefrA?

II क्या आपके मूत्राशय / गुर्दे में पथरी थी / है?
Kya aapke mutrashaya / gurde mein pathri thi / hai?

Have you ever had a kidney / urinary tract infection?

ES ¿Ha tenido infección renal / de las vías urinarias?

ZH 你有没有得过肾 / 尿道感染？
nĭ yŏu méi yŏu dé guò shèn / niào dào găn răn?

FR Avez-vous jamais eu une infection du rein / du tractus urinaire?

DE Hatten Sie jemals eine Nieren- / Harnwegsinfektion?

VI Quý vị đã bao giờ bị viêm đường niệu / thận chưa?

IT Ha mai avuto un'infezione renale / del tratto urinario?

KO 신장 / 요로관 감염이 있은 적 있으십니까?
Sin-jang / yo-ro-gwan gam-yeom-i i-seun jeo-gi-i-seu-sim-ni-kka?

RU У вас когда-нибудь было инфекционное заболевание почек /
мочевыводящих путей?
U vas kogda-nibud' bylo infektsionnoe zabolevanie pochek / mochevyvodyashchikh
putey?

PL Czy miał(a) Pan(i) kiedykolwiek zakażenie dróg moczowych?

AR هل سبق أن اصبت بالتهاب الكلى \ التهاب المسلك البولي؟
Hal sabaq an usibt bi-iltihaab al-kilaa / iltihaab al-maslak al-bauli?

PT Alguma vez teve uma infecção nos rins / no tracto urinário?

FK Eske ou te janm genyen yon infeksyon nan ren / vwa urine?

EL Είχατε ποτέ λοίμωξη των νεφρών / της ουροφόρου οδού;
EEhate potE IEEmoxee ton nefrOn / tees urofOru odU?

HI क्या आपको कभी गुर्दे / पेशाब का संक्रमण हुआ था?
Kya aapko kabhi gurde / peshaab ka sankramaN hua tha?

Did you receive treatment for the infection? Successfully?

S ¿Le dieron tratamiento para esa infección? ¿Le sirvió?

H 你有没有对这些感染做过治疗？效果好吗？
nǐ yǒu méi yǒu duì zhè xiē gǎn rǎn zuò guò zhì liáo? xiào guǒ hǎo ma?

R Avez-vous reçu un traitement pour cette infection? efficace?

E Wurde die Infektion behandelt? Erfolgreich?

T Quý vị có điều trị bệnh viêm đó không? Điều trị có hiệu quả không?

O È stato / a curato / a per tale infezione? La cura ha avuto successo?

O 이 감염에 대한 치료를 받으셨습니까? 성공적이었습니까?
I gam-yeom-e dae-han chi-ryo-reul ba-deun jeo-gii-seu-sim-ni-kka? Seong-gong-jeo-gi-eot-seum-ni-kka?

U Лечили ли вы это инфекционное заболевание? Удачно?
Lechili li vy eto infektsionnoe zabolevanie? Udachno?

L Czy był(a) Pan(i) leczony(a) na tę chorobę? Czy został Pan(i) wyleczony(a)?

R هل تلقيت علاجاً للإلتهاب؟ بالنجاح؟
Hal talaqqayt "ilaaj lil-iltihaab? Bin-najaah?

T Recebeu tratamento para a infecção? Com êxito?

K Eske ou resevwa trètman pou infeksyon sa? Byen reisi?

L Λάβατε θεραπεία για αυτήν τη μόλυνση; Επιτυχώς;
lAvate therapEEa geea aftEEn tee mOleensee? epeeteehOs?

II क्या आपने संक्रमण के लिए इलाज करवाया? सफलतापूर्वक?
Kya aapne sankramaN ke liye ilaaj karvaya? safaltapoorvak?

Are you having problems in the genital area?

ES ¿Tiene algún problema en la región genital?

ZH 你生殖器部位有什么问题吗？
nǐ shēng zhí qì bù wèi yǒu shén me wèn tí ma?

FR Avez-vous des problèmes dans la région génitale?

DE Haben Sie Beschwerden im Bereich der Geschlechtsorgane?

VI Quý vị có đang gặp vấn đề ở vùng sinh dục không?

IT Ha problemi alla zona genitale?

KO 생식기 부위에 문제가 있으십니까?
Saeng-sik-gi bu-wi-e mun-je-ga i-seu-sim-ni-kka?

RU У вас есть проблемы с половыми органами?
U vas est' problemy s polovymi organami?

PL Czy ma Pan(i) problemy z obszarem narządów płciowych?

AR هل تعاني \ تعانين من مشاكل في المنطقة التناسلية؟
Hal tu"aani / tu"aaneen min mashaakil fil-mantiqah at-tanaasuliyyah?

PT Tem problemas na zona genital?

FK Eske ou gen pwoblèm nan zon prive ou?

EL Έχετε προβλήματα στην περιοχή των γεννητικών οργάνων;
Ehete provlEEmata steen pereeohEE ton geneeteekOn orgAnon?

HI क्या आपको जननांग क्षेत्र में कोई समस्या है? ...
Kya aapko jannaang kShetra mein koi samasya hai?

burning / itching / pain / liquid discharge / bleedings

.S ardor / picazón (comezón) / dolor / secreciones / sangrado

H 烧灼感 / 痒 / 痛 / 液体外溢 / 出血
shāo zhuó gǎn / yǎng / tòng / yè tǐ wài yì / chū xiě

R brûlures / démangeaisons / douleur / pertes / saignements

E Brennen / Jucken / Schmerzen / Flüssigkeitsabsonderungen / Blutungen

I bỏng rát / ngứa / đau / tiết ra chất dịch lỏng / chảy máu

T bruciori / prurito / dolore / perdite liquide / perdite di sangue

O 쓰림 / 가려움 / 통증 / 액체 분비물 / 출혈
sseu-rim / ga-ryeo-um / tong-jeung / aek-che bun-bi-mul / chul-hyeol

U жжение / зуд / боль / водянистые выделения / кровотечение
zhzhenie / zud / bol' / vodyanistye vydeleniya / krovotechenie

L pieczenie / swędzenie / ból / płynna wydzielina / krwawienia

R الإحتراق \ الحك \ الألم \ إفراز سائل \ نزيف دم
Al-ihtiraaq / al-hakk / al-alam / ifraaz saa'il / nazeef damm

T sensação de ardor / comichão / dor / descarga líquida / sangramentos

K boule / grate w / doulè / bay likid / ran san

L καύσος / κνησμός / πόνος / υγρές εκκενώσεις / αιμορραγία
kAfsos / kneesmOs / pOnos / eegrEs ekenOsees / emoragEEa

H जलन / खुजली / दर्द / तरल स्राव / रक्तस्राव
jalan / khujli / dard / taral sraav / raktasraav

When was your last / first period? Day / month / year

ES ¿Cuándo tuvo su última / primera menstruación? Día / mes / año

ZH 你的最后一次 / 第一次月经时什么时间？某天 / 某月 / 某年
nǐ de zuì hòu yī cì / dì yī cì yuè jīng shí shén me shí jiā? mǒu tiān / mǒu yuè / mǒu nián

FR Quelle est la date de vos dernières / premières règles? Jour / mois / année

DE Wann war Ihre erste / letzte Periode? Tag: Monat: Jahr:

VI Quý vị bắt đầu có kinh nguyệt từ khi nào / lần có kinh nguyệt gần đây nhất là kh nào? Ngày / tháng / năm

IT Quando ha avuto l'ultimo / il primo ciclo? Giorno / mese / anno

KO 마지막 / 첫 월경이 언제 였습니까? 일 / 월 / 년
Ma-ji-mak / cheot wol-gyeong-i eon-je yeot-seum-ni-kka? Il / wol / nyeon

RU Когда у вас были последние / первые месячные? День / месяц / год
Kogda u vas byli poslednie / pervye mesyachnye? Den' / mesyats / god

PL Kiedy miała Pani ostatnią / pierwszą miesiączkę? Dzień / miesiąc / rok

AR متى كان محيضك الأخير \ الأول؟ اليوم \ الشهر \ السنة
Mattaa kaan maheedhik al-akheer \ al-awwal? Al-youm \ al-shahr \ as-sanah

PT Quando é que teve o seu último / primeiro período menstrual? Dia / mês / ano

FK Ki lè ou te gen reg ou denye fwa / premye fwa? Jou / mwa / ane

EL Πότε ήταν η τελευταία / πρώτη περίοδός σας; Ημέρα / Μήνας / Χρόνος
pOte EEtan ee telefteEa / prOtee perEEodOs sas? eemEra / mEEnas / hrOnos

HI आपको अंतिम / पहली बार माहवारी कब हुई? दिन / महीना / वर्ष
Aapko antim / pehli bar mahavaari kab hui? Din / Mahina / VarSh

Is your period regular? (approximately) every ... days

S ¿Su menstruación es regular? (aproximadamente) cada ... días

H 你的月经规律吗？（大约）多少天一次
nǐ de yuè jīng guī lǜ ma? (dà yuē) duō shǎo tiān yī cì

R Sont-elles régulières? (environ) tous les ... jours

E Ist Ihre Periode regelmäßig? (Ungefähr) Alle ... Tage

VI Chu kỳ kinh nguyệt của quý vị có đều không? (khoảng) ... ngày một chu kỳ

T Ha il ciclo regolare? (circa) ogni ... giorni

O 월경이 규칙적입니까? (대략) ... 일 마다
Wol-gyeong-i gyu-chik-jeo-gim-ni-kka? (dae-ryak) ... il ma Da

RU У вас месячные регулярные? (примерно) каждые ... дней
U vas mesyachnye regulyarnye? (primerno) kazhdye ... dney

PL Czy mieszczki Pani są regularne? (mniej więcej) co ... dni

AR هل يتكرر محيضك بشكل عادي؟ كل __ يوم (تقريباً)
Hal yitkarrir maheedhik bi-shekl "aadi? Kull __ youm (taqreeban)

PT O seu período menstrual é regular? (aproximadamente) cada ... dias

FK Eske reg ou regilye? (apepe) chak jou

EL Είναι τακτική η περίοδός σας; (περίπου) κάθε ... ημέρες
EEne takteekEE ee perEEodOs sas? (perEEpu) kAthe ... eemEres

HI क्या आपकी माहवारी नियमित है? (लगभग) प्रत्येक ... दिन
Kya aapki mahavaari niyamit hai? (lagbhag) pratyek ... din

Do you have cramps during your period?

ES	¿Tiene cólicos durante la menstruación?
ZH	月经时有绞痛感吗？ yuè jīng shí yǒu jiǎo tòng gǎn ma?
FR	Avez-vous des crampes au cours de vos règles?
DE	Haben Sie Krämpfe während Ihrer Periode?
VI	Quý vị có bị đau thắt trong thời gian có kinh không?
IT	Ha dolori mestruali durante il ciclo?
KO	월경할 때 급격한 복통을 경험하십니까? Wol-gyeong-hal ttae geup-gyeok-han bok-tong-eul gyeong-heom-ha-sim-ni-kka?
RU	Во время месячных вы испытываете боли внизу живота? Vo vremya mesyachnykh vy ispytyvaete boli vnizu zhivota?
PL	Czy w czasie miesiączki miewa Pani skurcze?
AR	هل تعانين من التشنجات أثناء المحيض؟ Hal tu"aaneen min at-tashannujaat athnaa' al-maheedh?
PT	Tem cólicas menstruais durante o seu período menstrual?
FK	Eske ou gen kramp lè ou gen reg ou?
EL	Έχετε κράμπες κατά τη διάρκεια της περιόδου σας; Ehete krAbes katA tee deeArkeea tees pereeOdu sas?
HI	क्या आपको माहवारी के दौरान मोच आई? Kya aapko mahavaari ke dauraan moch aayi?

Did you observe unusual bleeding / discharge?

ES ¿Ha observado sangrado / secreción anormal?

ZH 你有过不正常的出血 / 白带吗？
nǐ yǒu guò bù zhèng cháng de chū xiě / bái dài ma?

FR Avez-vous remarqué un saignement anormal / un écoulement?

DE Hatten Sie eine ungewöhnliche Blutung / Ausfluss?

VI Quý vị có bị chảy máu / tiết chất dịch bất thường không?

IT Ha notato insolite perdite di sangue / secrezioni?

KO 심상치 않은 출혈 / 분비물이 있었습니까?
Sim-sang-chi a-neun chul-hyeol / bun-bi-mu-ri i-seot-seum-ni-kka?

RU Замечали ли вы необычное кровотечение / необычные выделения?
Zamechali li vy neobychnoe krovotechenie / neobychnye vydeleniya?

PL Czy zauważyła Pani jakieś nietypowe krwawienie / wydzielinę?

AR هل لاحظت أي نزيف دم \ إفراز غير عادي؟
Hal laahadht ayyi nazeef damm / ifraaz gheyr "aadi?

PT Notou um sangramento / descarga invulgar?

FK Eske ou obseve ke seyman ou pa nomal / dechaj?

EL Παρατηρήσατε ασυνήθιστη αιμορραγία / εκκένωση;
parateerEEsate aseenEEtheestee emoragEEa / ekEnosee?

HI क्या आपने असामान्य रक्तस्राव / स्राव देखा?
Kya aapne A-saamanya raktasraav / sraav dekha?

Are you pregnant / is it possible that you are pregnant?

ES ¿Está embarazada? / ¿Cree que pueda estar embarazada?

ZH 你是否怀孕 / 有没有怀孕的可能？
nǐ shì fǒu huái yùn / yǒu méi yǒu huái yùn de kě néng?

FR Etes-vous enceinte / est-il possible que vous soyez enceinte?

DE Sind Sie schwanger / Ist es möglich, dass Sie schwanger sind?

VI Quý vị có đang mang thai không / có khả năng là quý vị đang mang thai không?

IT È incinta / potrebbe essere incinta?

KO 임신 중이십니까? / 임신 중일 가능성이 있습니까?
Im-sin jung-i-sim-ni-kka? / im-sin jung-il ga-neung-seong-i it-seum-ni-kka?

RU Вы беременны / возможно, что вы беременны?
Vy beremenny / vozmozhno, chto vy beremenny?

PL Czy jest Pani w ciąży / czy jest możliwe, żeby Pani była w ciąży?

AR هل انت حامل؟ هل يحتمل أنك حامل؟
Hal inti haamil? Hal yahtamil annik haamil?

PT Está grávida / é possível que esteja grávida?

FK Eske ou ansent / eske li posib ke ou ansent?

EL Είστε έγκυος / Είναι πιθανό να είστε έγκυος;
EEste Egeeos / EEne peethanO na EEste Egeeos?

HI क्या आप गर्भवती है / क्या आपके गर्भवती होने की संभावना है?
Kya aap garbhavati hain / Kya aapke garbhavati hone ki sambhavna hai?

When would be your due date? Day: month:

ES ¿Cuándo debería venir la menstruación? Día: mes:

ZH 预产期时什么时间？哪一天，哪一月
yù chǎn qī shí shén me shí jiān? nǎ yī tiān, nǎ yī yuè

FR Quelle serait la date attendue? Jour: mois:

DE Wann wäre der erwartete Geburtstermin? Tag: Monat:

VI Ngày dự liệu sinh nở của quý vị là ngày nào? Ngày: tháng:

IT Qual è la data presunta del parto? Giorno: mese:

KO 분만 예정일이 언제 입니까? 일. 월:
Bun-man ye-jeong-i-ri eon-je im-ni-kka? il. wol:

RU Когда вам рожать? День: месяц:
Kogda vam rozhat'? Den': mesyats:

PL Kiedy miałoby nastąpić rozwiązanie? Dzień: miesiąc:

AR متى يحتمل أن يكون يوم الولادة؟ اليوم: الشهر:
Mattaa yahtamil an yakoon youm al-wilaadah? Al-youm: Al-shahr:

PT Quando seria a data do parto? Dia: mês:

FK Ki dat ke w ap akouche? Jou mwa

EL Πότε είναι η αναμενόμενη ημερομηνία τοκετού σας; Ημέρα: Μήνας:
pOte EEne ee anamenOmenee eemeromeenEEa toketU sas? eemEra: mEEnas:

HI आपकी माहवारी की तय तिथि कब होगी? दिन: महीनाः
Aapki mahavaari ki teya tithi kab hogi? Din: Mahina:

How many days are you overdue? ... days

ES ¿Cuántos días se le ha atrasado? ... días

ZH 超过预产期几天了？？ ... 天
chāo guò yù chǎn qī jǐ tiān le? ... tiān

FR Combien de jours de retard avez-vous? ... jours

DE Wie lange sind Sie überfällig? ... Tage

VI Quý vị đã bị trễ bao nhiêu ngày? ... ngày

IT Quanto è il ritardo rispetto alla data presunta del parto? ... giorni

KO 분만 예정일을 얼마나 넘기셨습니까? ... 일
Bun-man ye-jeong-i-reul eol-ma-na neom-gi-syeot-seum-ni-kka? ... il

RU Сколько дней вы перенашиваете? ... дней
Skol'ko dney vy perenashivaete? ... dney

PL Ile dni jest po terminie? ... dni

AR كم يوم مرّ بعد يوم الولادة المتوقعة؟ ... يوم
Kam youm marr ba"d youm al-wilaadah al-mutawaqqa"ah? ... youm

PT Há quantos dias é que o seu período menstrual está atrasado? ... dias

FK Kombyen jou ke ou anreta? Jou

EL Πόσες ημέρες πέρασαν από την αναμενόμενη ημερομηνία τοκετού σας; ... ημέρες
pOses eemEres pErasan apO teen anamenOmenee eemeromeenEEa toketU sas? ... eemEres

HI कितने दिन विलंबित हैं? ... दिन
kitne din vilambit hain? ... din

Have you had an infection (German measles) during pregnancy?

ES ¿Ha tenido alguna infección (rubéola) durante el embarazo?

ZH 你怀孕期间有过感染（风疹）吗？
nǐ huái yùn qī jiān yǒu guò gǎn rǎn (fēng zhěn) ma?

FR Avez-vous eu une infection (rubéole) au cours de la grossesse?

DE Hatten Sie eine Infektion (Röteln) während der Schwangerschaft?

VI Quý vị có bị viêm nhiễm (bệnh ban đào) trong thời gian mang thai không?

IT Ha avuto un'infezione (la rosolia) durante la gravidanza?

KO 임신 중에 감염(풍진)이 있었습니까?
Im-sin jung-e gam-yeom(pung-jin)i i-seot-seum-ni-kka?

RU У вас была инфекция (краснуха) во время беременности?
U vas byla infektsiya (krasnukha) vo vremya beremennosti?

PL Czy przechodziła pani zakażenie (rózyczkę) podczas ciąży?

AR هل اصبت بإلتهاب (الحصبة الألمانية) أثناء الحمل؟
Hal usibt bi-iltihaab (al-hasbah al-almaaniyah) athnaa' al-haml?

PT Teve uma infecção (rubéola) durante a gravidez?

FK Eske ou te yon yon infeksyon (Rubeol) pandan ke ou te ansent?

EL Είχατε λοίμωξη (ερυθρά) κατά την εγκυμοσύνη;
EEhate IEEmoxee (ereethrA) katA teen egeemosEEnee?

HI क्या आपको गर्भावस्था के दौरान संक्रमण (जर्मन खसरा) हुआ?
Kya aapko garbhavastha ke dauraan sankramaN (German khasra) hua?

Did you take any medications? Please specify. For how long?

ES ¿Le dieron medicamentos? Dígame cuáles. ¿Por cuánto tiempo?

ZH 你当时用什么药了吗？具体是什么药？用了多久？
nǐ dāng shí yòng shén me yào le ma? jù tǐ shì shén me yào? yòng le duō jiǔ

FR Prenez-vous des médicaments? Veuillez spécifier s'il vous plaît. Depuis quand?

DE Haben Sie irgendwelche Medikamente genommen? Welche? Wie lange?

VI Quý vị có dùng thuốc men gì không? Xin trình bày rõ. Trong bao lâu?

IT Ha assunto farmaci? La prego di specificare. Per quanto tempo?

KO 약을 드셨습니까? 구체적으로 밝혀주십시오. 얼마나 오래?
Ya-geul deu-syeot-seum-ni-kka? Gu-che-jeo-geu-ro bal-kyeo-ju-sip-si-o. Eol-ma-na o-rae?

RU Вы принимали какие-либо лекарства? Пожалуйста, уточните. Как долго?
Vy prinimali kakie-libo lekarstva? Pozhaluysta, utochnite. Kak dolgo?

PL Czy przyjmowała Pani jakieś leki? Proszę bliżej określić. Jak długo?

AR هل أخذت اية أدوية؟ بينها مع مدة أخذها.
Hal akhadhti ayyi adwiyyah? Bayyineehaa ma" muddat akhdhihaa.

PT Tomou alguns medicamentos? Por favor, especifique. Durante quanto tempo?

FK Eske ou te pran okin medikaman? Tanpri spesifye Pandan konbyen tan?

EL Λάβατε κάποια φάρμακα; Παρακαλώ καθορίστε. Για πόσο καιρό;
lAvate kApeea fArmaka? parakal0 kathorEEste. geea pOso kerO?

HI क्या आपने कोई दवा ली? कृपया स्पष्ट करें। कितने समय तक?
Kya aapne koi davaa lee? Kripya spaST karein. Kitne samay tak?

Have you taken / are you taking sleeping pills during pregnancy?

S ¿Ha tomado / está tomando pastillas para dormir durante el embarazo?

H 你怀孕期间有没有吃过 / 在吃安眠药？
nǐ huái yùn qī jiān yǒu méi yǒu chī guò / zài chī ān mián yào?

R Avez-vous pris / ou prenez-vous des somnifères pendant la grossesse?

E Nahmen / nehmen Sie Schlafmittel während der Schwangerschaft?

VI Quý vị đã / có đang dùng thuốc ngủ trong thời gian mang thai không?

T Ha preso / sta prendendo pillole di sonnifero durante la gravidanza?

O 임신 중에 수면제를 드신 적이 있으십니까 / 현재 드시고 계십니까?
Im-sin jung-e su-myeon-je-reul deu-sin jeo-gi i-seu-sim-ni-kka / hyeon-jae deu-si-go gye-sim-ni-kka?

U Вы принимали / принимаете снотворное во время беременности?
Vy prinimali / prinimaete snotvornoe vo vremya beremennosti?

L Czy przyjmowała / przyjmuje Pani środki nasenne podczas ciąży?

R هل أخذت أية \ هل تأخذين حبات نوم أثناء الحمل؟
Hal akhadhti / ta'khudheen habbaat noum athnaa' al-haml?

T Tomou / está a tomar comprimidos para dormir durante a gravidez?

K Eske ou te pran / eske w ap pran gren pou ede w domi pandan ou ansent?

L Λάβατε / Λαμβάνετε υπνωτικά κατά την εγκυμοσύνη;
lAvate / lamvAnete eepnoteekA katA teen egeemosEEnee?

HI क्या आपने गर्भावस्था के दौरान नींद की गोलियां ली थी / लेती हैं?
Kya aapne garbhavastha ke dauraan neend ki goliyan lee thi / leti hain?

Did you drink alcohol during pregnancy?

ES	¿Ha bebido alcohol durante el embarazo?
ZH	你怀孕期间有没有喝过酒？ nǐ huái yùn qī jiān yǒu méi yǒu hē guò jiǔ?
FR	Buvez-vous de l'alcool pendant la grossesse?
DE	Haben Sie Alkohol während der Schwangerschaft getrunken?
VI	Quý vị có uống rượu trong thời gian mang thai không?
IT	Ha bevuto alcol durante la gravidanza?
KO	임신 중에 술을 마시셨습니까? Im-sin jung-e su-reul ma-sin jeo-gi i-seu-sim-ni-kka?
RU	Вы употребляли алкоголь во время беременности? Vy upotreblyali alkogol' vo vremya beremennosti?
PL	Czy piła Pani alkohol podczas ciąży?
AR	هل شربت الكحول أثناء الحمل؟ Hal sharabti il-kuhoul athnaa' al-haml?
PT	Consumiu bebidas alcoólicas durante a gravidez?
FK	Eske ou te bouwe tafya pandan ou te ansent?
EL	Ήπιατε αλκοόλ κατά την εγκυμοσύνη; EEpeeate alkoOl katA teen egeemosEEnee?
HI	क्या आपने गर्भावस्था के दौरान शराब पी थी? Kya aapne garbhavastha ke dauraan sharab pee thi?

Do you have diabetes / too high blood pressure?

¿Tiene diabetes / presión arterial muy alta?

你有没有糖尿病 / 非常高的血压 ?
nǐ yǒu méi yǒu táng niào bìng / fēi cháng gāo de xuè yā?

Avez-vous du diabète / une pression sanguine trop élevée?

Haben Sie Diabetes / einen zu hohen Blutdruck?

Quý vị có bị tiểu đường / huyết áp quá cao không?

Ha il diabete / la pressione troppo alta?

당뇨병 / 지나치게 높은 혈압이 있으십니까?
Dang-nyo-byeong / ji-na-chi-ge no-peun hyeo-ra-bi i-seu-sim-ni-kka?

У вас есть диабет / повышенное артериальное давление?
U vas est' diabet / povyshennoe arterial'noe davlenie?

Czy ma Pani cukrzycę / nadciśnienie?

هل تعانين من مرض السكر \ إرتفاع شديد في ضغط الدم؟
Hal tu"aaneen min maradh as-sukkar / irtifaa" shaded fi dhaght ad-damm?

Tem diabetes / tensão arterial demasiado alta?

Eske ou fè sik / tansyon w te two wo?

Έχετε διαβήτη / πολύ υψηλή αρτηριακή πίεση;
Ehete deeavEEtee / polEE eepseelEE arteereeakEE pEEesee?

क्या आपको म ध ुमेह / बहुत उच्च रक्तचाप है?
Kya aapko madhumeh / bahut uchch raktchap hai?

How many times have you been pregnant?

ES	¿Cuántas veces se ha embarazado?
ZH	你怀孕过几次了？ nǐ huái yùn guò jǐ cì le?
FR	Combien de fois avez-vous été enceinte?
DE	Wie viele Schwangerschaften hatten Sie?
VI	Quý vị đã mang thai bao nhiêu lần?
IT	Quante gravidanze ha avuto?
KO	임신을 몇 번이나 하셨습니까? Im-si-neul myeot beo-ni-na ha-syeot-seum-ni-kka?
RU	Сколько раз вы были беременны? Skol'ko raz vy byli beremenny?
PL	Ile razy była Pani w ciąży?
AR	كم مرة كنت حامل لحد الآن؟ Kam marrah kunti haamil li-hadd al-aan?
PT	Quantas vezes esteve grávida?
FK	Konbyen fwa ou te ansent?
EL	Πόσες φορές ήσασταν έγκυος; pOses forEs EEsastan Egeeos?
HI	आप कितनी बार गर्भवती हुई? Aap kitni baar garbhvati hui?

Did you have a miscarriage?

ES ¿Ha abortado?

ZH 你以前有过流产吗？
nǐ yǐ qián yǒu guò liú chǎn ma?

FR Avez-vous eu une fausse couche?

DE Hatten Sie eine Fehlgeburt?

VI Quý vị có bị sảy thai không?

IT Ha avuto un aborto spontaneo?

KO 유산하셨습니까?
Yu-san-ha-syeot-seum-ni-kka?

RU У вас были аборты?
U vas byli aborty?

PL Czy Pani poroniła?

AR هل سبق أن حدث عندك إسقاط؟
Hal sabaq an hadath "indik isqaat?

PT Teve um aborto natural?

FK Eske ou te pedi pitit la?

EL Είχατε αποβολή;
EEhate apovolEE?

HI क्या आपका गर्भपात हुआ?
Kya aapka garbhpaat hua?

Have you had any prenatal care? Type of provider?

ES ¿Ha recibido atención médica prenatal? ¿Qué tipo de atención?

ZH 你有没有做过产前护理？是哪一种护理？
nǐ yǒu méi yǒu zuò guò chǎn qián hù lǐ? shì nǎ yī zhǒng hù lǐ?

FR Avez-vous eu l'un ou l'autre soin prénatal? Quel type d'aide?

DE Sind Sie zur Mutterschaftsvorsorge gegangen? Zu wem?

VI Quý vị có được chăm sóc dưỡng thai không? Theo dạng dịch vụ nào?

IT Ha avuto assistenza medica durante la gravidanza? Che tipo di medico?

KO 산전 서비스를 받으신 적이 있으십니까? 어떤 곳에서 받으셨습니까?
San-jeon seo-bi-seu-reul ba-deu-sin jeo-gi i-seu-sim-ni-kka? Eo-tteon go-se-seo ba-deu-syeot-seum-ni-kka?

RU Вас наблюдали во время беременности? Какой специалист?
Vas nablyudali vo vremya beremennosti? Kakoy spetsialist?

PL Czy miała Pani opiekę prenatalną? Kto jej udzielał?

AR هل تلقيت أية عناية قبل الولادة؟ ما نوع الطبيب؟
Hal talaqqayt ayyi "inaayah qabl al-wilaadah? Maa nou" at-tabeeb?

PT Recebeu alguns cuidados pré-natais? Tipo de provedor?

FK Eske ou te gen okinn swen prenatal? Tip founisè?

EL Είχατε προγεννητική περίθαλψη; Είδος παροχέα;
EEhate progeneeteekEE perEEthalpsee? EEdos parohEa?

HI क्या आपकी प्रसव-पूर्व देखभाल हुई? प्रदाता का प्रकार?
Kya aapki prasav-poorv dekhbhal hui? pradata ka prakaar?

Have you had intercourse? With one / several partners?

ES ¿Ha tenido relaciones sexuales? ¿Con una pareja / varias parejas?

ZH 你有没有性交行为？与一个 / 几个性伴侣？
nǐ yǒu méi yǒu xìng jiāo xíng wéi? yǔ yī gè / jǐ gè xìng bàn lǚ?

FR Avez-vous des rapports sexuels? Avec un / plusieurs partenaire(s)?

DE Hatten Sie Geschlechtsverkehr? Mit einem / mehreren Partnern?

VI Quý vị có quan hệ tình dục không? Với một / nhiều người bạn tình?

IT Ha avuto rapporti sessuali? Con un partner / diversi partner?

KO 성교를 하신 적이 있습니까? 한 사람하고만 / 다수 동반자와?
Seong-gyo-reul ha-sin jeo-gi it-seum-ni-kka? Han sa-ram-ha-go-man / yeo-reo dong-ban-ja-wa?

RU У вас была половая связь? С одним / несколькими партнерами?
U vas byla polovaya svyaz'? S odnim / neskol'kimi partnerami?

PL Czy odbywała Pani stosunek seksualny? Z jednym partnerem / kilkoma partnerami?

AR هل قمت بالجماع؟ مع شخص واحد \ عدة أشخاص؟
Hal qumti bil-jimaa"? Ma" shakhs waahid / "iddat ashkaas?

PT Já teve relações sexuais? Com um parceiro / vários parceiros?

FK Eske ou te fè seks? Ak yon / plizye patnè?

EL Είχατε συνουσία; Με ένα εραστή / αρκετούς εραστές;
EEhate seenusEEa? Me Ena erastEE / arketUs erastEs?

HI क्या आपने सहवास किया? एक / अनेक साथियों के साथ?
Kya aapne sahvaas kiya? Ek / anek sathiyon ke saath?

Do you already have children? How many? Birth weight?

ES ¿Ya ha tenido hijos? ¿Cuántos? ¿Cuánto pesaron al nacer?

ZH 你有孩子吗？有几个？出生时重量是多少？
nǐ yǒu hái zǐ ma? yǒu jǐ gè? chū shēng shí zhòng liàng shì duō shǎo?

FR Avez-vous déjà des enfants? Combien? Poids à la naissance?

DE Haben Sie schon Kinder? Wie viele? Geburtsgewicht?

VI Quý vị đã có con chưa? Bao nhiêu người con? Cân nặng khi sinh?

IT Ha già figli? Quanti? Peso alla nascita?

KO 이미 자녀가 있으으십니까? 몇 명? 출생시 체중?
I-mi ja-nyeo-ga i-seu-sim-ni-kka? Myeot myeong? Chul-saeng-si che-jung?

RU У вас уже есть дети? Сколько? Их вес при рождении?
U vas uzhe est' deti? Skol'ko? Ikh ves pri rozhdenii?

PL Czy Pan(i) już ma dzieci? Ile? Waga przy narodzeniu?

AR هل لديك أطفال؟ كم طفل؟ كم كان وزنهم عند الولادة؟
Hal ladayk atfaal? Kam tifl? Kam kaan waznhum "ind al-wilaadah?

PT Já tem filhos? Quantos filhos tem? Peso ao nascer?

FK Eske ou gen pitit deja? Konbyen? Konbyen li te peze lè li fèt?

EL Έχετε ήδη παιδιά; Πόσα; Πόσο ζύγιζαν κατά τη γέννησή τους;
Ehete EEdee pedeeA? pOsa? pOso zEEgeezan katA tee gEneesEE tus?

HI क्या आपके पहले ही बच्चे हैं? कितने? जन्म के समय वज़न?
Kya aapke pehle hi bachche hain? Kitne? Janam ke samay vazan?

Do you want more children? How many? When?

S ¿Quiere tener más hijos? ¿Cuántos? ¿Cuándo?

H 你打算要更多的孩子吗？要几个？什么时候？
nǐ dǎ suàn yào gèng duō de hái zǐ ma? yào jǐ gè? shén me shí hòu?

R Souhaitez-vous avoir davantage d'enfants? combien? quand?

DE Möchten Sie noch mehr Kinder? Wie viele? Wann?

VI Quý vị có muốn đẻ thêm không? Đẻ thêm bao nhiêu? Khi nào?

IT Desidera altri figli? Quanti? Quando?

KO 자녀를 더 원하십니까? 몇 명이나? 언제?
Ja-nyeo-reul deo won-ha-sim-ni-kka? Myeot myeong-i-na? Eon-je?

RU Вы ещё хотите детей? Сколько? Когда?
Vy eshchyo khotite detey? Skol'ko? Kogda?

PL Czy chce Pani mieć więcej dzieci? Ile? Kiedy?

AR هل ترغبين فى المزيد من الأطفال؟ كم منهم؟ متى؟
Hal targhabeen fil-mazeed min al-atfaal? Kam minhum? Mattaa?

PT Quer ter mais filhos? Quantos? Quando?

FK Eske ou vle gen plis timoun? Konbyen? Ki lè?

EL Θέλετε περισσότερα παιδιά; Πόσα; Πότε;
thElete pereesOtera pedeeA? pOsa? pOte?

HI क्या आप और बच्चें चाहती हैं? कितने? कब?
Kya aap aur bachche chahti hain? Kitne? Kab?

Are you taking contraceptives? Which ones?

ES ¿Usa anticonceptivos? ¿De qué tipo?

ZH 你在吃避孕药吗？哪一种？
nǐ zài chī bì yùn yào ma? nǎ yī zhǒng?

FR Prenez-vous des contraceptifs? Lesquels

DE Nehmen Sie Kontrazeptiva? Welche?

VI Quý vị có đang sử dụng các biện pháp ngừa thai không? Những biện pháp nào?

IT Fa uso di contraccettivi? Quali?

KO 피임하고 계십니까? 어떤 겁니까?
Pi-im-ha-go gye-sim-ni-kka? Eo-tteon geom-ni-kka?

RU Вы используете противозачаточные средства? Какие?
Vy ispol'zuete protivozachatochnye sredstva? Kakie?

PL Czy używa Pani środków antykoncepcyjnych? Jakich?

AR هل تستعملين وسائل تحديد النسل؟ اي نوع منها؟
Hal tasta"mileen wasaa'il tahdeed an-nasl? Ayyi nou" minhaa?

PT Está a usar anticoncepcionais? Quais?

FK Eske w ap fè planinn? Ki les ladan yo?

EL Λαμβάνετε αντισυλληπτικά; Ποια;
lamvAnete anteeseeleepteekA? peeA?

HI क्या आप गर्भनिरोधक ६ ।क ले रही हैं? कौन-सा? ...
Kya aap garbhanirodhak le rahi hain? Kaun sa?

pill / coil / diaphragm / suppository / foam / condoms

píldora / espiral / diafragma / supositorio / espuma / condones

药片 / 节育环 / 隔膜 / 避孕栓 / 泡沫 / 安全套
yào piàn / jié yù huán / gé mó / bì yùn shuān / pào mò / ān quán tào

pilule / stérilet / diaphragme / suppositoire / gelée / préservatifs

Pille / Intrauterinpessar / Diaphragma / Zäpfchen / Schaum / Kondome

thuốc viên / đặt vòng / màng chắn / thuốc đạn / bọt / bao cao su

pillola / spirale / diaframma / supposta spermicida / schiuma spermicida / preservativi

약 / 코일 / 격막 / 좌약 / 폼 / 콘돔
yak / ko-il / gyeong-mak / jwa-yak / pom / kon-dom

таблетки / спираль / диафрагма / свечи / пена / презервативы
tabletki / spiral' / diafragma / svechi / pena / prezervativy

tabletki / krążek maciczny / czopki / pianka / prezerwatywy

حبة منع الحمل \ حلزون منع الحمل \ الحجاب الحاجز \ التحميلة \ الرغوة \ واقيات جنسية
Habbat mana" al-haml / halazon mana" al-haml / al-hijaab al-haajiz / at-tahmeelah / ar-raghwah / waaqiyaat jinsiyyah

pílula / dispositivo intra-uterino / diafragma / supositório / espuma / preservativos

gren / diafram / supozitwa / mous / kapot

χάπι / σπειράλ / διάφραγμα / υπόθετο / αφρός / προφυλακτικά
hApee / speerAl / deeAfragma / eepOtheto / afrOs / profeelakteekA

गोली / डायफ्राम / सपोजिटरी / फोम / कंडोम
Goli / diaphragm / suppository / foam / condom

Did you undergo tubal ligation?

ES ¿Tiene ligadas las trompas?

ZH 你做过结扎吗？
nǐ zuò guò jiē zā ma?

FR Avez-vous subi une ligature des trompes?

DE Wurde bei Ihnen eine Tubenligatur durchgeführt?

VI Quý vị có làm giải phẫu thắt vòi trứng không?

IT Si è sottoposta a legatura delle tube?

KO 난관 봉합을 하셨습니까?
Nan-gwan bong-ha-beul ha-syeot-seum-ni-kka?

RU Вам выполняли перевязку труб?
Vam vypolnyali perevyazku trub?

PL Czy poddała się Pani zabiegowi podwiązania jajowodów?

AR هل اجري عليك عملية ربط القنوات الفالوبية؟
Hal ujree "alayk "amaliyah rabt al-qanaawaat al-faalobiyah?

PT Submeteu-se a uma ligação das trompas uterinas?

FK Eske ou te fè operasyon pou mare tib ou?

EL Υποβληθήκατε σε σαλπιγγική απολίνωση;
eepovleethEEkate se salpeegeekEE apolEEnosee?

HI क्या आपने ट्यूब बंधन कराया था?
Kya aapne tube bandhan karaaya tha?

Did you have a vasectomy performed? Have you undergone sterilization?

¿Se hizo la vasectomía? ¿Se sometió a esterilización?

你做过输精管切除手术吗？你做过绝育手术吗？
nǐ zuò guò shū jīng guǎn qiē chú shǒu shù ma? nǐ zuò guò jué yù shǒu shù ma?

Avez-vous subi une vasectomie? avez-vous subi une stérilisation?

Hatten Sie eine Vasektomie? Sind Sie sterilisiert?

Quý vị có làm giải phẫu thắt ống dẫn tinh không? Quý vị có làm giải phẫu triệt sản không?

Si è sottoposto a vasectomia? Si è sottoposto a sterilizzazione?

정관절제수술을 하셨습니까? 불임 수술을 하셨습니까?
Jeong-gwan-jeol-je-su-su-reul ha-syeot-seum-ni-kka? Bu-rim su-su-reul ha-syeot-seum-ni-kka?

Вам делали вазэктомию? Вам делали стерилизацию?
Vam delali vazektomiyu? Vam delali sterilizatsiyu?

Czy poddał się Pan wazektomii? Czy poddał się Pan sterylizacji?

هل اجري عليك عملية قطع القناة المنوية؟ هل اجري عليك عملية تعقيم؟
Hal ujree "alaik "amaliyah qata" al-qanaah al-manawiyah? Hal ujree "alaik "amaliyah ta"qeem?

Submeteu-se a uma vasectomia? Submeteu-se a esterilização?

Eske ou te fè operasyon vasektomi? Eske ou fè operasyon pou sterilize w?

Σας έγινε αφαίρεση του σπερματικού πόρου; Υποβληθήκατε σε στείρωση;
sas Egeene afEresee tu spermateekU pOru? eepovleethEEkate se stEErosee?

क्या आपने वाहिका संकुचन कराया था? क्या आपने विसंक्रमण कराया था?
Kya aapne vahika sankuchan karaaya tha? Kya aapne visankramaN karaaya tha?

When was your last cancer check-up?

ES	¿Cuándo fue su último examen de cáncer?
ZH	你上一次做癌症检查是什么时间？ nǐ shàng yī cì zuò ái zhèng jiǎn chá shì shén me shí jiān?
FR	De quand date votre dernier dépistage d'un cancer?
DE	Wann war die letzte Krebsvorsorge?
VI	Lần khám kiểm tra ung thư gần đây nhất của quý vị là khi nào?
IT	Quando ha fatto l'ultimo controllo contro il cancro?
KO	마지막으로 암 검사를 하신 게 언제 입니까? Ma-ji-ma-geu-ro am geom-sa-reul ha-sin ge eon-je im-ni-kka?
RU	Когда последний раз вы проходили онкологический осмотр? Kogda posledniy raz vy prokhodili onkologicheskiy osmotr?
PL	Kiedy miał(a) Pan(i) ostatni test na raka?
AR	متى كان فحصك الأخير للسرطان؟ Mattaa kaan fahsak al-akheer lis-sirataan?
PT	Quando se realizou o seu último exame médico contra o cancro?
FK	Ki denye fwa ou fè egzamin kanse a?
EL	Πότε έγινε ο τελευταίος έλεγχος για καρκίνο; pOte Egeene o teleftEos Eleghos geea karkEEno?
HI	आपकी अंतिम कैंसर जांच कब हुई थी? Aapki antim cancer jaanch kab hui thi?

When did you have your last mammogram / breast examination?

S ¿Cuándo se hizo mamografía / examen de mama la última vez?

H 你上一次做乳房造影 / 乳房检查是什么时候？
nǐ shàng yī cì zuò rǔ fáng zào yǐng / rǔ fáng jiǎn chá shì shén me shí hòu?

R Quand avez-vous subi votre dernière mammographie / dernier examen des seins?

E Wann war bei Ihnen die letzte Mammographie / Brustuntersuchung?

VI Lần khám vú / chụp khám ung thư vú gần đây nhất của quý vị là khi nào?

T Quando ha fatto l'ultima mammografia / l'ultimo esame del seno?

O 유방 검사를 마지막으로 하신 게 언제 입니까?
Yu-bang geom-sa-reul ma-ji-ma-geu-ro ha-sin ge eon-je im-ni-kka?

U Когда последний раз вам делали маммографию / обследование молочных желез?
Kogda posledniy raz vam delali mammografiyu / obsledovanie molochnykh zhelez?

L Kiedy miała Pani ostatnie badanie mammograficzne / badanie piersi?

R متى كان عندك آخر فحص الصدر؟
Mattaa kaan "indak aakhir fahs as-sadr?

T Quando se realizou a sua última mamografia / o seu último exame da mama?

K Ki denye fwa ou fè tès mammogram ou / egzamin tete w?

L Πότε είχατε την τελευταία μαστογραφία / εξέταση μαστών;
pOte EEhate teen teleftEa mastografEEa / exEtasee mastOn?

HI आपकी अंतिम मेमोग्राम/स्तन जांच कब हुई थी?
Aapki antim mammogram / stan jaanch kab hui thi?

Have you noticed any changes in your breast?

ES ¿Se ha notado algún cambio en los pechos?

ZH 你注意到乳房有什么变化吗？
nǐ zhù yì dào rǔ fáng yǒu shén me biàn huà ma?

FR Avez-vous remarqué le moindre changement dans vos seins?

DE Haben Sie Veränderungen bei Ihren Brüsten bemerkt?

VI Quý vị có thấy thay đổi gì ở vú không?

IT Ha notato cambiamenti al seno?

KO 유방에 변화가 생긴 게 있습니까?
Yu-bang-e byeon-hwa-ga saeng-gin ge it-seum-ni-kka?

RU Вы заметили какие-нибудь изменения в молочных железах?
Vy zametili kakie-nibud' izmeneniya v molochnykh zhelezakh?

PL Czy zauważył Pani jakieś zmiany w swoich piersiach?

AR هل لاحظت أيّ تغييرات في ثديك؟
Hal laahadht ayyi taghyeeraat fi thadyik?

PT Notou algumas alterações na sua mama?

FK Eske ou remake okinn chanjman nan tete w?

EL Παρατηρήσατε οποιεσδήποτε αλλαγές στο στήθος σας;
parateerEEsate opee-esdEEpote alagEs sto stEEthos sas?

HI क्या आपने अपने स्तनों में कोई बदलाव नोट किया? ....
Kya aapne apne stanon mein koi badlaav note kiya?

skin changes / redness / pain / lumps

ES cambios de la piel / enrojecimiento / dolor / bolitas

ZH 皮肤改变 / 发红 / 痛 / 肿块
pí fū gǎi biàn / fā hóng / tòng / zhǒng kuài

FR changements de la peau / rougeur / douleur / masses

DE Hautveränderungen / Rötung / Schmerzen / Knoten

VI thay đổi màu da / đỏ tấy / đau / có u

IT cambiamenti della pelle / rossore / dolore / noduli

KO 피부 변화 / 빨개짐 / 통증 / 덩어리
pi-bu byeon-hwa / ppal-gae-jim / tong-jeung / deong-eo-ri

RU изменение кожи / покраснение / боль / уплотнения
izmenenie kozhi / pokrasnenie / bol' / uplotneniya

PL zmiany skórne / zaczerwienienie / ból / guzy

AR تغيرات في الجلد \ الإحمرار \ الآلام \ الكتل
Taghyeeraat fil-jild \ al-ihmiraar \ al-aalaam \ al-kutal

PT alterações da pele / vermelhidão / dor / nódulos

FK po w chanje / li wouj / doulè / boul gres

EL δερματικές αλλαγές / ερυθρότητα / πόνος / σβώλοι
dermateekEs alagEs / ereethrOteeta / pOnos / svOlee

HI त्वचा परिवर्तन / लालिमा / दर्द / गांठें ...
twacha parivartan / lalima / dard / gaanThein

release of fluid from the nipples / nipple inflammation

ES	escape de líquido por los pezones / inflamación de los pezones
ZH	乳头溢液 / 乳头发炎 rǔ tóu yì yè / rǔ tóu fā yán
FR	perte de liquide par les mamelons / inflammation du mamelon
DE	Flüssigkeit aus der Brustwarze / Entzündung der Brustwarze
VI	núm vú tiết ra chất dịch / núm vú sưng viêm
IT	fuoriuscita di fluido dai capezzoli / infiammazione dei capezzoli
KO	젖꼭지에서 액체가 나옴 / 젖꼭지 염증 jeot-kkok-ji-e-seo aek-che-ga na-om / jeot-kkok-ji yeom-jeung
RU	жидкое отделяемое из сосков / воспаление сосков zhidkoe otdelyaemoe iz soskov / vospalenie soskov
PL	wyciek płynu z brodawki sutkowej / zapalenie brodawek sutkowych
AR	إفراز السائل من الحلمات \ إلتهاب الحلمة Ifraaz as-saa'il min al-halamaat / iltihaab al-halamah
PT	descarga de líquido dos mamilos / inflamação dos mamilos
FK	likid ki soti nan pwint tete w / pwint tete w anfle
EL	έκλυση υγρού από τις θήλες / φλεγμονή θηλών Ekleesee eegrU apO tees thEEles / flegmonEE theelOn
HI	चूचक से तरल स्राव / चूचक में जलन chuchak se taral sraav / chuchak mein jalan

Are you suffering from erectile dysfunction?

¿Está padeciendo disfunción eréctil?

你阴茎勃起有问题吗？
nǐ yīn jìng bó qǐ yǒu wèn tí ma?

Souffrez-vous d'un dysfonctionnement érectile?

Leiden Sie unter Potenzschwierigkeiten?

Quý vị có gặp bị rối loạn cường dương không?

Soffre di disfunzione erettile?

발기 기능 이상이 있으십니까?
Bal-gi gi-neung i-sang-i i-seu-sim-ni-kka?

Вы страдаете нарушением эрекции?
Vy stradaete narusheniem erektsii?

Czy cierpi Pan na zaburzenia erekcji?

هل تعاني من عطل الإنتصاب؟
Hal tu"aani min "atal il-intisaab?

Sofre de disfunção erétil?

Eske w ap soufri disfonksyon band?

Υποφέρετε από στυτική δυσλειτουργία;
eepofErete apO steeteekEE deesleeturgEEa?

क्या आप उत्थापनीय अक्षमता से पीड़ित हैं?
Kya aap utthaapniya a-kShamta se peeDit hain?

Have you noticed changes (in your testes / your penis)?

ES ¿Ha notado cambios (en los testículos / el pene)?

ZH 你发现（睾丸／阴茎）有什么变化吗？
nǐ fā xiàn (gāo wán / yīn jìng) yǒu shén me biàn huà ma?

FR Avez-vous remarqué des changements (dans vos testicules / votre pénis)?

DE Haben Sie Veränderung (an Ihren Hoden / Ihrem Penis) festgestellt?

VI Quý vị có thấy thay đổi gì (ở tinh hoàn / dương vật) không?

IT Ha notato cambiamenti (ai testicoli / al pene)?

KO (고환 / 성기)에 변화가 생긴 것이 있습니까?
(Go-hwan / seong-gi)-e byeon-hwa-ga saeng-gin geo-si it-seum-ni-kka?

RU Заметили ли вы изменения (в яичках / половом члене)?
Zametili li vy izmeneniya (v yaichkakh / polovom chlene)?

PL Czy zauważył Pan zmiany (w swoich jądrach / prąciu)?

AR هل لاحظت التغيرات (فى خصياتك / قضيبك)؟
Hal laahadht at-taghyeeraat (fi khisyaatak / qadheebak)?

PT Notou algumas alterações (nos seus testículos / no seu pénis)?

FK Eske ou remake okinn chanjman (nan testikil ou /

EL Παρατηρήσατε αλλαγές (στους όρχεις σας / στο πέος σας);
parateerEEsate alagEs (stus Orhees sas / sto pEos sas)?

HI क्या आपने (अपने अंडकोष／अपने लिंग में) कोई परिवर्तन नोट किया? ...
Kya aapne (apne andkoSh / apne ling mein) koi parivartan note kiya?

swelling / inflammation / ulcer / skin changes / discharge / pain

hinchazón / inflamación / úlcera / cambios de la piel / secreción / dolor

肿胀 / 发炎 / 溃疡 / 皮肤改变 / 有分泌物 / 痛
zhǒng zhàng / fā yán / kuì yáng / pí fū gǎi biàn / yǒu fēn mì wù / tòng

gonflement / inflammation / ulcère / modifications cutanées / pertes / douleur

Schwellung / Entzündung / Geschwür / Hautveränderungen / Ausfluss / Schmerz

sưng / sưng viêm / loét / thay đổi về da / tiết dịch / đau

gonfiore / infiammazione / ulcerazione / cambiamenti della pelle / secrezioni / dolore

부음 / 염증 / 궤양 / 피부 변화 / 분비물 / 통증
bu-um / yeom-jeung / gwe-yang / pi-bu byeon-hwa / bun-bi-mul / tong-jeung

опухание / воспаление / язва / изменения кожи / выделения / боль
opukhanie / vospalenie / yazva / izmeneniya kozhi / vydeleniya / bol'

obrzmienie / zapalenie / wrzód / zmiany skórne / wydzielinę / ból

التورم / الإلتهاب / القرحات / التغيرات في الجلد \ إفراز سائل \ الألم
At-tawarrum / al-iltihaab / al-qurhaat / at-taghyeeraat fil-jild / ifraaq saa'il / al-alam

inchaço / inflamação / úlcera / mudanças da pele / prurido / dor

anfle / inflamasyon / ulsè / chanjman nan po / dechaj / doulè

οίδημα / φλεγμονή / έλκος / δερματικές αλλαγές / εκκένωση / πόνος
EEdeema / flegmonEE / Elkos / dermateekEs alagEs / ekEnosee / pOnos

सूजन / जलन / छाले / त्वचा बदलाव / साव / दर्द
Soojan / jalan / Chale / twacha badlaav / sraav / dard

Have you ever had a genital disease?

ES	¿Ha tenido enfermedades de los genitales?
ZH	你的过性病吗？ nǐ dé guò xìng bìng ma?
FR	Avez-vous jamais eu une maladie génitale?
DE	Hatten Sie jemals eine Geschlechtskrankheit?
VI	Quý vị đã bao giờ mắc bệnh về đường sinh dục chưa?
IT	Ha mai avuto una malattia genitale?
KO	생식기 질환이 있은 적이 있으십니까? Saeng-sik-gi jil-hwa-ni i-seun jeo-gi i-seu-sim-ni-kka?
RU	У вас когда-нибудь были заболевания половых органов? U vas kogda-nibud' byli zabolevaniya polovykh organov?
PL	Czy przechodził(a) Pan(i) kiedykolwiek chorobę narządów płciowych?
AR	هل سبق أن اصبت بمرض تناسلي؟ Hal sabaq an usibt bi-maradh tanaasuli?
PT	Alguma vez teve uma doença genital?
FK	Eske ou te janm gen yon maladi jenital?
EL	Είχατε ποτέ ασθένεια των γεννητικών οργάνων; EEhate potE asthEneea ton geneeteekOn orgAnon?
HI	क्या आपको कभी जनन–संबंधी बीमारी हुई? Kya aapko kabhi janan-sambandhi beemari hui?

Syphilis / gonorrhea / the clap / HIV / AIDS

ES Sífilis / gonorrea / blenorragia / HIV / SIDA

ZH 梅毒 / 淋球菌感染 / 淋病 / HIV阳性 / 艾滋病
méi dú / lìn qiú jùn gǎn rǎn / lìn bìng / HIV yáng xìng / ài zī bìng

FR Syphilis / gonorrhée / blennorragie / chaude-pisse / VIH / sida

DE Syphilis / Gonorrhö / Tripper / HIV / AIDS

VI Giang mai / lậu / bệnh lậu / HIV / AIDS

IT Sifilide / gonorrea / blenorragia / HIV / AIDS

KO 매독 / 임질 / 인체 면역 결핍 바이러스(HIV) / 에이즈
mae-dok / im-jil / in-che myeon-nyeok gyeol-pip ba-i-reo-seu(HIV) / e-i-ieu

RU Сифилис / гонорея / триппер / ВИЧ / СПИД
Sifilis / gonoreya / tripper / VICh / SPID

PL syfilis / rzeżączkę / HIV / AIDS

AR مرض الزهري / مرض السيلان / مرض الأتش آي في / الأيدز
Maradh az-zuhari / maradh as-saylaan / maradh al-HIV / al-AIDS

PT sífilis / gonorreia / esquentamento / VIH / SIDA

TK Syfilis" gonore / "clap" / VIH / SIDA

EL σύφιλη / βλεννόρροια / γονόρροια / HIV / EITZ
sEEfeelee / vlenOreea / gonOreea /

HI सिफीलिस / गोनोरिया / क्लैप / एचआईवी / एड्स
Syphilis / gonorrhea / clap / HIV / AIDS

Was the treatment successful?

ES ¿Resultó útil el tratamiento?

ZH 治疗的效果好吗？
zhì liáo de xiào guǒ hǎo ma?

FR Le traitement fut-il efficace?

DE War die Behandlung erfolgreich?

VI Biện pháp điều trị có hiệu quả không?

IT La terapia ha avuto successo?

KO 치료가 성공적이었습니까?
Chi-ryo-ga seong-gong-jeo-gi-eot-seum-ni-kka?

RU Было лечение успешным?
Bylo lechenie uspeshnym?

PL Czy leczenie miało pomyślny wynik?

AR ؟هل نجح العلاج
Hal najah al-"ilaaj?

PT O tratamento foi bem sucedido?

FK Eske trètman an reisi?

EL Ηταν επιτυχής η θεραπεία;
EEtan epeeteehEEs ee therapEEa?

HI क्या इलाज सफल रहा?
Kya ilaaj safal raha?

Do you have joint pain / skin rashes?

S ¿Le duelen las articulaciones / tiene erupciones en la piel?

H 你有没有关节痛 / 皮肤红疹？
nǐ yǒu méi yǒu guān jié tòng / pí fū hóng zhěn?

R Avez-vous des douleurs articulaires / des éruptions cutanées?

E Haben Sie Gelenkschmerzen / Hautausschläge?

I Quý vị có bị đau khớp / nổi mẩn trên da không?

T Ha dolore alle articolazioni / eruzioni cutanee?

O 관절 통증 / 피부 발진이 있으십니까?
Gwan-jeol tong-jeung / pi-bu bal-ji-ni i-seu-sim-ni-kka?

RU У вас есть боль в суставах / кожная сыпь?
U vas est' bol' v sustavakh / kozhnaya syp'?

PL Czy cierpi Pan(i) na ból stawów / wysypki skórne?

AR هل تعاني \ تعانين من ألم فى المفاصل؟ \ ١ طفح جلدي؟
Hal tu"aani / tu"aaneen min alam fil-mafaasil? / tafah jildi?

PT Tem dores nas articulações / erupções cutâneas?

EK Eske ou gen doulè nan jo / po w wouj ak grate w?

EL Έχετε πόνο στις αρθρώσεις / δερματικά εξανθήματα;
Ehete pOno stees arthrOsees / dermateekA exanthEEmata?

HI क्या आपको जोड़ों में दर्द / त्वचा पर खरोंचे हैं?
Kya aapko joDon mein dard / twacha par khronche hain?

14 Musculoskeletal System

Did you have an accident?

ES ¿Tuvo un accidente?

ZH 有过外伤吗？
yǒu guò wài shāng ma?

FR Avez-vous eu un accident?

DE Hatten Sie einen Unfall?

VI Quý vị có bị tai nạn không?

IT Ha avuto un incidente?

KO 사고를 입으셨습니까?
Sa-go-reul i-beu-syeot-seum-ni-kka?

RU У вас была травма?
U vas byla travma?

PL Czy miał(a) Pan(i) wypadek?

AR هل كنت (male) / كنتِ (female) في حادث؟
Hal kunta (male) / kunti (female) fi haadith?

PT Teve um acidente?

FK Eske ou te fè yon aksidan?

EL Είχατε ατύχημα;
EEhate atEEheema?

HI क्या आपका अकस्मात हुआ है ?
Kya aapkaa akasmaat hua hai?

Do you have pain? Where does it hurt?

ES ¿Siente dolor? ¿Dónde le duele?

ZH 痛吗？哪里痛？
tòng ma? nǎ lǐ tòng?

FR Avez-vous mal? Où avez-vous mal?

DE Haben Sie Schmerzen? Wo?

VI Quý vị có bị đau không? Đau ở vùng nào?

IT Ha dolori? Dove Le fa male?

KO 통증이 있으십니까? 어디가 아프십니까?
Tong-jeung-i is-eu-sim-ni-kka? Eo-di-ga a-peu-sim-ni-kka?

RU Испытываете ли вы боль? Где болит?
Ispytyvaete li vy bol'? Gde bolit?

PL Czy czuje Pan(i) ból? Co Pana (Panią) boli?

AR هل لديك ألم؟ \ أين الألم؟
Hal ladayk alam? / Ayn al-'alam?

PT Tem dores? Onde é que lhe dói?

FK Eske ou gen doulè? Ki bò kap fè w mal ?

EL Έχετε πόνο; Πού πονάτε;
Ehete pOno? pu ponAte?

HI क्या आपको दर्द होता है ? कहां पर दर्द होता है ? ...
Kya aapko dard hota hai? Kahan per dard hota hai?

Joints / muscles / nerves / back / shoulders

ES	Articulaciones / músculos / nervios / espalda / hombros

ZH 关节 / 肌肉 / 神经 / 背部 / 肩膀
guān jié / jī ròu / shén jīng / bēi bù / jiān bǎng

FR Articulations / muscles / nerfs / dos / épaules

DE Gelenke / Muskel / Nerven / Rücken / Schultern

VI Khớp / cơ / các dây thần kinh / lưng / vai

IT Articolazioni / muscoli / nervi / schiena / spalle

KO 관절 / 근육 / 신경 / 등 / 어깨
gwan-jeol / geun-yuk / sin-gyeong / deung / eo-kkae

RU Суставы / мышцы / нервы / спина / плечи
Sustavy / myshtsy / nervy / spina / plechi

PL Stawy / mięśnie / nerwy / plecy / ramiona

AR في المفاصل \ في العضلات \ في الأعصاب \ في الظهر \ في الأكتاف
Fil-mafaasil / fil-"adhalaat / fil-a"saab / fidh-dhahr / fil-aktaaf

PT Articulações / músculos / nervos / costas / ombros

FK Jwinti / misk / nè / do / zepòl

EL αρθρώσεις / μύες / νεύρα / πλάτη / ὠμοι
arthrOsees / mEes / nEvra / plAtee / Omee

HI जोड़ / स्नायु / तंत्रिका / पीठ / कंधे
jod / snayu / tantrika / peeth / kandhe

When do you feel the pain?

S ¿Cuándo le viene el dolor?

H 什么时间痛？
shén me shí jiān tòng?

R Quand ressentez-vous la douleur?

E Wann spüren Sie den Schmerz?

VI Quý vị cảm thấy đau lúc nào?

T Quando prova dolore?

O 언제 아프십니까?
Eon-je a-peu-sim-ni-kka?

U Когда вы испытываете боль?
Kogda vy ispytyvaete bol'?

PL Kiedy odczuwa Pan(i) ten ból?

R متى تشعر \ تشعرين بالألم؟
Mattaa tash"ur / tash"ureen bil-alam?

T Quando é que sente a dor?

K Ki lè ou santi doulè a ?

L Πότε νιώθετε τον πόνο;
pOte neeOthete ton pOno?

HI आपको दर्द कब होता है ? ... ...
Aapko dard kab hota hai?

before / after getting up / in the morning / when I perform specific movements / always

ES antes / después de levantarse / por la mañana / con ciertos movimientos / siempre

ZH 起床前 / 起床后 / 早上 / 做特殊活动时 / 一直是
qǐ chuáng qián / qǐ chuáng hòu / zǎo shàng / zuò té shú huó dòng shí / yì zhí shì

FR Avant / après le lever / le matin / lorsque vous faites des mouvements précis / toujours

DE vor / nach dem Aufstehen / morgens / bei bestimmten Bewegungen / immer

VI trước / sau khi ngủ dậy / vào buổi sáng / khi tôi có những cử động cụ thể / lúc nào cũng thấy đau

IT prima di alzarmi / dopo essermi alzato / la mattina / quando faccio movimenti specifici / sempre

KO 일어나기 전 / 후 / 아침에 / 특정한 움직임을 행할 때 / 항상
i-reo-na-gi jeon / hu / a-chim-e / teuk-jeong-han um-ji-gi-meul haeng-hal ttae / hang-sang

RU до / после подъема / утром / при определённых движениях / всегда
do / posle pod"ema / utrom / pri opredelyonnykh dvizheniyakh / vsegda

PL przed wstaniem / po wstaniu z łóżka / rano / przy wykonywaniu specyficznych ruchów / stale

AR قبل او بعد الإستيقاظ \ في الصباح \ عندما اقوم بحركات معينة \ دائماً
Qabla aw ba"d il-istiyqaadh / fis-sabaah / "indama aqoom bi-harakaat mu"ayyanah / daa'iman

PT antes / depois do levantar / de manhã / quando faço determinados movimentos / sempre

FK avan / apre ou leve nan matin / lè map fè setin mouvman / tout tan

EL πριν / αφού σηκωθώ / το πρωί / όταν κάνω συγκεκριμένες κινήσεις / πάντα
preen / afU seekothO / to proEE / Otan kAno seegekreemEnes keenEEsees / pAnda

HI सुबह / उठने के पहले / उठने के बाद / जब मैं विशेष कार्य करता हूँ / हमेशा
subah / uthne ke pahle / uthne ke baad / jab main vishesh karya karta hun / hamesha

Did you ever have a bone / joint injury? In which area?

S ¿Se ha lesionado alguna vez un hueso / articulación? ¿En qué parte?

H 你骨骼／关节受过伤吗？那个部位？
nǐ gǔ gé / guān jié shòu guò shāng ma? nǎ gè bù wèi?

R Avez-vous jamais eu une fracture / une lésion articulaire? Dans quelle région?

E Hatten Sie jemals eine Knochen- / Gelenkverletzung? Wo?

I Quý vị có bao giờ bị chấn thương xương / khớp không? Ở vùng nào?

T Ha mai avuto lesioni ad un osso / ad una articolazione? In quale area?

O 뼈 / 관절 상해를 입으신 적이 있습니까? 어디 입니까?
Ppyeo / gwan-jeol sang-hae-reul i-beu-sin jeo-gi it-seum-ni-kka? Eo-di im-ni-kka?

U У вас когда-либо была травма костей / суставов? В каком месте?
U vas kogda-libo byla travma kostei / sustavov? V kakom meste?

PL Czy doznał(a) Pan(i) kiedykolwiek uszkodzenia kości / stawu? W którym miejscu?

AR هل سبق لك الإصابة بجرح في العظام او المفاصل؟ وفي أي مكان؟
Hal sabaq lak al-isaabah bi-jurh fil-"idhaam au al-mafaasil? Wa fi ayyi makaan?

PT Alguma vez sofreu de uma lesão óssea / lesão na articulação? Em que zona?

K Eske ou andomaje nan zò / jwenti ? Ki bò ?

EL Είχατε ποτέ τραυματισμό οστού / άρθρωσης; Σε ποια περιοχή;
EEhate potE travmateesmO ostU / Arthosees? Se peea pereeohEE?

HI क्या आपको कभी भी हड्डी/जोड़ में चोट पहुँची है ? किस क्षेत्र में ?
Kya aapko kabhi bhi haddi / jod mein chot lagi hai? Kis kshetra mein?

Have you noticed any changes on yourself?

ES ¿Ha notado cambios en su salud?

ZH 发现自己有什么变化吗？
fā xiàn zì jǐ yǒu shén me biàn huà ma?

FR Avez-vous, par vous-même, remarqué l'un ou l'autre changement?

DE Haben Sie Veränderungen bei sich bemerkt?

VI Quý vị có nhận thấy thay đổi nào trong người không?

IT Ha notato cambiamenti in Lei?

KO 본인한테 변화가 생긴 것을 느끼셨습니까?
Bo-nin-han-te byeon-hwa-ga saeng-gin geo-seul neu-kki-syeot-seum-ni-kka?

RU Заметили ли вы у себя какие-нибудь изменения?
Zametili li vy u sebya kakie-nibud' izmeneniya?

PL Czy zauważył Pan(i) u siebie jakieś zmiany?

AR هل لاحظت اية تغيرات فى نفسك؟
Hal laahadhta ayyati taghyeeraat fi nafsak?

PT Notou em si algumas alterações?

FK Eske ou remake okinn chanjman sou ou?

EL Παρατηρήσατε οποιεσδήποτε αλλαγές στον εαυτό σας;
parateerEEsate opee-esdEEpote alagEs ston eaftO sas?

HI क्या आपको अपने अंदर कुछ बदलाव दिखे ?
Kya aapko apne andar kuchh badlaav dikhe?

swollen legs / varicose veins / sensation of tightness in the calf muscles

ES piernas hinchadas / várices / tensión en las pantorrillas

ZH 腿肿 / 静脉曲张 / 小腿后发紧
tuǐ zhǒng / jìng mài qū zhāng / xiǎo tuǐ hòu fā jǐn

FR jambes gonflées / varices / sensation de raideur dans les muscles du mollet

DE geschwollene Beine / Krampfadern / Spannungsgefühl in den Waden

VI sưng chân / giãn tĩnh mạch / cảm thấy căng ở cơ bắp chân ..

IT gambe gonfie / vene varicose / sensazione di rigidità nei muscoli del polpaccio

KO 부은 다리 / 정맥류 정맥 / 종아리 근육이 당기는 느낌
bu-eun dari / jeong-maeng-nyu jeong-maek / jong-ari geun-yu-gi dang-gi-neun neu-kkim

RU отек ног / варикозное расширение вен / напряжение икроножных мышц
otek nog / varikoznoe rasshirenie ven / napryazhenie ikronozhnykh myshts

PL obrzęk nóg / żylaki / uczucie ściśnięcia w mięśniach łydek

AR الرجلان منتفختان \ ظهور العروق الدوالية \ أحساس الضيق في عضلات بطن الساق
Ar-rijlaan muntafikhataan / zhuhour al-"urouq ad-duwaaliyah / ahsaas adh-dheeq fil-"adhalaat batn as-saaq

PT pernas inchadas / veias varicosas / sensação de rigidez nos músculos da barriga da perna

FK janb anfle / ven gonfle nan janb / sensasyon ke misk jarèt o rèd

EL πρησμένα κάτω άκρα / κιρσοί φλεβών / αίσθημα σφίξιματος στους γαστροκνημίους μύες
preesmEna kAto Akra / kirsEE flevOn / Esteema sfeexEEmatos stus gastrokneemEEus mEEes

HI पैरों में सूजन /नसों में सूजन /पिंडली के स्नायुओं में सख्ती की संवेदना ... ...
pairon mein soojan / nason mein soojan / pindli ke snayuon mein sakhti ki samvedna

cold feet / tingling sensation in the arms, legs, hands, feet

ES pies fríos / hormigueo en los brazos, piernas, manos, pies

ZH 脚冷 / 四肢有刺痛感
jiǎo lěng / sì zhī yǒu cì tòng gǎn

FR pieds froids / sensation de picotement dans les bras, les jambes, les mains, les pieds

DE kalte Füße / Kribbeln in Armen, Beinen, Händen, Füßen

VI bàn chân lạnh / cảm giác ngứa ran ở cánh tay, chân, bàn tay, bàn chân

IT piedi freddi / formicolio alle braccia, alle gambe, alle mani, ai piedi

KO 차가운 발 / 팔, 다리, 손, 발이 욱신거리는 느낌
cha-ga-un bal / pal, dari, son, ba-ri uk-sin-geo-ri-neun neu-kkim

RU похолодание стоп / покалывание в руках, ногах, кистях и стопах
pokholodanie stop / pokalyvanie v rukakh, nogakh, kistyakh i stopakh

PL zimne stopy / uczucie mrowienia w rękach, nogach, dłoniach, stopach

AR شعور البرد في القدمين \ أحساس التوخز في الأذرع او الرجلين او اليدين او القدمين
Shu"oor al-bard fil-qadamayn / ahsaas at-tawakkhuz fil-adhru" au ar-rijleyn au al-yaddeyn au alqadameyn

PT pés frios / sensação de formigueiro nos braços, nas pernas, nas mãos e nos pés

FK pye w fret / pikotman nan bra, janb, men, pye

EL κρύα πόδια / αίσθημα μυρμηκίασης στα άνω άκρα, κάτω άκρα, χέρια, πόδια
krEEa pOdeea / Estheema meermeekEEasees sta Ano Akra, kAto Akra, hEreea, pOdeea

HI ठंडे पैर / हाथ, पैर, पंजों और उंगलियों में सूनापन
Thande pair / haath, pair, panjon aur ungaliyon mein soonapan

swollen joints / stiff joints

ES articulaciones hinchadas / rígidas

ZH 关节肿胀 / 僵硬
guān jié zhǒng zhàng / jiāng yìng

FR articulations gonflées / articulations raides

DE geschwollene Gelenke / steife Gelenke

VI sưng khớp / cứng khớp

IT articolazioni gonfie / articolazioni rigide

KO 부은 관절 / 뻐근한 관절
bu-eun gwan-jeol / ppeo-geun-han gwan-jeol

RU опухшие суставы / тугоподвижные суставы
opukhshie sustavy / tugopodvizhnye sustavy

PL obrzęk stawów / sztywność w stawach

AR مفاصل متنفخة \ مفاصل صلبة
Mafaasil muntafikhah / mafaasil sulbah

PT articulações inchadas / articulações rígidas

FK jwenti anfle / jwenti ki rèd

EL πρησμένες αρθρώσεις / άκαμπτες αρθρώσεις
preesmEnes arthrOsees / Akamptes arthrOsees

HI जोड़ों में सूजन / सख्त जोड़
Jaudon mein soojan / sakth jod

Do you have calf pain? Always? When moving?

ES ¿Le duelen las pantorrillas? ¿Siempre? ¿Cuándo se mueve?

ZH 感觉小腿肚痛么？一直痛？走路时痛？
gǎn jué xiǎo tuǐ dù tòng ma? yì zhí tong? zǒu lù shí tong?

FR Avez-vous mal dans le mollet? Toujours? En marchant?

DE Haben Sie Wadenschmerzen? Immer? Nach Bewegung?

VI Quý vị có bị đau bắp chân không? Lúc nào cũng đau? Khi di chuyển?

IT Ha dolori ai polpacci? Sempre? Quando si muove?

KO 종아리가 아프십니까? 항상 그렇습니까? 움직일 때 아프십니까?
Jong-a-ri-ga a-peu-sim-ni-kka? Hang-sang geu-reo-sseum-ni-kka? Um-ji-gil ttae a-peu-sim-ni-kka?

RU У вас болит задняя часть голени? Всегда? При движении?
U vas bolit zadnyaya chast' goleni? Vsegda? Pri dvizhenii?

PL Czy bolą Pana(Panią) łydki? Stale? Gdy jest Pan(i) w ruchu?

AR هل عندك ألم في بطن الساق؟ دائماً؟ عند التحرك؟
Hal "indak alam fi batn as-saaq? Daa'iman? "Ind at-taharruk?

PT Tem dores na barriga da perna? Sempre? Quando se movimenta?

FK Eske ou gen doulè nan jaret ou? Pandan ou ap fè movman?

EL Έχετε πόνο στη γαστροκνημία; Πάντα; Όταν κινείστε;
Ehete pOno stee gastrokneemEEa? pAnda? Otan keenEEste?

HI क्या आपको पिंडलियों में दर्द होता है ? हमेशा ? चलते समय ?
Kya aapko pindliyon mein dard hota hai? Hamesha? Chalte samay?

How far can you walk until you start to have pain? ... meters

S ¿Qué tanto puede caminar antes de que le duela? ... metros

H 在你感觉痛之前，能走多远？... 多少米？
zài nǐ gǎn jué tòng zhī qián, néng zǒu duō yuǎn? ... duō shǎo mǐ?

R Sur quelle distance savez-vous marcher jusqu'à ce que la douleur revienne? ... mètres

E Wie weit können Sie gehen bis Sie Schmerzen haben? ... Meter

VI Quý vị có thể đi được bao xa kể từ khi quý vị bắt đầu bị đau? ... mét

T Quanto riesce a camminare prima di iniziare a sentire dolore? ... metri

O 어느 정도 걸어야 아프기 시작합니까? ... 미터
Eo-neu jeong-do geo-reo-ya a-peu-gi si-jak-ham-ni-kka? ... mi-teo

U Сколько вы можете пройти до того, как начнете испытывать боль? ... метров
Skol'ko vy mozhete proyti do togo, kak nachnete ispytyvat' bol'? ... metrov

L Jak długo jest Pan(i) w stanie chodzić zanim odczuje Pan(i) ból? ... metrów

R كم مسافة تستطيع \ تستطيعين مشيها حتى تبدأ الشعور بالألم؟ ... متراً
Kam masaafah tastatee' / tastatee"een mashyihaa hattaa tabda' ash-shu"oor bil-'alam? ... mitran?

T Que distância percorre até começar a sentir dor? ... metros

K Ki distans ke ou ka mache avan ou komanse gen doulè ? ... . Mèt

L Πόσο μακριά μπορείτε να περπατήσετε έως ότου αρχίσετε να έχετε πόνο; ... μέτρα
pOso makreeA borEEte na permatEEsete Eos Otu arhEEsete na Ehete pOno? ... mEtra

NI आपको कितना दूर चलने के बाद दर्द होता है ? ... मीटर
Aapko kitna door chalne ke baad dard hota hai? ... meters

Can you move your feet / toes / legs / hands / fingers / arms?

ES ¿Mueve bien los pies / dedos del pie / las piernas / manos / los dedos / brazos?

ZH 你能活动你的脚 / 脚趾 / 腿 / 手 / 手指 / 胳膊么？
nǐ néng huó dòng nǐ de jiǎo / jiǎo zhǐ / tuǐ / shǒu / shǒu zhǐ / gē bó me?

FR Savez-vous bouger les pieds / les orteils / les jambes / les mains / les doigts / les bras?

DE Können Sie die Füße / Zehen / Beine / Hände / Finger / Arme bewegen?

VI Quý vị có thể cử động bàn chân / ngón chân / chân / ngón tay / tay không?

IT Riesce a muovere piedi / dita dei piedi / gambe / mani / dita / braccia?

KO 발 / 발가락 / 다리 / 손 / 손가락 / 팔을 움직일 수 있으십니까?
Bal / bal-ga-rak / da-ri / son / son-ga-rak / pa-reul um-ji-gil su i-seu-sim-ni-kka?

RU Вы можете двигать стопами / пальцами ног / ногами / кистями / пальцами рук / руками?
Vy mozhete dvigat' stopami / pal'tsami nog / nogami / kistyami / pal'tsami ruk / rukami?

PL Czy jest Pan(i) w stanie poruszać stopami / palcami u nóg / nogami / dłońmi / palcami u rąk / rękami?

AR هل تستطيع \ تستطيعين أن تحرك \ تحركي قدميك \ قدميك \ أطراف قدميك \ رجليك \ يديك \ أصابعك \ راعيك؟

Hal tastatee" / tastatee"een an tuharrik / tuharrikee qadamayk / atraaf qadamayk / rijleyk / yaddayk / asaabi"ak / dhiraa"ayk?

PT Pode movimentar os seus pés / dedos dos pés / pernas / mãos / dedos / braços?

FK Eske ou ka bouje pye w / zotey yo / men w yo / dwet yo / bra w?

EL Μπορείτε να κουνήσετε τα πόδια / δάχτυλα ποδιών / κάτω άκρα / χέρια / δάχτυλα χεριών / άνω άκρα σας;
borEEte na kunEEsete ta pOdeea / dAhteela podeeOn / kAto Akra / hEEreea / dAhteela hereeOn / Ano Akra sas?

HI क्या आप अपने पैर की उंगलियाँ / पैर के अंगूठे / पैर / पंजे / उंगलि याँ / हाथ चला सकते हैं ?
Kya aap apne pair ki ungliyaan / pair ke angoothe / pair / panje / ungliyaan / haath chalaa sakte hain?

5 Neurology, Psychiatry

Have you noticed any of the following changes on yourself?

S ¿Ha notado alguno de estos cambios en su salud?

H 你有没有发现自己有以下的变化？
nǐ yǒu méi yǒu fā xiàn zì jǐ yǒu yǐ xià de biàn huà?

R Avez-vous noté l'un des changements suivants sur vous-mêmes?

DE Haben Sie folgende Veränderungen bei sich bemerkt?

VI Quý vị có nhận thấy thay đổi nào sau đây trong người không?

T Ha mai notato qualcuno dei seguenti cambiamenti in Lei?

KO 다음의 변화 중 본인한테 일어났다고 생각하는 것이 있습니까?
Da-eu-mui byeon-hwa jung bo-nin-han-te i-reo-nat-da-go saeng-gak-ha-neun geo-si it-seum-ni-kka?

RU Заметили ли вы у себя следующие изменения?
Zametili li vy u sebya sleduyushchie izmeneniya?

L Czy zauważył Pan(i) u siebie następujące zmiany?

AR هل لاحظت أية من التغييرات التالية على نفسك؟
Hal laahadht ayyi min at-taghyeeraat at-taaliyah "alaa nafsak?

PT Notou, em si, algumas das seguintes alterações?

EK Eske ou wè ninpòt nan chanjman swivan ou nan ou menm?

EL Παρατηρήσατε οποιεσδήποτε από τις ακόλουθες αλλαγές στον εαυτό σας;
parateerEEsate opee-esdEEpote apO tees akOluthes alagEs ston eaftO sas?

HI क्या आपने स्वयं में निम्नलिखित में से कोई बदलाव नोट किया? ...
Kya aapne swayam mein nimnlikhit mein se koi badlaav note kiya?

dizziness / disturbances of balance / seizures

ES mareos / trastornos del equilibrio / convulsiones

ZH 眩晕 / 站立不稳 / 抽搐
xuàn yūn / zhàn lì bù wěn / chōu chù

FR vertiges, étourdissements / troubles de l'équilibre / attaque d'apoplexie

DE Schwindel / Gleichgewichtsstörungen / Krampfanfälle

VI chóng mặt / rối loạn thăng bằng / những cơn co giật

IT capogiri / disturbi dell'equilibrio / convulsioni

KO 현기증 / 균형 감각 장애 / 간질 발작
hyeon-gi-jeung / gyun-hyeong gam-gak jang-ae / gan-jil bal-jak

RU головокружение / нарушения равновесия / припадки
golovokruzhenie / narusheniya ravnovesiya / pripadki

PL zawroty głowy / zaburzenia równowagi / drgawki

AR الدوخة / الإضطرابات فى التوازن / النوبات الفجائية
Ad-doukhah / al-idhtiraabaat fit-tawaazun / an-nowbaat al-fajaa'iyyah

PT tonturas / perturbações do equilibrio / crises ou ataques

FK vetij / chanjman nan balans ou / kriz

EL ζάλη / διαταραχές ισορροπίας / σπασμοι
zAlee / deeatarahEs eesoropEEas / spasmEE

HI चक्कर आना / संतुलन बिगड़ना / दौरे पड़ना ...
chakkar aana / santulan bigaDna / daure paDna

weakness / paralysis / muscle wasting / involuntary movements

ES debilidad / parálisis / pérdida de músculo / movimientos involuntarios

ZH 虚弱 / 麻痹 / 肌肉萎缩 / 不自主的动
xū ruò / má bì / jī ròu wěi suō / bù zì zhǔ de dòng

FR faiblesse / paralysie / atrophie musculaire / mouvements involontaires

DE Schwächen / Lähmungen / Muskelschwund / unwillkürliche Bewegungen

VI suy nhược / liệt / teo cơ / cử động ngoại ý

IT debolezza / paralisi / indebolimento muscolare / movimenti involontari

KO 힘이 없음 / 마비 / 근육이 없어지는 것 / 불수의 운동
Hi-mi eop-seum / ma-bi / geun-yu-gi eop-seo-ji-neun geot / bul-su-ui un-dong

RU слабость / паралич / атрофия мышц / непроизвольные движения
slabost' / paralich / atrofiya myshts / neproizvol'nye dvizheniya

PL osłabienie / paraliż / utrata mięśni / odruchy niezamierzone

AR الضعف / الشلل / تهدر العضلات / حركات جسمية غير إرادية
Adh-dha"f / ash-shalal / tahaddur al-"adhalaat / harakaat jismiyyah ghayr iraadiyyah

PT fraqueza / paralisia / definhamento muscular / movimentos involuntários

FK febles / paralyze / misk kap pedi fos yo / movman ou paka kontwole

EL αδυναμία / παράλυση / εξασθένιση μυών / ακούσιες κινήσεις
adeenamEEa / parAleesee / exasthEneesee meeOn / akUsee-es keenEEsees

HI कमजोरी / लकवा / मांसपेशी ह्रास / अनैच्छिक हरकतें ...
kamzori / lakva / maanspeshi hraash / anaiChik harkatein

pain / disturbances of sensation / shivering / insecure gait

ES dolor / trastornos de la sensibilidad / temblores / marcha inestable

ZH 痛 / 感觉异常 / 颤抖 / 走路不稳
tòng / gǎn jué yì cháng / chàn dǒu / zǒu lù bù wěn

FR douleur / troubles des sensations / tremblement / démarche incertaine

DE Schmerzen / Empfindungsstörungen / Zittern / Gangunsicherheit

VI đau / rối loạn cảm giác / run rẩy / đi không vững

IT dolore / disturbi delle sensazioni / tremori / andatura incerta

KO 통증 / 감각 장애 / 떨림 / 불안정한 걸음
tong-jeung / gam-gak jang-ae / tteol-lim / bu-ran-jeong-han geo-reum

RU боль / нарушение чувствительности / дрожь / шаткая походка
bol' / narushenie chuvstvitel'nosti / drozh' / shatkaya pokhodka

PL ból / zaburzenia czucia / dreszcze / niepewny chód

AR الألم / إضطرابات في الإحساس / الرعشات / عدم الإستواء في المشي
Al-alam / idhtiraabaat fil-ihsaas / ar-ra"shaat / "adam al-istiwaa' fil-mashiy

PT dor / perturbações da sensação / calafrios / marcha insegura

FK doulè / chanjman nan sensasyon / la tranblad / ensekirite demach ou

EL πόνος / διαταραχές αίσθησης / ρίγος / ασταθής βηματισμός
pOnos / deeatarahEs Estheesees / reegos / astathEEs veemateesmOs

HI दर्द / संवेदना में परेशानी / कंपकंपी / असुरक्षित चाल...
dard / samvedna mein pareshani / kampkampi / A-surakshit chaal

disturbances of coordination / head aches / memory problems

S problemas de coordinación / dolores de cabeza / problemas de memoria

H 动作不协调 / 头痛 / 记忆力不好
dòng zuò bù xié tiáo / tóu tòng / jì yì lì bù hǎo

FR troubles de la coordination / maux de tête / problèmes de mémoire

DE Koordinationsstörungen / Kopfschmerz / Gedächtnisstörung

VI rối loạn về phối hợp vận động / đau đầu / các vấn đề về trí nhớ

IT disturbi di coordinazione / mal di testa / problemi di memoria

KO 운동 능력 부조화 / 두통 / 기억력 문제
Un-dong neung-nyeok bu-jo-hwa / du-tong / gi-eong-nyeok munje

RU нарушения координации / головные боли / нарушение памяти
narusheniya koordinatsii / golovnye boli / narushenie pamyati

PL zaburzenia koordynacji / bóle głowy / kłopoty z pamięcią

AR اضطرابات في التنسيق / صداعات / مشاكل في الذاكرة
Idhtiraabaat fit-tansiiq / sudaa"aat / mashaakil fidh-dhaakirah

PT perturbações da coordenação / dores de cabeça / problemas da memória

FK chanjman koordinasyon / mal tèt / pwoblèm memwa

EL διαταραχές συντονισμού / κεφαλαλγίες / προβλήματα μνήμης
deeatarahEs seedoneesmU / kefalalgEEes / provlEEmata mnEEmees

HI तालमेल में परेशानी / सिर में दर्द / याददाश्त में कमी ...
talmail mein pareshani / sir mein dard / yaddaSht mein kami

concentration problems / problems when reading / writing / speaking

ES problemas de concentración / problemas para leer / escribir / hablar

ZH 注意力不集中 / 读书报有困难 / 书写困难 / 说话困难
zhù yì lì bù jí zhōng / dú shū bào yǒu kùn nán / shū xiě kùn nán / shuō huà kùn nán

FR problèmes de concentration / problèmes de lecture / d'écriture / de parole

DE Konzentrationsstörung / Probleme beim Lesen / Schreiben / Sprechen

VI các vấn đề về tập trung chú ý / các vấn đề khi đọc / viết / nói

IT problemi di concentrazione / problemi quando legge / scrive / parla

KO 정신 집중 문제 / 읽기 / 쓰기 / 말하기 문제
jeong-sin jip-jung mun-je / ik-gi / sseu-gi / mal-ha-gi mun-je

RU нарушения концентрации / проблемы, связанные с чтением / письмом / речью
narusheniya kontsentratsii / problemy, svyazannye s chteniem / pis'mom / rech'yu

PL kłopoty z koncentracją / problemy z czytaniem / pisaniem / mówieniem

AR مشاكل في التركيز / صعوبات في القراءة او الكتابة او الحديث
Mashaakil fit-tarkiiz / su"oobat fil-qaraa'ah au al-kitaabah au al-hadith

PT problemas de concentração / problemas da leitura / da escrita / da fala

FK pwoblèm konsentrasyon / pwoblè lè ou ap li / ekri / pale

EL προβλήματα στη συγκέντρωση / προβλήματα κατά την ανάγνωση / γραφή / ομιλία
provlEEmata stee seegEntrosee / provlEEmata katA teen anAgnosee / grafEE / omeelEEa

HI एकाग्रता में परेशानी / पढ़ते / लिखते / बोलते समय परेशानी
ekagrata mein pareshani / paDhte / likhte / bolte samay pareshani

Are you experiencing / have you experienced disturbances of sensory perception? Specify

ES ¿Tiene / ha tenido trastornos de la percepción sensorial? Especifique

ZH 你是不是有／或以前有过感觉异常？具体是什么？
nǐ shì bù shì yǒu / huò yǐ qián yǒu guò gǎn jué yì cháng? jù tǐ shì shén me?

FR Avez-vous / avez-vous eu des troubles de la perception sensorielle? spécifiez

DE Sind / waren Ihre Sinneswahrnehmungen gestört? wo?

VI Quý vị có đang / đã gặp phải tình trạng rối loạn nhận thức giác quan không? Trình bày rõ

IT Ha / ha avuto disturbi delle percezioni sensoriali? Specificare

KO 감각 능력 장애를 현재 경험하시고 있거나 경험하신 적이 있습니까? 구체적으로 명시하십시오.
Gam-gak neung-nyeok jang-ae-reul hyeon-jae gyeong-heom-ha-si-go it-geo-na gyeong-gheom-ha-sin jeo-gi it-seum-ni-kka? Gu-che-jeo-geu-ro myeung-si-ha-sip-si-o

RU У вас есть / когда-нибудь были нарушения чувственного восприятия? Уточните
U vas est' / kogda-nibud' byli narusheniya chuvstvennogo vospriyatiya? Utochnite

PL Czy doznaje Pan(i) zaburzeń w odbiorze wrażeń? Proszę to bliżej opisać

AR هل تواجهك / واجهتك إضطرابات حسّية؟ بيّن بالتفصيل
Hal tuwaajihak / waajahatak idhtiraabaat hissiyyah? bayyin (male) / bayyinee (female) bit-tafseel

PT Sente / já sentiu algumas perturbações da percepção sensorial? Especifique

FK Eske ou remake / te remake yon chanjman nan persepsyon sensasyon ou? Spesifye

EL Έχετε / Είχατε διαταραχές της αισθητήριας αντίληψης; Καθορίστε
Ehete / EEhate deeatarahEs tees estheetEEreeas adEEleepsees? kathorEEste

HI क्या आप संवेदना अनुभूति में परेशानी अनुभव कर रहे हैं/थे? .... स्पष्ट करें
Kya aap sanvedna anubhuti mein pareshani anubhav kar rahein hain / The? spaSt karein

numbness / tingling

ES entumecimiento / hormigueo

ZH 麻木感 / 刺痛感
má mù gǎn / cì tòng gǎn

FR engourdissement / picotements

DE Gefühllosigkeit / Kribbeln

VI tê cứng / ngứa ran

IT intorpidimento / formicolio

KO 저림 / 욱신거림
jeo-rim / uk-sin-geo-rim

RU онемение / покалывание
onemenie / pokalyvanie

PL drętwienie / cierpnięcie

AR التخدر \ التوخز
At-takhaddur / at-tawakhkhuz

PT Adormecimento / formigueiro

FK pèt sensasypikotman

EL μούδιασμα / μυρμηκίαση
mUdeeasma / meermeekEEasee

HI अचेतना / झनझनाहट
achetna / jhanjhanaahat

When did the symptoms first appear?

¿Cuándo empezó a tener esos síntomas?

这些症状最早出现是什么时候？
zhè xie zhèng zhuàng zuì zǎo chū xiàn shì shén me shí hòu?

Quand ces symptômes sont-ils apparus pour la première fois?

Wann haben die Symptome begonnen?

Các triệu cứng này bắt đầu xuất hiện từ khi nào?

Quando sono apparsi i primi sintomi?

언제 증상이 처음 나타났습니까?
Eon-je jeung-sang-i cheo-eum na-ta-nat-seum-ni-kka?

Когда эти симптомы впервые появились?
Kogda eti simptomy vpervye poyavilis'?

Kiedy pojawiły się te objawy?

متى ظهرت هذه الأعراض لأول مرة؟
Mattaa dhaharat hadhihil-aa"raadh li'awwal marrah?

Quando é que os sintomas apareceram pela primeira vez?

Ki lè sintòm sa yo parèt pou premye fwa?

Πότε παρουσιάστηκαν τα συμπτώματα για πρώτη φορά;
pOte paruseeAsteekan ta seemptOmata geea prOtee forA?

पहली बार लक्षण कब प्रकट हुए थे?
Pehli baar lakshaN kab prakat hue the?

hours / days / weeks / years ago

ES	hace horas / días / semanas / años
ZH	几小时前 / 几天前 / 几周前 / 几年前 jǐ xiǎo shí qián / jǐ tiān qián / jǐ zhōu qián / jǐ nián qián
FR	il y a des heures / jours / semaines / années
DE	vor Stunden / Tagen / Wochen / Jahren
VI	giờ / ngày / tuần / năm trước đây
IT	ore / giorni / settimane / anni fa
KO	시간 / 일 / 주 / 년 / 전 si-gan / il / ju / nyeon / jeon
RU	часов / дней / недель / лет тому назад chasov / dney / nedel' / let tomu nazad
PL	godzin / dni / tygodni / lat temu
AR	ساعات \ أيام \ أسابيع \ قبل سنوات Sa"aat / ayyaam / asaabee" / qabl sanawaat
PT	Há horas / dias / semanas / anos
FK	hètan / jou / semen / plizye ane
EL	ώρες / ημέρες / εβδομάδες / χρόνια πριν Ores / eemEres / evdomAdes / hrOneea preen
HI	घंटे / दिन / हफ्ते / वर्ष पहले ghante / din / hafte / varS pehle

Are you forgetful?

¿Se le olvidan las cosas?

你健忘吗？
nǐ jiàn wàng ma?

Etes-vous oublieux?

Können Sie sich an alles erinnern?

Quý vị có mắc chứng hay quên không?

Si distrae facilmente?

기억력이 없으십니까?
Gi-eong-nyeo-gi eop-seu-sim-ni-kka?

Вы забывчивы?
Vy zabyvchivy?

Czy ma Pan(i) tendencję do zapominania?

هل أنت كثير \ كثيرة النسيان؟
Hal inta katheer (male) / inti katheerah (female) an-nisyaan?

Está esquecido?

Eske ou distre / kon bliye?

Ξεχνάτε;
xehnAte?

क्या आप भुलक्कड़ हैं?
Kya aap bhulakkaD hain?

What day / month is today? Please write down

ES ¿En qué día / mes estamos? Anótelo, por favor

ZH 今天是几月几日？请写下来
jīn tiān shì jǐ yuè jǐ rì? qǐng xiě xia lai

FR Quel jour de quel mois, sommes-nous, aujourd'hui? S'il vous plaît, écrivez

DE Welcher Tag / Monat ist heute? Bitte aufschreiben

VI Hôm nay là ngày bao nhiêu / tháng mấy? Xin viết ra

IT Che giorno / mese è oggi? Lo scriva, per favore

KO 오늘은 무슨 요일 / 몇 월 달 입니까? 써 주십시오
O-neu-reun mu-seun yo-il / myeot wol dal im-ni-kka? Sseo Ju-sip-si-o

RU Какой сегодня день / месяц? Пожалуйста, напишите
Kakoy segodnya den' / mesyats? Pozhaluysta, napishite

PL Jaki jest dzisiaj dzień / miesiąc? Proszę to zapisać

AR ما هو اليوم \ الشهر الحالي؟ الرجاء إكتبه \ اكتبه
Ma huwa al-youm? Ash-shahr al-haali? Ar-rajaa' uktubhu / uktubeeh

PT Que dia / mês do ano é hoje? Responda por escrito, por favor

FK Ki jou / mwa ke li ye jodya? Tanpri ekri l

EL Τι ημέρα / μήνας είναι σήμερα; Παρακαλώ γράψτε το
tee eemEra / mEEnas EEne sEEmera? parakalO grApste to

HI आज कौन–सा दिन / महीना है? कृपया नीचे लिखें
Aaj kaun-sa din / mahina hai? Kripya niche likhein

Do you know where you presently are? In the hospital / doctors office

¿Me puede decir dónde estamos ahora? En el hospital / consultorio

你知道自己现在在在哪里吗？在医院 / 医生办公室
nǐ zhī dao zì jǐ xiàn zài zài nǎ li ma? zài yī yuàn / yī shēng bàn gōng shì

Savez-vous où nous sommes, en ce moment? À l'hôpital / dans le bureau d'un médecin

Wissen Sie, wo Sie sind? Sie sind in der Klinik / Arztpraxis

Quý vị có biết mình hiện đang ở đâu không? Trong bệnh viện / phòng mạch bác sĩ

Sa dove si trova ora? In ospedale / in uno studio medico

지금 어디에 계시는 지 아십니까? 병원에 / 의사 사무실에
Ji-geum eo-di-e gye-si-neun ji a-sim-ni-kka? Byeong-won-e / ui-sa sa-mu-si-re

Вы знаете, где вы сейчас находитесь? В больнице / кабинете у врача
Vy znaete, gde vy seychas nakhodites'? V bol'nitse / kabinete u vracha

Czy wie Pan(i) gdzie się Pan(i) obecnie znajduje? W szpitalu / gabinecie lekarskim

هل تعرف \ تعرفين مكان تواجدك في الوقت الحاضر؟ في المستشفى \ عند مكتب الطبيب
Hal ta"rif / ta"rifeen / makaan tawaajudak fil-waqt il-haadhir? Fil-mustashfaa / "ind maktab at-tabeeb

Sabe onde se encontra presentemente? No hospital / consultório médico

Eske ou kon kote ou ye kounye la? Nan lopital / klinik doktè a

Γνωρίζετε πού είστε τώρα; Σε νοσοκομείο / ιατρείο
grorEEzete pU EEste tOra? se nosokomEEo / eeatrEEo

क्या आप जानते हैं कि आप अभी कहां हैं? अस्पताल / डॉक्टर के कार्यालय में
Kya aap jaante hain ki aap abhi kahan hain? Aspataal / Doctor ke karyaalay mein

Do you feel ill? Did you vomit?

ES ¿Se ha sentido enfermo? ¿Ha vomitado?

ZH 你觉得有病吗？有没有想吐？
nǐ jué de yǒu bìng ma? yǒu méi yǒu xiǎng tù?

FR Vous sentez-vous malade? Avez-vous vomi?

DE Fühlen Sie sich krank? Haben Sie erbrochen?

VI Quý vị có cảm thấy đau yếu không? Quý vị có bị ói mửa không?

IT Si sente male? Ha vomitato?

KO 아프십니까? 토하셨습니까?
A-peu-sim-ni-kka? To-ha-syeot-seum-ni-kka?

RU Вы чувствуете себя больным? У вас была рвота?
Vy chuvstvuete sebya bol'nym? U vas byla rvota?

PL Czy czuje się Pan(i) chory(a)? Czy Pan(i) wymiotował(a)?

AR هل تشعر\ تشعرين بالمرض؟ هل تقيّأت؟
Hal tish"ur / tish"ureen bil-maradh? Hal taqayya't?

PT Sente-se doente? Vomitou?

FK Eske ou santi w malad? Eske ou vomi ?

EL Νιώθετε άρρωστοι; Κάνατε εμετό;
neeOthete Arostee? kAnate emetO?

HI क्या आप बीमार महसूस कर रहे हैं? क्या आपने उल्टी की थी?
Kya aap bimar mehsoos kar rahe hain? kya apne ulti ki thi?

Do you have diabetes / high blood pressure / epilepsy / seizures?

¿Tiene diabetes / hipertensión / epilepsia / convulsiones?

你有没有糖尿病 / 高血压 / 颠痫 / 抽搐？
nǐ yǒu méi yǒu táng niào bìng / gāo xuè yā / diān xián / chōu chù?

Avez-vous du diabète / une pression sanguine élevée / de l'épilepsie / une attaque d'apoplexie

Haben Sie Diabetes / Bluthochdruck / Epilepsie / Krampfanfälle?

Quý vị có bị bệnh tiểu đường / huyết áp cao / chứng động kinh / co thắt không?

Soffre di diabete / pressione alta / epilessia / convulsioni?

당뇨병 / 고혈압 / 간질 / 간질 발작이 있으십니까?
Dang-nyo-byeong / go-hyeo-rap / gan-jil / gan-jil bal-ja-gi i-seu-sim-ni-kka?

У вас есть диабет / повышенное кровяное давление / эпилепсия / припадки?
U vas est' diabet / povyshennoe krovyanoe davlenie / epilepsiya / pripadki?

Czy ma Pan(i) cukrzycę / nadciśnienie / padaczkę / drgawki?

هل تعاني \ تعانين من مرض السكّر \ ضغط دمّ عالٍ \ مرض الصرع \ النوبات الفجائية؟
Hal tu"aani / tu"aaneen min maradh as-sukkar / dhaght damm "aali / maradh as-sar"a / an-noubaat al-fajaa'iyah?

Sofre de diabetes / tensão arterial alta / epilepsia / crises ou ataques?

Eske ou fè / gen sik / tansyon / epilepsy / kriz?

Έχετε διαβήτη / υψηλή αρτηριακή πίεση / επιληψία / σπασμούς;
Ehete deeaVEEtee / eepseeIEE arteereeakEE pEEsee / epeeleepsEEa / spasmUs?

क्या आपको म ६ ुमेह / उच्च रक्तचाप / मिरगी / दौरे पड़ने की बीमारी है?
Kya aapko madhumeh / uchch raktchaap / mirgi / daure paDne ki bimari hai?

When did you experience your last seizure? Days / weeks / months / years ago

ES ¿Cuándo tuvo convulsiones por última vez? Hace días / semanas / meses / años

ZH 你最近一次抽搐时什么时候？几天前 / 几周前 / 几月前 / 几年前
nǐ zuì jìn yī cì chōu chù shí shén me shí hòu? jǐ tiān qiá / n jǐ zhōu qián / jǐ yuè qián / jī nián qián

FR Quand avez-vous présenté votre dernière attaque d'apoplexie? Il y a des jours / semaines / mois / années

DE Wann war der letzte Krampfanfall? Tage / Wochen / Monate / Jahre

VI Lần gần đây nhất quý vị bị tai biến mạch máu não là khi nào? Ngày / tuần / tháng / năm trước đây

IT Quando ha avuto l'ultimo attacco? Giorni / settimane / mesi / anni fa

KO 마지막으로 언제 간질 발작이 있었습니까? 일 / 주 / 달 / 년 전
Ma-ji-ma-geu-ro eon-je gan-jil bal-ja-gi i-seot-seum-ni-kka? Il / ju / dal / nyeon jeor

RU Когда у вас был последний припадок? Дней / недель / месяцев / лет тому назад
Kogda u vas byl posledniy pripadok? Dney / nedel' / mesyatsev / let tomu nazad

PL Kiedy miał miejsce ostatni atak padaczki? Dni / tygodni / miesięcy / lat temu

AR متى اصبت بنوبتك الفجائية الأخيرة؟ أيام \ أسابيع \ شهور \ قبل سنوات
Mattaa usibt bi-noubatak al-fajaa'iyah al-akhiirah? Ayyam / asaabee" / shuhoor / qabl sanawaat

PT Quando é que teve o seu último ataque? Há dias / semanas / meses / anos

FK Ki denye fwa ou te gen yon kriz? Jou / semen / mwa / plize ane

EL Πότε πάθατε τον τελευταίο σπασμό σας; Ημέρες / εβδομάδες / μήνες / χρόνια πριν
pOte pAthate ton telefteo spasmO sas? eemEres / evdomAdes / mEEnes / hrOneea preen

HI आपको अंतिम बार दौरा कब पड़ा था? दिन / हफ्ते / महीने / वर्ष पहले
aapko antim baar daura kab paDa tha? Din / Hafte / Mahine / VarS pehle

Did you lose consciousness?

¿Perdió el conocimiento?

当时失去知觉了吗？
dāng shí shī qù zhī jué le ma?

Avez-vous perdu connaissance?

Haben Sie das Bewusstsein verloren?

Quý vị có bị bất tỉnh không?

Ha perso conoscenza?

의식을 잃으셨습니까？
Ui-si-geul i-reu-syeot-seum-ni-kka?

Вы теряли сознание?
Vy teryali soznanie?

Czy stracił(a) Pan(i) przytomność?

هل فقدت / فقدتِ وعيك؟
Hal faqadta / faqadti wa"iyak?

Perdeu os sentidos?

Eske ou te pedi konesans?

Χάσατε τις αισθήσεις σας;
hAsate tees esthEEsees sas?

क्या आपने होश खोया था?
Kya aapne hosh khoya tha?

Did you experience loss of control over urination / defecation (urinary and fecal incontinence)?

ES ¿Perdió el control de la orina / intestinos (incontinencia urinaria y fecal)?

ZH 以前有没有过小便 / 大便失禁?
yǐ qián yǒu méi yǒu guò xiǎo biàn / dà biàn shī jìn?

FR Avez-vous perdu le contrôle de la miction / défécation (incontinence urinaire et fécale)?

DE Haben Sie Urin / die Darmkontrolle verloren?

VI Quý vị có gặp tình trạng không kiểm soát được tiểu tiện / đại tiện (không kiểm chế được việc tiểu tiện và đại tiện) không?

IT Ha perso il controllo dell'urina / delle feci (incontinenza urinaria e fecale)?

KO 대소변을 못가리는 경험을 하셨습니까 (대소변 실금)?
Dae-so-byeo-neul mot-ga-ri-neun gyeong-heo-meul ha-syeot-seum-ni-kka (dae so-byeon sil-geum)?

RU Теряли ли вы когда-нибудь контроль над мочеиспусканием и испражнение (недержание мочи и кала)?
Teryali li vy kogda-nibud' kontrol' nad mocheispuskaniem i isprazhneniem (nederzhanie mochi i kala)?

PL Czy doznał(a) Pan(i) kiedykolwiek utraty kontroli nad oddawaniem moczu / kału (nietrzymania moczu / kału)?

AR هل واجهتك فقدان السيطرة على التبوّل \ التغوّط (السلس التبولي والبرازي)؟
Hal waajahatak fuqdaan as-saytara "alaat-tabawwul / at-taghawwut (as-salis it-tabawwuliy wal-baraaziy)?

PT Perdeu o controlo sobre a micção / evacuação (incontinência urinária e fecal)?

FK Eske ou pedi kontwol pipi w / watè (paka kanbe pipi oswa wate w)?

EL Είχατε απώλεια του ελέγχου της ούρησης / αφόδευσης (ακράτεια ούρων και κοπράνων)?
EEhate apOleea tu elEnhu tees Ureesees / afOdefsees (akrAteia Uron ke koprAnon)?

HI क्या आपने मूत्र / मल अनियंत्रित होना (मूत्र और मल असंयमता) अनुभव किया?
Kya aapne mutra / mal aniyantrit hona (mutra aur mal Asanyamta) anubhav kiya?

For how long did you lose consciousness? Seconds / minutes

S ¿Cuánto tiempo estuvo inconsciente? Segundos / minutos

H 当时失去知觉多长时间？ 几秒钟 / 几分钟
dāng shí shī qù zhī jué duō cháng shí jiān? jǐ miǎo zhōng / jǐ fēn zhōng

R Pendant combien de temps avez-vous perdu connaissance? Secondes / minutes

E Wie lange waren Sie bewusstlos? Sekunden / Minuten

VI Quý vị đã bất tỉnh trong bao lâu? Giây / phút

T Per quanto tempo ha perso conoscenza? Secondi / minuti

O 얼마 동안 의식을 잃으셨습니까? 초 / 분
Eol-ma dong-an ui-si-geul i-reu-syeot-seum-ni-kka? cho / bun

U Как долго вы были без сознания? Секунды / минуты
Kak dolgo vy byli bez soznaniya? Sekundy / minuty

L Na jak długo stracił(a) Pan(i) przytomność? sekund / minut

R لكم مدة فقدت وعيك؟ ثواني \ دقائق
Li-kam muddah faqadt wa"iyak? Thawaani / Daqaa'iq

T Durante quanto tempo perdeu os sentidos? Segundos / minutos

K Pandan konbyen tan ou te pedi konesans? Segond / minit

EL Για πόση ώρα χάσατε τις αισθήσεις σας; Δευτερόλεπτα / Λεπτά
geea pOsee Ora hAsate tees esthEEsees sas? defterOlepta / leptA

HI आपने कितने समय के लिए होश खोया था? सेकंड /मिनट
Aapne kitne samay ke liye hosh khoya tha? Seconds / minutes

Did you bite your tongue / hurt yourself?

ES ¿Se mordió la lengua / se golpeó o lastimó?

ZH 你当时有没有咬伤舌头 / 弄伤自己？
nǐ dāng shí yǒu méi yǒu yǎo shāng shé tóu / nòng shāng zì jǐ?

FR Avez-vous mordu votre langue? Vous êtes-vous blessé(e)?

DE Haben Sie sich auf die Zunge gebissen / sich verletzt?

VI Quý vị có tự cắn lưỡi / tự làm tổn thương mình không?

IT Si è morso la lingua / si è ferito?

KO 혀를 깨무셨습니까 / 다치셨습니까?
Hyeo-reul kkae-mu-syeot-seum-ni-kka? / da-chi-syeot-seum-ni-kka?

RU Вы прикусили язык / ушиблись?
Vy prikusili yazyk / ushiblis'?

PL Czy przygryzł(a) Pan sobie język / zrobił(a) sobie krzywdę?

AR هل عضضت لسانك ام آذيت نفسك؟
Hal "adhadht lisaanak am aadheyt nafsak"

PT Mordeu a língua / magoou-se?

FK Eske ou mode lang ou / blese tet ou?

EL Δαγκώσατε τη γλώσσα σας / Τραυματιστήκατε;
dagOsate tee glOsa sas / travmateestEEkate?

HI क्या आपने अपनी जीभ काटी / स्वयं को नुकसान पहुंचाया?
Kya aapne apni jeebh kaati / swayam ko nuksaan pahunchaya?

Are you presently taking any medications? Which ones / regularly?

ES ¿Toma actualmente medicamentos? ¿Cuáles / regularmente?

'H 你目前吃什么药吗？哪一种／天天吃吗？
nǐ mù qián chī shén me yào ma? nǎ yī zhǒng / tiān tiān chī ma?

FR Actuellement, prenez-vous des médicaments? Lesquels? régulièrement?

DE Nehmen Sie zur Zeit Medikamente? Welche / regelmäßig?

VI Quý vị hiện có đang dùng loại thuốc nào không? Loại thuốc nào / có thường xuyên không?

IT Al momento attuale sta prendendo farmaci? Quali / regolarmente?

KO 현재 드시는 약이 있습니까? 약 이름이 무엇입니까 / 정기적으로?
Hyeon-jae deu-si-neun ya-gi it-seum-ni-kka? yak i-reu-mi mu-eo-sim-ni-kka / jeong-gi-jeo-geu-ro?

RU Вы сейчас принимаете какие-нибудь лекарства? Какие / регулярно?
Vy seychas prinimaete kakie-nibud' lekarstva? Kakie / regulyarno?

PL Czy przyjmuje Pan(i) obecnie jakiekolwiek leki? Jakie / regularnie?

AR هل تأخذ \ تأخذين آية أدوية في الوقت الحاضر؟ اية أدوية هي؟ \ تأخذها \ تأخذيها بشكل متكرر؟
Hal ta"khudh / ta"khudheen ayy adwiyyah fil-waqt il-haadhir? Ayyi adwiyah hiya? Ta"khudh-haa / ta'khudheehaa bi-shekl mutakarrir?

PT Presentemente, está a tomar alguns medicamentos? Quais são / regularmente?

EK Eske ou ap pran okinn medikan kounye la? Ki les / regilyeman?

EL Λαμβάνετε επί του παρόντος οποιαδήποτε φάρμακα; Ποια / Τακτικά;
lamvAnete epEE tu parOdos opeeadEEpote fArmaka? peeA / takteekA?

HI क्या आप अभी कोई दवा ले रहे हैं? कौन सी／नियमित रूप से?
Kya aap abhi koi dava le rahe hain? kaun si / niyamit roop se?

Has there been a recent change in dosage?

ES	¿Le han cambiado recientemente la dosis?
ZH	最近有没有变更剂量？ zuì jìn yǒu méi yǒu biàn gēng jì liáng?
FR	Y a-t-il eu un changement récent dans le dosage?
DE	Wurde die Dosierung kürzlich verändert?
VI	Gần đây liều lượng thuốc có thay đổi không?
IT	Ha recentemente cambiato il dosaggio?
KO	최근에 약의 정량이 달라졌습니까? Choe-geu-ne ya-gui jeong-nyang-i dal-la-jyeot-seum-ni-kka?
RU	Изменилась ли доза в последнее время? Izmenilas' li doza v posledneye vremya?
PL	Czy zmieniono Panu(Pani) ostatnio dawkę?
AR	هل تم تغيير جرعة دوائك في الوقت الأخير؟ Hal tam taghyeer jur"at dawaa'ak fil-waqt il-akheer?
PT	Tem havido alguma alteração na dosagem?
FK	Eske yo resamman chanje doz la?
EL	Υπήρχε πρόσφατη αλλαγή στη δοσολογία; eepEErhe prOsfatee alagEE stee dosologEEa?
HI	क्या हाल में खुराक में कोई बदलाव हुआ है? Kya haal mein khuraak mein koi badlaav hua hai?

Did you recently suffer a head injury?

ES ¿Sufrió recientemente una lesión en la cabeza?

ZH 你最近有没有头部受伤？
nǐ zuì jìn yǒu méi yǒu tóu bù shòu shāng?

FR Avez-vous souffert récemment d'un traumatisme crânien?

DE Haben Sie sich kürzlich am Kopf verletzt?

VI Gần đây quý vị có bị chấn thương ở đầu không?

IT Ha recentemente avuto una lesione alla testa?

KO 최근에 머리를 다치셨습니까?
Choe-geu-ne meo-ri-reul da-chi-syeot-seum-ni-kka?

RU Была ли у вас недавно травма головы?
Byla li u vas nedavno travma golovy?

PL Czy doznał(a) Pan(i) ostatnio obrażeń głowy?

AR هل اصبت مؤخراً بجرح للرأس؟
Hal usibt mu'akhkharan bi-jarh lir-ra's?

PT Recentemente, sofreu alguma lesão traumática da cabeça?

FK Resamman eske ou andomaje nan tèt?

EL Υποφέρατε πρόσφατα από τραυματισμό κεφαλιού;
eepofErate prOsfata apO travmateesmO kefaleeU?

HI क्या हाल में आपके सिर में कोई चोट लगी?
Kya haal mein aapke sir mein koi chot lagi?

Are you pregnant / a diabetic / an alcoholic?

ES ¿Está usted embarazada / padece diabetes / alcoholismo?

ZH 你有没有怀孕 / 糖尿病 / 酗酒 ？
nǐ yǒu méi yǒu huái yùn / táng niào bìng / xù jiǔ?

FR Etes-vous enceinte / diabétique / alcoolique?

DE Sind Sie schwanger / Diabetiker / Alkoholiker?

VI Quý vị có đang mang thai / mắc bệnh tiểu đường / nghiện rượu không?

IT È incinta / soffre di diabete / alcolismo?

KO 임신 중 / 당뇨 환자 / 알콜 중독자 이십니까?
Im-sin jung / dang-nyo hwan-ja / al-kol jungdok-ja i-sim-ni-kka?

RU Вы беременны / диабетик / алкоголик?
Vy beremenny / diabetik / alkogolik?

PL Czy jest Pani w ciąży / ma cukrzycę / jest alkoholiczką?

AR هل أنت حامل \ مريض \ مريضة بالسكر \ مدمن \ مدمنة خمور؟
Hal inti haamil / maridh / maridhah bis-sukkar / mudmin / mudminat khumoor?

PT Está grávida / é diabético(a) / é alcoólico(a)?

FK Eske ou ansent / fè sik / tafyatè ?

EL Είστε έγκυος / διαβητικός / αλκοολικός;
EEste Egeeos / deeaveeteekOs / alkooleekOs?

HI क्या आप गर्भवती / म ६ ुमेह से पीड़ित / शराब पीने वाली महिला हैं?
Kya aap garbhvati / madhumeh se peeDit / sharaab peene wali mahila hain?

Have you ever suffered a stroke?

¿Alguna vez ha tenido embolia (apoplejía)?

你曾经有过中风吗？
nǐ céng jīng yǒu guò zhòng fēng ma?

Avez-vous souffert d'une apoplexie?

Hatten Sie schon einmal einen Schlaganfall?

Quý vị đã bao giờ bị đột quỵ chưa?

Ha mai avuto un ictus?

뇌졸증이 있은 적 있습니까?
Noe-jol-jeung-i i-seun jeok it-seum-ni-kka?

Вы когда-нибудь переносили инсульт?
Vy kogda-nibud' perenosili insul't?

Czy doznał(a) Pan(i) kiedykolwiek udaru?

هل سبق أن اصبت بسكتة دماغية؟
Hal sabaq an usibt bi-saktah dimaaghiyah?

Alguma vez sofreu um acidente vascular cerebral?

Eske ou jan fè yon estwok?

Υποφέρατε ποτέ από εγκεφαλικό επεισόδιο;
eepofErate potE apO egefaleekO epeesOdeeo?

क्या आपको कभी दौरा पड़ा है?
Kya aapko kabhi daura padaa hai?

Have you ever received psychiatric treatment?

ES ¿Ha recibido alguna vez tratamiento psiquiátrico?

ZH 你曾经接受过心理治疗吗？
nǐ céng jīng jiē shòu guò xīn lǐ zhì liáo ma?

FR Avez-vous jamais reçu un traitement psychiatrique?

DE Waren Sie jemals in psychiatrischer Behandlung?

VI Quý vị đã bao giờ được trị liệu tâm thần chưa?

IT Ha mai ricevuto cure psichiatriche?

KO 정신과 치료를 받은 적 있습니까?
Jeong-sin-gwa chi-ryo-reul ba-deun jeok it-seum-ni-kka?

RU Вы когда-нибудь получали психиатрическое лечение?
Vy kogda-nibud' poluchali psikhiatricheskoe lechenie?

PL Czy był(a) Pan(i) kiedykolwiek poddana leczeniu psychiatrycznemu?

AR هل سبق أن تلقيت علاجاً نفسانياً؟
Hal sabaq an talaqqayt "ilaaj nafsaani?

PT Alguma vez recebeu tratamento psiquiátrico?

FK Eske ou janm resevwa tretman sikyatri?

EL Λάβατε ποτέ ψυχιατρική θεραπεία;
lAvate potE pseeheeatreekEE therapEEa?

HI क्या आपने कभी मनोचिकित्सक से इलाज कराया है?
Kya aapne kabhi manochikitsak se ilaaz karaya hai?

Have you noticed the following changes on yourself?

S ¿Ha notado los siguientes cambios en usted?

H 你最近有没有发现自己有以下变化？
nǐ zuì jìn yǒu méi yǒu fā xiàn zì jǐ yǒu yǐ xià biàn huà?

R Avez-vous noté les changements suivants en vous-mêmes?

E Haben Sie folgende Veränderungen bei sich bemerkt?

VI Quý vị có nhận thấy các thay đổi sau đây trong cơ thể không?

T Ha notato in Lei i seguenti cambiamenti?

O 본인에게 다음의 변화가 생긴 것을 느끼셨습니까?
Bo-ni-ne-ge da-eu-mui byeon-hwa-ga saeng-gin geo-seul neu-kki-syeot-seum-ni-kka?

U Заметили ли вы у себя следующие изменения?
Zametili li vy u sebya sleduyushchie izmeneniya?

'L Czy zauważył Pan(i) u siebie następujące zmiany?

'R هل لاحظت التغيرات التالية في نفسك؟
Hal laahadht at-taghyeeraat it-taaliyah fi nafsak?

T Notou em si algumas das seguintes alterações?

K Eske ou janm remake okinn nan chanjman swivan yo nan ou menm?

L Παρατηρήσατε τις ακόλουθες αλλαγές στον εαυτό σας;
parateerEEsate tees akOluthes alagEs ston eaftO sas?

II क्या आपने स्वयं में निम्नलिखित बदलाव नोट किए हैं? ...
Kya aapne swayam mein nimnlikhit badlaav note kiye hain?

mood changes / sadness / depression / anger

ES cambios de humor (estado de ánimo) / tristeza / depresión / enojo

ZH 情绪不稳 / 沮丧 / 抑郁 / 易生气
qíng xù bù wěn / jǔ sàng / yì yù / yì shēng qì

FR changements d'humeur / tristesse / dépression / irascibilité

DE Stimmungsänderungen / Trauer / Depression / Wut

VI các thay đổi về cảm xúc / buồn chán / trầm cảm / giận dữ

IT cambiamenti d'umore / tristezza / depressione / rabbia

KO 기분 변화 / 슬픔 / 우울증 / 분노
gi-bun byeon-hwa / seul-peum / u-ul-jeung / bun-no

RU изменения настроения / грусть / депрессия / гнев
izmeneniya nastroeniya / grust' / depressiya / gnev

PL zmiany nastroju / smutek / depresję / gniew

AR تغيرات فى المزاج \ الحزن \ الكآبة \ الغضب
Taghyeeraat fil-mizaaj / al-huzn / al-ka'aabah / al-ghadhab

PT alterações do humor / tristeza / depressão / ira

FK tanperaman w chanje / tristes / depresyon / kolè

EL αλλαγές διάθεσης / λύπη / κατάθλιψη / θυμό
alagEs deeAthesees / lEEpee / katAthleepsee / theemO

HI मूड बदलाव / उदासी / तनाव / गुस्सा ...
mood badlaav / udasi / tanaav / gussa

confusion / sleeplessness / anxiety

confusión / insomnio / ansiedad

分辨能力不好 / 失眠 / 焦虑
fēn biàn néng lì bù hǎo / shī mián / jiāo lǜ

confusion / somnolence / anxiété

Verwirrung / Schlaflosigkeit / Angst

lẫn lộn / mất ngủ / lo âu

confusione / insonnia / ansia

혼동(의식 장애) / 졸림 / 불안
hon-dong(eui-sik-jang-ae) / jol-lim / bu-ran

спутанность / бессонница / страх
sputannost' / bessonnitsa / strakh

dezorientację / bezsenność / lęk

التحير \ عدم النوم \ القلق
At-tahayyur / "adam an-noum / al-qalaq

confusão / insónia / ansiedade

konfusyon / paka domi / angwas

σύγχυση / αϋπνία / άγχος
sEEnheesee / aeepnEEa / Anhos

भ्रम / अनिद्रा / चिंता
bhram / A-nidra / chinta

Do you feel the urge to hurt yourself / others?

ES ¿Siente el impulso de lastimarse / lastimar a otros?

ZH 你有没有要去伤害自己 / 别人的冲动？
nǐ yǒu méi yǒu yào qù shāng hài zì jǐ / bié rén de chōng dòng?

FR Avez-vous l'impression d'être poussé à vous blesser ou à blesser d'autres?

DE Verspüren Sie das Bedürfnis sich / andere zu verletzen?

VI Quý vị có cảm thấy muốn làm tổn thương bản thân / người khác không?

IT Sente l'impulso a far male a sé / ad altri?

KO 스스로를 / 타인을 해치고 싶은 충동을 느끼십니까?
seu-seu-ro-reul / ta-i-neul hae-chi-go si-peun chung-dong-eul neu-kki-sim-ni-kka?

RU Вы чувствуете позыв причинить боль себе / другим?
Vy chuvstvuete pozyv prichinit' bol' sebe / drugim?

PL Czy czuje Pan(i) potrzebę zadawania bólu sobie / innym?

AR هل تشعر\ تشعرين برغبة ملحّة لإيذاء نفسك \ آخرين؟
Hal tash"ur / tash"ureen bi-raghbah mulihhah li-eedhaa' nafsak / aakhareen?

PT Sente uma vontade incontrolável de se magoar ou ferir a si ou aos outros?

FK Eske ou santi ke ou anvi fè tèt ou / lòt moun mal?

EL Νιώθετε την ανάγκη να βλάψετε τον εαυτό σας / άλλους;
neeOthete teen anAgee na vlApsete ton eaftO sas / Alus?

HI क्या आप स्वयं / दूसरों को नुकसान पहुंचाने के लिए प्रेरित महसूस करते हैं?
Kya aap swayam / dusron ko nuksaan pahunchane ke liye prerit mehsoos karte hain?

Do you have suicidal thoughts?

¿Ha pensado alguna vez en el suicidio?

你有没有要自杀的想法？
nǐ yǒu méi yǒu yào zì shā de xiǎng fǎ?

Avez-vous des idées de suicide?

Verspüren Sie das Bedürfnis sich umzubringen?

Quý vị có ý nghĩ muốn tự tử không?

Ha pensieri suicidi?

자살하고 싶다는 생각을 하십니까?
Ja-sal-ha-go sip-da-neun saeng-ga-geul ha-sim-ni-kka?

У вас есть мысли о самоубийстве?
U vas est' mysli o samoubiystve?

Czy miewa Pan(i) samobójcze myśli?

هل تفكر \ تفكرين في الإنتحار؟
Hal tufakkir / tufakkireen fil-intihaar?

Tem pensamentos suicidas?

Eske ou janm gen lide touye tet ou?

Έχετε σκέψεις αυτοκτονίας;
Ehete skEpsees aftoktonEEas?

क्या आपको आत्महत्या के विचार आते हैं?
Kya aapko aatamhatya ke vichaar aate hain?

Are you experiencing / have you experienced hallucinations?

ES ¿Tiene / ha tenido alucinaciones?

ZH 你是否有 / 以前有过幻觉？
nǐ shì fǒu yǒu / yǐ qián yǒu guò huàn jué?

FR Avez-vous ou avez-vous eu des hallucinations?

DE Haben / hatten Sie Halluzinationen?

VI Quý vị có đang / đã gặp phải tình trạng ảo giác không?

IT Ha / ha avuto allucinazioni?

KO 환각을 경험하고 있으십니까? / 환각을 경험한 적이 있습니까?
Hwan-ga-geul gyeong-heom-ha-go i-seu-sim-ni-kka / hwan-ga-geul gyeong-heom-han jeo-gi it-seum-ni-kka?

RU У вас сейчас есть / когда-нибудь были галлюцинации?
U vas seychas est' / kogda-nibud' byli gallyutsinatsii?

PL Czy doświadcza / doświadczał (a) Pan(i) halucynacji?

AR هل تتعرض \ تتعرضين \ تعرضت للهلوسة؟
Hal tit"arridh / tit"arridheen / ta"arradht lil-halwasah?

PT Actualmente sente / tem sentido alucinações?

FK Eske ou janm soufri / te janm soufri halusynasyon ?

EL Έχετε / Είχατε παραισθήσεις;
Ehete / EEhate paresthEEsees?

HI क्या आप भ्रमित महसूस कर रहे हैं / थे?
Kya aap bhramit mehsoos kar rahe hain / the?

Have you seen / heard / smelled anything?

Ha visto / oído / olido cosas?

你是否看见 / 听见 / 闻见什么东西？
nǐ shì fǒu kàn jiàn / tīng jiàn / wén jiàn shén me dōng xī?

Avez-vous vu / entendu / senti quelque chose?

Haben Sie etwas gesehen / gehört / gesehen / gerochen?

Quý vị có nhìn / nghe / ngửi thấy bất kỳ cái gì không?

Ha visto / sentito / odorato qualcosa?

무언가를 본 / 들은 / 냄새 맡은 게 있습니까?
Mu-eun-ga-reul bon / deu-reun / naem-sae ma-teun ge it-seum-ni-kka?

Вы видели / слышали / чувствовали запах чего-нибудь?
Vy videli / slyshali chto-nibud' / chuvstvovali zapakh chego-nibud'?

Czy widzi / słyszy / czuje Pan(i) cokolwiek?

هل رأيت \ سمعت \ شممت اي شيء؟
Hal ra'ayt / sami"t / shamamt ayy shey'?

Tem visto / ouvido / cheirado algo?

Eske ou te janm wè / tande / pran sant okinn bagay ?

Είδατε / Ακούσατε / Μυρίσατε κάτι;
EEdate / akUsate / meerEEsate kAtee?

क्या आपने कुछ देखा / सुना / सूंघा है?
Kya aapne kuCh dekha / sunaa / soongha hai?

Are you taking medications / psychopharmaceuticals? Which ones?

ES ¿Toma actualmente medicamentos / psicofármacos? ¿Cuáles?

ZH 你是否在用药 / 精神药物？什么药？
nǐ shì fōu zài yòng yào / jīng shén yào wù? shén me yào?

FR Prenez-vous des médicaments / à usage psychiatrique? Lesquels?

DE Nehmen Sie Medikamente / Psychopharmaka? Welche?

VI Quý vị có đang dùng thuốc / thuốc chữa tâm thần không? Đó là các loại thuốc nào?

IT Sta prendendo farmaci / psicofarmaci? Quali?

KO 약 / 정신과 약을 드시는 게 있습니까? 이름이 뭡니까?
Yak / jeong-sin-gwa ya-geul deu-si-neun ge it-seum-ni-kka? I-reu-mi mwom-ni-kka?

RU Вы сейчас принимаете лекарства / психофармакологические средства? Какие?
Vy seychas prinimaete lekarstva / psikhofarmakologicheskie sredstva? Kakie?

PL Czy przyjmuje Pan(i) obecnie leki / środki psychofarmakologiczne? Jakie?

AR هل تأخذ \ تأخذين أدوية عادية \ أدوية للعلاج النفساني؟ أي نوع منها؟
Hal ta'khudh / ta'khudheen adwiyah "aadiyah / adwiyah lil-"ilaaj in-nafsaani? Ay nou" minha?

PT Está a tomar medicamentos / psicofármacos? Quais?

FK Eske ou ap pran medikaman / sykofarmasetik ? Ki les ladan yo ?

EL Λαμβάνετε φάρμακα / ψυχοφάρμακα; Ποια;
lamvAnete fArmaka / pseehofArmaka? peeA?

HI क्या आप कोई दवा/फिजिकोफार्मास्युटीकल्स ले रहे हैं? कौन सी? ... क्यूक्यू एसए
Kya aap koi davaa / psychopharmaceuticals le rahe hain? kaun si?

Are you regularly taking drugs? Which ones?

¿Consume drogas regularmente? ¿De qué tipo?

你经常吸毒吗？哪一种？
nǐ jīng cháng xī dú ma? nǎ yī zhǒng?

Prenez-vous régulièrement des médicaments? Lesquels?

Nehmen Sie regelmäßig Drogen? Welche?

Quý vị có uống thuốc đều đặn không? Đó là những loại thuốc nào?

Assume regolarmente farmaci? Quali?

정기적으로 드시는 마약이 있습니까? 이름이 뭡니까?
Jeong-gi-jeo-geu-ro deu-si-neun ma-ya-gi it-seum-ni-kka? I-reu-mi mwom-nikka?

Вы регулярно принимаете лекарства? Какие?
Vy regulyarno prinimaete lekarstva? Kakie?

Czy stosuje Pan(i) regularnie jakieś leki? Jakie?

هل تأخذ \ تأخذين أدوية بشكل متكرر؟ اي نوع منها؟
Hal ta'khudh / ta'khudheen adwiyah bi-shekl mutakarrir? Ay nou" minha?

Está a tomar medicamentos com regularidade? Que medicamentos?

Eske ou pran dwog sou yon baz regilye? Ki les ladan yo?

Λαμβάνετε τακτικά φάρμακα; Ποια;
lamvAnete takteekA fArmaka? peeA?

क्या आप नियमित रूप से दवाएं ले रहे हैं? कौन सी? ... क्यूक्यू एसए
Kya aap niyamit roop se davaayein le rahe hain? kaun si?

Have you undergone detoxification treatment? When?

ES ¿Se ha sometido a tratamiento de desintoxicación? ¿Cuándo?

ZH 你有没有接受过解毒治疗？是什么时间？
nĭ yŏu méi yŏu jiē shòu guò jiĕ dú zhì liáo? shì shén me shí jiān?

FR Avez-vous suivi une cure de désintoxication? Quand?

DE Haben Sie eine Drogen-Entziehungskur gemacht? Wann?

VI Quý vị có điều trị cai nghiện không? Khi nào?

IT Ha subito un trattamento detossificante? Quando?

KO 약물 중독 치료를 받은 적이 있습니까? 언제입니까?
Yang-mul jung-dok chi-ryo-reul ba-deun jeo-gi it-seum-ni-kka? Eon-je-im-ni-kka?

RU Вы когда-нибудь проходили детоксикационное лечение? Когда?
Vy kogda-nibud' prokhodili detoksikatsionnoe lechenie? Kogda?

PL Czy przechodził(a) Pan(i) leczenie detoksykacyjne? Kiedy?

AR هل اجري عليك علاجاً لإنهاء الإدمان على المخدرات؟ متى؟
Hal oojree "alayk "ilaaj li-inhaa' al-idmaan "alaa al-mukhaddiraat? Mattaa?

PT Já se submeteu a algum tratamento de desintoxicação? Quando?

FK Eske ou te janm fè tretman detoksifikasyon ? Ki lè ?

EL Υποβληθήκατε σε θεραπεία αποτοξίνωσης; Πότε;
eepovleethEEkate se therapEEa apotoxEEnosees? pOte?

HI क्या आपने कभी जहर उतारने का इलाज करवाया है? कब?
Kya aapne kabhi zehar utaarne ka ilaaz karvaaya hai? kab?

Have you lost a family member / loved one?

¿Ha perdido a algún miembro de la familia / ser querido?

你有没有失去家庭成员 / 你爱的人？
nǐ yǒu méi yǒu shī qù jiā tíng chéng yuán / nǐ ài de rén?

Avez-vous perdu un membre de votre famille / un être cher?

Haben Sie ein Familienmitglied / geliebten Menschen verloren?

Quý vị có người nhà / người thân qua đời không?

Ha perso un familiare / una persona amata?

가족 일원 / 사랑하는 사람을 잃은 적이 있습니까?
Ga-jok ir-won / sa-rang-ha-neun sa-ra-meul i-reun jeo-gi it-seum-ni-kka?

Вы потеряли кого-нибудь из членов семьи / любимого человека?
Vy poteryali kogo-nibud' iz chlenov sem'i / lyubimogo cheloveka?

Czy stracił(a) Pan(i) członka rodziny / bliską osobę?

هل مات احد من أفراد عائلتك او احد عزيز عندك؟
Hal maat ahad min afraad "aa'ilatak aw ahad "azeez "indak?

Perdeu algum familiar / ente querido?

Eske ou pedi yon manb fanmi w / moun ou renmin?

Χάσατε οικογενειακό μέλος / αγαπημένο πρόσωπο;
hAsate eekogeneeakO mElos / agapeemEno prOsopo?

क्या आपने कोई पारिवारिक सदस्य / प्रिय खो दिया है? ... क्यूक्यू एफए
Kya aapne koi paarivaarik sadasya / priya kho diya hai?

Did you lose your job?

ES	¿Perdió su trabajo?
ZH	你有没有失业？ nǐ yǒu méi yǒu shī yè?
FR	Avez-vous perdu votre emploi?
DE	Haben Sie Ihre Arbeit verloren?
VI	Quý vị có bị mất việc làm không?
IT	Ha perso il lavoro?
KO	직장을 잃으셨습니까? Jik-jang-eul i-reu-syeot-seum-ni-kka?
RU	Вы потеряли работу? Vy poteryali rabotu?
PL	Czy stracił(a) Pan(i) pracę?
AR	هل فقدت شغلك؟ Hal faqadta / faqadti shughlak?
PT	Perdeu o seu emprego?
FK	Eske ou pedi travay ou?
EL	Χάσατε τη δουλειά σας; hAsate tee duleeA sas?
HI	क्या आपने अपनी नौकरी खो दी? Kya aapne apni naukri kho di?

16 Blood Diseases

Have you noticed any changes in yourself?

ES ¿Ha notado algún cambio en usted?

ZH 你有没有发现自己有何 变化？
nǐ yǒu méi yǒu fā xiàn zì jǐ yǒu hé biàn huà?

FR Avez-vous remarqué des changements en vous-mêmes?

DE Haben Sie Veränderungen an sich bemerkt?

VI Quý vị có nhận thấy thay đổi gì trong người không?

IT Ha notato nessun cambiamento nelle sue condizioni?

KO 스스로에 변화를 느끼신 게 있습니까?
seu-seu-ro-e byeon-hwa-reul neu-kki-sin ge it-seum-ni-kka?

RU Заметили ли вы какие-нибудь изменения в себе?
Zametili li vy kakie-nibud' izmeneniya v sebe?

PL Czy zauważył Pan(i) u siebie jakieś zmiany?

AR هل لاحظت اية تغيرات في نفسك؟
Hal laahadht ayyi taghyeeraat fi nafsak?

PT Notou algumas alterações em si?

FK Eske ou remake okenn chanjman lakay ou?

EL Παρατηρήσατε οποιεσδήποτε αλλαγές στον εαυτό σας;
parateerEEsate opee-esdEEpote alagEs ston eaftO sas?

HI क्या आपने स्वयं में कोई परिवर्तन नोट किया है? ...
Kya aapne swayam mei koi parivartan note kiya hai? .

Fatigue / weakness / swellings (location?)

ES	Fatiga / debilidad / hinchazón (¿dónde?)
ZH	疲劳 / 虚弱 / 肿胀（在哪里？） pí láo / xū ruò / zhǒng zhàng（zài nǎ lǐ？）
FR	de la fatigue / de la faiblesse / des gonflements (localisation?)
DE	Müdigkeit / Schwäche / Schwellungen (wo?)
VI	Mệt mỏi / ốm yếu / sưng (ở đâu?)
IT	Stanchezza / debolezza / gonfiori (dove?)
KO	피곤 / 허약 / 붓기(장소?) pi-gon / heo-yak / but-gi(jang-so?)
RU	Усталость / слабость / опухоли (где именно?) Ustalost' / slabost' / opukholi (gde imenno?)
PL	Zmęczenie / osłabienie / obrzęk (gdzie?)
AR	الإرهاق \ الضعف \ التضخمات (مكانها؟) Al-irhaaq / adh-dha"f / at-tadhakhkhumaat (makaanhaa?)
PT	Fadiga / debilidade / inchaços (local?)
FK	Fatig / fèbles / enflamasyon (ki bo?)
EL	Κούρασση / αδυναμία / διογκώσεις (σε ποιο σημείο;) kUrasee / adeenamEEa / deeogkOsees (se peeO seemEEo?)
HI	थकान / कमजोरी / सूजन (स्थिति?) Thakaan / kamjori / soojan (isthiti?)

Have you noticed blood? Where did you see it?

ES ¿Ha notado sangre? ¿En qué parte?

ZH 你有没有发现血？哪里发现的？
nǐ yǒu méi yǒu fā xiàn xiě? nǎ lǐ fā xiàn de?

FR Avez-vous remarqué la présence de sang? Où l'avez-vous vu?

DE Haben Sie Blut bemerkt? Wo?

VI Quý vị có thấy máu không? Quý vị thấy máu ở đâu?

IT Ha notatao presenza di sangue? Dove l'ha notato?

KO 피가 나온 데가 있습니까? 어디서 보셨습니까?
pi-ga na-on de-ga it-seum-ni-kka? Eo-di-seo bo-syeot-seum-ni-kka?

RU Вы заметили кровь? Где вы её видели?
Vy zametili krov'? Gde vy eyo videli?

PL Czy zauważył(a) Pan(i) krew? Gdzie ją Pan(i) zaobserwował(a)?

AR هل لاحظت دماً؟ اين لاحظت الدم؟
Hal laahadht damman? Ayna laahadht ad-damm?

PT Notou sangue? Onde viu o sangue?

FK Eske ou remake san? Ki bo ou wè l?

EL Παρατηρήσατε αίμα; Πού το είδατε;
parateerEEsate Ema? pu to EEdate?

HI क्या आपने रक्तस्राव नोट किया? आपने उसे कहां देखा? ...
Kya aapne raktsraav note kiya? Aapne use kahan dekha?

coming out of my nose / in my urine / in my feces

ES	por la nariz / en la orina / en las heces
ZH	我鼻子里 / 尿里 / 大便里 wǒ bí zǐ lǐ / niào lǐ / dà biàn lǐ
FR	s'échappant de mon nez / dans mes urines / dans mes selles
DE	aus der Nase / im Urin / im Stuhl
VI	mũi chảy máu / trong nước tiểu / trong phân
IT	dal naso / nelle urine / nelle feci
KO	코에서 나왔음 / 소변에서 / 대변에서 ko-e-seo na-wa-seum / so-byeon-e-seo / dae-byeon-e-seo
RU	шла из носа / в моче / в кале shla iz nosa / v moche / v kale
PL	ciekła mi z nosa / w moczu / w stolcu
AR	خارج من انفي \ في بولي \ في غائطي Khaarij min anfi / fi bauli / fi ghaa'iti
PT	A sair do nariz / na urina / nas fezes
FK	soti nan nen mwen / nan pipi m / nan watè m
EL	να βγαίνει από τη μύτη μου / στα ούρα μου / στα κόπρανα μου na vgEnee apO tee mEEtee mu / sta Ura mu / sta kOprana mu
HI	मेरी नाक से / अपने मूत्र में / मेरे मल से निकलता हुआ Meri naak se / apne mootra mein / mere mal se nikalta hua

Have you vomited blood?

S ¿Ha vomitado usted sangre?

H 你吐血了吗？
nǐ tù xiě le ma?

R Avez-vous vomi du sang?

DE Haben Sie Blut erbrochen?

VI Quý vị có ói ra máu không?

IT Ha vomitato sangue?

KO 피를 토하신 적이 있습니까?
pi-reul to-ha-sin jeo-gi it-seum-ni-kka?

RU Вы рвали кровью?
Vy rvali krov'yu?

PL Czy wymiotował(a) Pan(i) krwią?

AR هل تقيأت بالدم؟
Hal taqayya't bid-damm?

PT Vomitou sangue?

FK Eske ou vomi san?

EL Κάνατε εμετό με αίμα;
kAnate emetO me Ema?

HI क्या आपको रक्त की उल्टी हुई?
Kya aapko rakt ki ulti hui?

Have you noticed bloody mucus?

ES ¿Ha notado usted moco sanguinolento?

ZH 你有没有发现带血的粘液？
nǐ yǒu méi yǒu fā xiàn dài xiě de nián yè?

FR Avez-vous remarqué du mucus sanguinolent?

DE Haben Sie Schleim mit Blutspuren bemerkt?

VI Quý vị có thấy máu trong chất nhầy không?

IT Ha notato del muco sanguinolento?

KO 침에 피가 섞인 것을 보셨습니까?
chi-me pi-ga seo-kkin geo-seul bo-syeot-seum-ni-kka?

RU Вы заметили кровь в мокроте?
Vy zametili krov' v mokrote?

PL Czy zauważył(a) Pan(i) krwawy śluz?

AR هل لاحظت البلغم الدامي عندك؟
Hal laahadht il-balgham ad-daami "indak / "indik?

PT Notou alguma mucosidade sanguinolenta?

FK Eske ou remake mukus ki gen san?

EL Παρατηρήσατε αιματώδη βλέννη;
parateerEEsate ematOdee vlEnee?

HI क्या आपने बलगम में रक्त नोट किया?
Kya aapne balgam mein rakt note kiya?

Do you bleed extensively for an unusually long time?

S ¿Sangra usted mucho y por mucho tiempo?

SH 你有没有出血时间较长？
nǐ yǒu méi yǒu chū xiě shí jiān jiào cháng?

FR Avez-vous saigné fort pendant un temps anormalement long?

Bluten Sie ungewöhnlich lange und viel?

IT Quý vị có bị ra nhiều máu trong khoảng thời gian quá dài không?

Ha delle perdite di sangue accentuate per lunghi periodi di tempo?

Q 지나치게 오랫 동안 출혈을 심하게 하십니까?
ji-na-chi-ge o-raet dong-an chul-hyeo-reul sim-ha-ge ha-sim-ni-kka?

U У вас бывают обильные кровотечения в течение очень длительного времени?
U vas byvayut obil'nye krovotecheniya v techenie ochen' dlitel'nogo vremeni?

L Czy krwawi Pan(i) często i nadzwyczaj długo?

R هل ينزف دمك بشدة لفترة طويلة غير عادية؟
Hal yanzif dammak bishiddah li-fatrah taweelah ghayr "aadiyah?

T Sangra consideravelmente durante um período de tempo excepcionalmente longo?

K Eske ou senyen anpil pandan yon bon bout tan ki pa normal?

L Αιμορραγείτε σε μεγάλο βαθμό για ασυνήθιστα μεγάλη χρονική περίοδο;
emoragEEte se megAlo vathmO geea aseenEEtheesta megAlee hroneekEE perEEodo?

HI क्या आपको असाधारण रूप से लंबे समय तक बहुत अधिक रक्तस्राव हुआ?
Kya aapko asadharaN roop se lambe samay tak bahut adhik raktasraav hua?

Do you bruise easily?

ES ¿Se le hacen moretones fácilmente?

ZH 有没有经常有淤血斑？
yǒu méi yǒu jīng cháng yǒu yū xiě bān?

FR Est-ce que vous vous cognez facilement?

DE Bekommen Sie leicht blaue Flecken?

VI Quý vị có dễ bị bầm tím không?

IT Tende ad avere facilmente ematomi?

KO 멍이 쉽게 드십니까?
meong-i swip-ge deu-sim-ni-kka?

RU У вас легко образуются синяки?
U vas legko obrazuyutsya sinyaki?

PL Czy łatwo tworzą się u Pana(i) siniaki?

AR هل تصاب \ تصابين بالكدمات بسهولة؟
Hal tusaab / tusabeen bil-kadmaat bi-suhoulah?

PT Tem tendência para fazer nódoas negras?

FK Eske li fasil pou ou gen san kaye? [Blese]

EL Μελανιάζετε εύκολα;
melaneeAzete Efkola?

HI क्या आपको आसानी से खरोंच लग जाती है?
Kya aapko aasani se kharonch lag jaati hai?

Do you take coumarin / aspirin / heparin?

¿Toma usted warfarina / aspirina / heparina?

你用华发令 / 阿斯匹林 / 肝素吗 ?
nǐ yòng huá fā lìng / a sī pī lín / gān sù ma?

Avez-vous pris de la coumarine / de l'aspirine / de l'héparine?

Nehmen Sie Cumarin / Aspirin / Heparin?

Quý vị có dùng coumarin / aspirin / heparin không?

Assume cumarina / aspirina / eparina

쿠마린 / 아스피린 / 헤파린을 복용하십니까?
ku-ma-rin / a-seu-pi-rin / he-pa-ri-neul bo-gyong-ha-sim-ni-kka?

Вы принимаете кумарин / аспирин / гепарин?
Vy prinimaete kumarin / aspirin / geparin?

Czy przyjmuje Pan(i) kumarynę / aspirynę / heparynę?

هل تأخذ \ تأخذين الكومارين \ الأسبرين \ الهيبارين؟
Hal ta'khudh / ta'khudheen al-coumarin / al-aspirin / al-heparin?

Toma cumarina / aspirina / heparina?

Eske ou pran koumarin / aspirin / heparin?

Λαμβάνετε κουμαρίνη / ασπιρίνη / ηπαρίνη;
lamvAnete kumarEEnee / aspeerEEnee / eeparEEnee?

क्या आप कोमरिन / एस्पिरिन / हेपरिन लेते हैं?
Kya aap coumarin / aspirin / heparin lete hain?

Do you have sickle cell anemia?

ES	¿Tiene usted anemia de células falciformes (drepanocítica)?
ZH	你有镰刀形贫血吗？ nǐ yǒu lián dāo xíng pín xiě ma?
FR	Souffrez-vous de thalassémie?
DE	Leiden Sie an Sichelzellanämie?
VI	Quý vị có mắc bệnh thiếu máu tế bào hình liềm không?
IT	È affetto da anemia falciforme?
KO	겸상 적혈구성 빈혈이 있으십니까? gyeom-sang jeok-hyeol-gu-seong bin-hyeo-ri i-seu-sim-ni-kka?
RU	Вы болеете серповидноклеточной анемией? Vy boleyete serpovidnokletochnoy anemiey?
PL	Czy ma Pan(i) sierpowicę?
AR	هل تعاني \ تعانين من فقر الدم المنجلي؟ Hal tu"aani / tu"aaneen min faqr ad-damm al-munjali?
PT	Tem anemia de células falciformes?
FK	Eske ou gen anemi falsifòm?
EL	Έχετε δρεπανοκυτταρική αναιμία; Ehete drepanokeetareekEE anemEEa?
HI	क्या आपको हंसिया कोषाणु एनीमिया है? Kya aapko hansiya koShaNu anemia hai?

Intoxications, Overdose

Did you take drugs? Which ones?

¿Tomó usted alguna medicina o droga? ¿Cuál o cuáles?

你吸毒吗？哪 一种？
nǐ xī dú ma? nǎ yī zhǒng?

Prenez-vous des drogues? lesquelles?

Haben Sie Drogen genommen? Welche?

Quý vị có dùng thuốc không? Quý vị dùng loại thuốc nào?

Assume farmaci? Quali?

마약 하셨습니까? 어떤 것을요?
ma-yak ha-syeot-seum-ni-kka? Eo-tteon geo-seur-yo?

Вы принимаете лекарства? Какие?
Vy prinimaete lekarstva? Kakie?

Czy przyjmował(a) Pan(i) lekarstwa? Jakie?

هل تعاطيت اية مخدرات؟ ما هي؟
Hal ta"aatayt ayyi mukhaddiraat? Maa hiya?

Tomou drogas? Quais?

Eske ou pran dwog? Ki les?

Πήρατε ναρκωτικές ουσίες; Ποιες;
pEErate narkoteekEs usEEes? peeEs?

क्या आपने दवा ली थी? कौन सी? ...
Kya aapne davaa lee thee? Kaun si?

What did the child eat / drink?

ES ¿Qué comió / bebió el niño?

ZH 孩子吃了 / 喝了什么吗？
hái zǐ chī le / hē le shén me ma?

FR Qu'est-ce que votre enfant a mangé / bu?

DE Was hat das Kind gegessen / getrunken?

VI Đứa trẻ đã ăn / uống gì?

IT Cosa ha mangiato / bevuto il bambino?

KO 아이가 뭘 먹었습니까? / 마셨습니까?
a-i-ga mwol meo-geot-seum-ni-kka? / ma-syeot-seum-ni-kka?

RU Что ребёнок проглотил / выпил?
Chto rebyonok proglotil / vypil?

PL Co dziecko jadło / piło?

AR ماذا أكل \ شرب الطفل؟
Maadha akal / sharab at-tifl?

PT O que é que a criança comeu ou bebeu?

FK Kisa timoun lan manje / bouwè?

EL Τι έφαγε / ήπιε το παιδί;
tee Efage / EEpee-e to pedEE?

HI बच्चे ने क्या खाया / पीया? ...
Bachche ne kya khaya / peeya?

medications / aspirin / drain opener / toilet cleaner / lye

S
medicamentos / aspirina / destapacaños / limpiador de baños / lejía

H
药物 / 阿斯匹林 / 管道疏通剂 / 马桶清洗剂 / 染料
yào wù / ā sī pī lín / guǎn dào shū tōng jì / mǎ tǒng qīng xǐ jì / rán liào

R
Des médicaments / de l'aspirine / un produit pour déboucher / un nettoyant pour toilette / une lessive

E
Medikamente / Aspirin / Abfluss- / Toilettenreiniger / Lauge

VI
thuốc / aspirin / dung dịch thông cống / thuốc tẩy rửa bồn vệ sinh / thuốc giặt quần áo

T
farmaci / aspirina / acido muriatico / detersivo per toilette / liscivia

O
약 / 아스피린 / 하수구 뚫는 약 / 변기 청소약 / 잿물
yak / a-seu-pi-rin / ha-su-gu ttul-leun yak / byeon-gi cheong-so-yak / jaen-mul

U
лекарства / аспирин / средство для удаления засоров в трубах / средство для чистки унитазов / щёлок
lekarstva / aspirin / sredstvo dlya udaleniya zasorov v trubakh / sredstvo dlya chistki unitazov / shchyolok

L
leki / aspirynę / środek do udrażniania rur kanalizacyjnych / środek do czyszczenia muszli toaletowej / ług

AR
الأدوية \ الأسبرين \ محلول فتح المجاري المسدودة \ سائل تنظيف المرحاض \ الغسول
Al-adwiyah / al-aspirin / mahloul fat'h al-majaari al-masdoudah / saa'il tandheef al-mirhaadh / al-ghusool

PT
Medicamentos / aspirina / produto para desentupir canos / produto para limpar a sanita / lixívia

K
medikaman / aspirin / pwodwi ki debouche tiyo / pwodwi netwaye twalet / lesiv

EL
φάρμακα / ασπιρίνη / αποφρακτικό αποχετεύσεων / καθαριστικό τουαλέτας / καυστική ουσία
fArmaka / aspeerEEnee / apofrakteekO apohetEfseon / kathareesteekO tualEtas / kafsteekEE usEEa

HI
दवाएं / एस्प्रिन / नाली खोलने वाला / प्रसाधन साफ करने वाला / क्षार मिला पानी
davayein / aspirin / naali kholne wala / prasaadhan saaf karne wala / kShar mila paani

bleach / cleaning detergent / paint thinner / gasoline

ES blanqueador / detergente / diluyente de pintura / gasolina

ZH 漂白剂 / 洗涤剂 / 油漆稀释剂 / 汽油
piāo bái jì / xǐ dí jì / yóu qī xī shī jì / qì yóu

FR un produit blanchissant / un décolorant / un détergent / un diluant pour peinture / de l'essence pour voiture

DE Bleicher / Reinigungsmittel / Farbverdünner / Benzin

VI thuốc tẩy / bột giặt / chất làm loãng sơn / xăng

IT varecchina / detersivo / vernice / benzina

KO 표백약 / 세제 / 페인트 신나 / 가솔린
pyo-baeg-yak / se-je / pe-in-teu sin-na / ga-sol-lin

RU отбеливатель / моющее средство / разбавитель для краски / бензин
otbelivatel' / moyushchee sredstvo / razbavitel' dlya kraski / benzin

PL chlorek / środek do prania / rozcieńczalnik do farby / benzynę

AR السائل القاصر (البليج) \ مسحوق غسيل \ مخفف الدهان \ البنزين
As-saa'il al-qaasir (al-bleach) / mas'hooq ghaseel / mukhaffif ad-dihaan / al-benzin

PT Cloro / detergente para limpeza / diluente de tintas / gasolina

FK kloroks / savon lesiv / pwodwi ki rafinen penti / gazolin

EL χλωρίνη / καθαριστικό / διαλυτικό μπογιάς / βενζίνη
hlorEEnee / kathareesteekO / deealeeteekO bogeeAs / venzEEnee

HI ब्लीच / सफाई डिटरजेंट / पेंट वाला थिनर / गैसोलीन
bleech / safaai deterjent / paint wala thinner / gasoline

Which tablets have you (has he / she) ingested?

S ¿Qué pastillas tomó usted (él / ella)?

H 你(他 / 她)吞咽了哪一种药片？
nǐ (tā / tā) tūn yàn le nǎ yī zhǒng yào piàn?

R Quels comprimés avez-vous (a-t-il / elle) ingéré?

E Welche Tabletten haben Sie (hat er / sie) genommen?

VI Quý vị (anh ta / cô ta) đã uống viên thuốc nào?

T Quali compresse ha ingerito?

O 당신은 (그는 / 그녀는) 어떤 정제를 드셨습니까?
dang-si-neun (geu-neun / geu-nyeo-neun) eo-tteon jeong-je-reul deu-syeot-seum-ni-kka?

U Какие таблетки вы (он / она) проглотили?
Kakie tabletki vy (on / ona) proglotili?

L Jakie tabletki Pan połknął (on) połknął / Pani (ona) połknęła?

R ما هي الحبات التي اكلتها (التي اكلها \ اكلتها)؟
Maa hiya al-habbat alati akalthaa (alati akalhaa / akalathaa)?

T Que comprimidos é que você (ele / ela) ingeriu?

K Ki grenn ke ou (ke li) vale?

L Ποια δισκία έχετε (έχει) καταπιεί;
peea deeskEEa Ehete (Ehee) katapeeEE?

I आपने (उसने) कौन–सी गोलियां खाई थीं?
Aapne (usne) kaun si goliyan khayi thee?

When did you (he / she) take the tablets?

ES ¿Cuándo tomó usted (él / ella) las pastillas?

ZH 你(他 / 她) 是什么时间吞咽药片的？
nǐ (tā / tā) shì shén me shí jiān tūn yàn yào piàn de?

FR Quand avez-vous (a-t-il / elle) pris ces comprimés?

DE Wann haben Sie (hat er / sie) die Tabletten genommen?

VI Quý vị (anh ta / cô ta) đã dùng các viên thuốc đó khi nào?

IT Quando ha preso queste compresse?

KO 당신은 (그는 / 그녀는) 언제 정제를 드셨습니까?
dang-si-neun (geu-neun / geu-nyeo-neun) eon-je jeong-je-reul deu-syeot-seum-ni-kka?

RU Когда вы (он / она) приняли эти таблетки?
Kogda vy (on / ona) prinyali eti tabletki?

PL Kiedy je Pan (on) połknął / Pani (ona) połknęła?

AR متى أخذت (أخذ / أخذت) الحبات؟
Mattaa akhadht (akhadh / akhadhat) al-habbat?

PT Quando é que você (ele / ela) tomou os comprimidos?

FK Ki lè ke ou (li) te pran grenn sa a?

EL Πότε πήρατε (πήρε) τα δισκία;
pOte pEErate (pEEre) ta deeskEEa?

HI आपने (उसने) गोलियाँ कब खाई थीं?
Aapne (usne) goliyan kab khayee thee?

What was the color and shape of the tablets?

ES ¿De qué color y forma eran las pastillas?

ZH 药片的颜色和形状是什么？
yào piàn de yán sè hé xíng zhuàng shì shén me?

FR Quelle couleur et quelle forme avaient ces comprimés?

DE Welche Farbe und Form hatten die Tabletten?

VI Viên thuốc đó có màu sắc và hình dạng như thế nào?

IT Di che colore e di che forma erano le compresse?

KO 정제의 색깔과 모양은 어땠습니까?
jeong-je-ui sae-kkkal-gwa mo-yang-eun eo-ttaet-seum-ni-kka?

RU Какого цвета и формы были эти таблетки?
Kakogo tsveta i formy byli eti tabletki?

PL Jakiego koloru i kształtu były te tabletki?

AR ما هو لون الحبات وشكلها؟
Ma huwa laun al-habbat wa shaklhaa?

PT Qual era a cor e a forma dos comprimidos?

FK Ki koulè ak ki fòm grenn sa?

EL Τι χρώμα και σχήμα είχαν τα δισκία;
tee hrOma ke shEEma EEhan ta deeskEEa?

HI गोलियों का रंग और आकार क्या था? ...
Goliyon ka rang aur aakar kya tha?

white / blue / green / red / brown / pink and round / oval / square

ES blancas / azules / verdes / rojas / cafés / rosas y redondas / ovaladas / cuadradas

ZH 白色 / 蓝色 / 绿色 / 红色 / 棕色 / 粉红 和圆形 / 椭圆 / 方形
bái sè / lán sè / lǜ sè / hóng sè / zōng sè / fén hóng sè hé yuán xíng / tuó yuán xíng / fāng xíng

FR blanc / bleu / vert / rouge / brun / rose et rond / ovale / carré

DE weiß / blau / grün / rot / braun / rosa und rund / oval / eckig

VI màu trắng / màu xanh lơ / màu xanh lá cây / màu đỏ / màu nâu / màu hồng và có hình tròn / bầu dục / vuông

IT bianco / blu / verde / rosso / marrone / rosa e rotonde / ovali / quadrate

KO 흰색 / 푸른색 / 녹색 / 빨간색 / 갈색 / 분홍색이고 동그란 / 타원형 / 정사각형
huin-saek / pu-reun-saek / nok-saek / ppal-gan-saek / gal-saek / bun-hong-sae-gigo dong-geu-ran / ta-won-hyeong / jeong-sa-ga-khyeong

RU белые / голубые / зеленые / красные / коричневые / розовые и круглые / овальные / квадратные
belye / golubye / zelenye / krasnye / korichnevye / rozovye i kruglye / oval'nye / kvadratnye

PL białe / niebieskie / zielone / brązowe / różowe i okrągłe / owalne / kwadratowe

AR ابيض \ ازرق \ اخضر \ احمر \ بني \ وردي ومستدير الشكل \ بيضوي الشكل \ مربع الشكل
Abyadh / azraq / akhdhar / ahmar / bunni / wardi wa mustadeer ash-shakl / baydhawi ash-shakl / murabba' ash-shakl

PT Branco / azul / verde / vermelho / castanho / cor-de-rosa e redondo / oval / quadrado

FK blan / ble / vet / wouj / mawon / woz ak won / oval / kare

EL άσπρο / μπλε / πράσινο / κόκκινο / καφέ / ροζ και στρογγυλό / οβάλ / τετράγωνο
Aspro / ble / prAseeno / kOkeeno / kafE / roz ke strogeelO / ovAl / tetrAgono

HI सफेद / नीला / हरा / लाल / भूरा / गुलाबी और गोल / अंडाकार / वर्गाकार
safed / neela / haraa / laal / bhoora / gulabi aur gol / andaakaar / vargakaar

How many did you (he / she) take?

ES ¿Cuántas tomó usted (él / ella)?

CH 你(他 / 她)吞咽了多少 ？
nǐ (tā / tā) tūn yàn le duō shǎo?

FR Combien en avez-vous (en a-t-il / elle) pris?

DE Wie viele haben Sie (hat er / sie) genommen?

VI Quý vị (anh ta / cô ta) đã dùng bao nhiêu viên?

IT Quante ne ha prese?

KO 당신은 (그는 / 그녀는) 몇 알 드셨습니까?
dang-si-neun (geu-neun / geu-nyeo-neun) myeot al deu-syeot-seum-ni-kka?

RU Сколько вы (он / она) приняли?
Skol'ko vy (on / ona) prinyali?

PL Ile ich Pan (on) wziął / Pani (ona) wzięła?

AR كم حبة اخذت (اخذ \ اخذت) ؟
Kam habbah akhadht (akhadh / akhadhat)?

PT Quantos é que você (ele / ela) tomou?

HK Konbyen ke ou (li) te pran?

EL Πόσα πήρατε (πήρε);
pOsa pEErate (pEEre)?

HI आपने (उसने) कितनी ली? …
Aapne (usne) kitni lee?

(not) many / the whole package / I do not know

ES	(no) muchas / todo el envase / no sé
ZH	(不) 多 / 整个包装 / 不清楚 (bù) duō / zhěng gè bāo zhuāng / bù qīng chǔ
FR	(pas) beaucoup / tout le paquet / Je ne sais pas
DE	(nicht) viele / die ganze Packung / ich weiß es nicht
VI	(không) nhiều / cả gói / tôi không biết
IT	(non) molte / l'intera scatola / non lo so
KO	(안)많이 / 한 통 다 / 모른다 (an)ma-ni / han tong da / mo-reun-da
RU	(не)много / всю упаковку / я не знаю (ne)mnogo / vsyu upakovku / ya ne znayu
PL	(nie)wiele / całe opakowanie / nie wiem
AR	(ليس) كثيرة \ كل الحبات \ لا ادري (Laysa) katheerah / kull al-habbaat / laa adri
PT	(não) muitos / a embalagem inteira / não sei
FK	(pa) anpil / tout paket la / mwen pa konnen
EL	(όχι) πολλά / ολόκληρη τη συσκευασία / Δεν γνωρίζω (Ohee) polA / olOkleeree tee seeskevasEEa / den gnorEEzo
HI	(नहीं) कई / पूरा पैकेट / मैं नहीं जानता (nahin) kayin / pura packet / main nahi jaanta

Do you have the packaging / container with you?

¿Trae usted la caja / el envase?

你有没有带来包装盒 / 瓶子？
nǐ yǒu méi yǒu dài lái bāo zhuāng hé / píng zǐ ?

Avez-vous l'emballage / la boite avec vous?

Haben Sie die Packung / den Behälter dabei?

Quý vị có mang theo gói / lọ thuốc đó không?

Ha portato la confezione / scatola con sè?

포장지 / 통을 가지고 오셨습니까?
po-jang-ji / tong-eul ga-ji-go o-syeot-seum-ni-kka?

У вас есть упаковка / контейнер с собой?
U vas est' upakovka / konteiner s soboy?

Czy ma Pan(i) to opakowanie / pojemnik przy sobie?

هل معك غلاف الحبات؟
Hal ma"ak ghilaaf al-habbaat?

Trouxe a embalagem / frasco consigo?

Eske ou te gen paket la / bwat la avèk ou?

Έχετε τη συσκευασία / το δοχείο μαζί σας;
Ehete tee seeskevasEEa / to dohEEo mazEE sas?

क्या आपके पास पैकेट / कंटेनर है?
Kya aapke paas packet / container hai?

Did you (he / she) vomit (the tablets)?

ES ¿Vomitó usted (él / ella) (las pastillas)?

ZH 你(他 / 她)有没有呕吐出（这些药片）？
nǐ (tā / tā) yǒu méi yǒu ǒu tù chū (zhè xiē yào piàn)?

FR Avez-vous (a-t-il / elle) vomi (les comprimés)?

DE Haben Sie (er / sie) (Tabletten) erbrochen?

VI Quý vị (anh ta / cô ta) có ói mửa (các viên thuốc) không?

IT Ha vomitato (le compresse)?

KO 당신은(그 / 그녀는) (정제들을) 토하셨습니까?
dang-si-neun(geu-neun / geu-nyeo-neun) (jeong-je-deu-reul) to-ha-syeot-seum-ni-kka?

RU Вы (он / она) вырвали (таблетки)?
Vy (on / ona) vyrvali (tabletki)?

PL Czy Pan (on) zwymiotował / Pani (ona) zwymiotowała (te tabletki)?

AR هل تقيأت (تقيأ \ تقيأت) بعد أخذ الحبات؟
Hal taqayya't (taqayya' / taqayya'at) ba"d akhdh al-habbat?

PT Você (ele / ela) vomitou (os comprimidos)?

FK Eske ou (li) te vomi (grenn lan)?

EL Κάνατε (έκανε) εμετό (τα δισκία);
kAnate (Ekane) emetO (ta deeskEEa)?

HI क्या आपने (उसने) उल्टी (गोलियाँ) की?
Kya aapne (usne) ulti (goliyan) ki?

Did you have him / her take something?

¿Le hizo tomar algo a él / ella?

你(他 / 她)有没有进食有什么？
nǐ (tā / tā) yǒu méi yǒu jìn shí shén me?

A-t-il / elle pris quelque chose?

Haben Sie ihm / ihr irgendetwas gegeben?

Quý vị có cho anh ta / cô ta dùng thứ gì không?

Ha preso qualcosa?

그 / 그녀가 뭔가를 먹도록 하셨습니까?
geu / geu-nyeo-ga mwon-ga-reul meok-do-rok ha-syeot-seum-ni-kka?

Вы давали ему / ей что-нибудь?
Vy davali emu / ey chto-nibud'?

Czy podał(a) mu / jej Pan(i) jakiś środek?

هل جعلته \ جعلتها يأخذ \ تأخذ شيئاً؟
Hal ja"althu / ja"althea ya'khudh / ta'khudh shay'an?

Deu alguma coisa para ele / ela tomar?

Eske ou fè l pran yon bagay?

Του / Της δώσατε να πάρει κάτι;
tu / tees dOsate na pAree kAtee?

क्या उसने कुछ खाया?
Kya Usne KuCh khaya?

water / milk / ipecac syrup / coal

ES	agua / leche / jarabe de ipecacuana / carbón
ZH	水 / 奶 / 吐根糖酱 / 活性碳 shuǐ / nǎi / tǔ gēn táng jiàng / huó xìng tàn
FR	de l'eau / du lait / du sirop d'ipéca / du charbon de bois
DE	Wasser / Milch / Brechwurz / Kohle
VI	Nước / sữa / xi-rô ipecac / than
IT	acqua / latte / sciroppo di ipecacuana / carbone
KO	물 / 우유 / 토근 시럽 / 석탄 mul / u-yu / to-geun si-reop / seok-tan
RU	вода / молоко / сироп рвотного корня / активированный уголь voda / moloko / sirop rvotnogo kornya / aktivirovannyi ugol'
PL	wodę / mleko / syrop z korzenia wymiotnego / węgiel
AR	الماء \ الحليب \ شراب الإيبيكاك \ الفحم Al-maa' / al-haliib / sharaab al-ipecac / al-fahhm
PT	Água / leite / xarope de ipecacuanha / carvão medicinal
FK	dlo / lèt / siwo ipecac / chabon
EL	νερό / γάλα / σιρόπι ιπεκακουάνας / ενεργό άνθρακα nerO / gAla / seerOpee eepekakuAnas / energO Anthraka
HI	पानी / दूध / आईपीकेक सीरप / कोयला paani / dudh / ipecac syrup / koyla

Do you (does he / she) have the following symptoms?

¿Tiene usted (él / ella) los síntomas siguientes?

你(他 / 她)有没有以下症状？
nǐ (tā / tā) yǒu méi yǒu yǐ xià zhèng zhuàng?

Avez-vous (a-t-il / elle) eu les symptômes suivants?

Haben Sie (er / sie) folgende Symptome?

Quý vị (anh ta / cô ta) có các triệu chứng sau đây không?

Ha i seguenti sintomi?

당신은 (그는 / 그녀는) 다음의 증상이 있습니까?
dang-si-neun (geu-neun / geu-nyeo-neun) da-eu-mui jeung-sang-i it-seum-ni-kka?

У вас (него / неё) есть следующие симптомы?
U vas (nego / neyo) est' sleduyushchie simptomy?

Czy Pan(i) (on / ona) ma następujące objawy?

هل تعاني \ تعانين (يعاني \ تعاني) من الأعراض التالية؟
Hal tu"aani / tu"aaneen (yu"aani / tu"aani) min al-a"araadh at-taaliyah?

Você (ele / ela) tem os seguintes sintomas?

Eske ou (eske li) gen youn nan sintòm swivan yo?

Έχετε (έχει) τα ακόλουθα συμπτώματα;
Ehete (Ehee) ta akOlutha seemptOmata?

क्या आपको (उसको) निम्नलिखित लक्षण हैं? ...
Kya aapko (usko) nimnlikhit lakShan hain?

dizziness attacks / headaches / abdominal pain

ES	mareos / dolor de cabeza / dolor abdominal
ZH	眩晕 / 头痛 / 腹痛 xuàn yūn / tóu tòng / fù tòng
FR	des vertiges / des maux de tête / des douleurs abdominales
DE	Schwindelanfälle / Kopfschmerzen / Bauchschmerzen
VI	các cơn chóng mặt / đau đầu / đau bụng
IT	attacchi di vertigine / mal di testa / dolore addominale
KO	현기증 발작 / 두통 / 복통 hyeon-gi-jeung bal-jak / du-tong / bok-tong
RU	приступы головокружения / головные боли / боль в животе pristupy golovokruzheniya / golovnye boli / bol' v zhivote
PL	zawroty głowy / ból głowy / ból brzucha
AR	حملات الدوخة \ الصداعات \ الأوجاع البطنية Hamlaat ad-doukhah / as-sudaa"aat / al-awjaa" al-batniyah
PT	Ataques de tonturas / dores de cabeça / dor abdominal
FK	vetij / maltèt / doulè nan vant
EL	κρίσεις ζάλης / πονοκέφαλους / κοιλιακό πόνο krEEsees zAlees / ponokEfalus / keeleeakO pOno
HI	चक्कर आना / सिर दर्द / पेट में दर्द Chakkar aana / sir dard / pet mein dard

8 Burns

What caused the burn?

S ¿Cómo se causó la quemadura?

H 是什么烧伤的？
shì shén me shāo shāng de?

R Qu'est-ce qui a causé cette brûlure?

E Was hat die Verbrennung verusacht?

T Quý vị bị bỏng do đâu?

O Cosa ha provocato l'ustione?

U 화상의 원인은 무엇입니까?
Hwa-sang-ui wo-ni-neun mu-eo-sim-ni-kka?

U Чем вызван ожог?
Chem vyzvan ozhog?

L Co spowodowało to oparzenie?

R ما هو الذي سبب الإحتراق؟
Maa huwa aladhi sabbab al-ihtiraaq?

T O que causou a queimadura?

K Ki sa ki lakòz ke ou boule?

L Τι προκάλεσε το έγκαυμα;
tee prokAlese to Egavma?

HI जलने का कारण क्या था? ...
Jalne ka kaaraN kya tha?

fire / the oven / hot water / chemicals

ES	fuego / el horno / agua caliente / productos químicos
ZH	火 / 炉子 / 热水 / 化学 huǒ / lú zǐ / rè shuǐ / huà xué
FR	le feu / le four / de l'eau chaude / des produits chimiques
DE	Feuer / der Ofen / heißes Wasser / Chemikalien
VI	lửa / lò hấp / nước nóng / hóa chất
IT	fuoco / forno / acqua calda / prodotti chimici
KO	불 / 오븐 / 뜨거운 물 / 화학물질 bul / o-beun / tteu-geo-un mul / hwa-hag-mul-jil
RU	пламенем / печкой / кипятком / химикатами plamenem / pechkoy / kipyatkom / khimikatami
PL	ogień / piekarnik / gorąca woda / środki chemiczne
AR	النار \ الفرن \ الماء الحار \ المواد الكيماوية An-naar / Al-furn / al-maa' al-haarr / al-mawwaad al-kimaawiyyah
PT	fogo / fogão / água quente / produtos químicos
FK	dife / fou / dlo cho / pwodwi chimik
EL	φωτιά / φούρνος / καυτό νερό / χημικά foteeA / fUrnos / kaftO nerO / heemeekA
HI	आग / ओवन / गर्म पानी / रसायन ... aag / oven / garam pani / rasaayan

lye / acid / hot fat / electric current

S lejía / ácido / grasa caliente / electricidad

H 碱 / 酸 / 热油 / 电击
jiǎn / suān / rè yóu / diàn jī

R une lessive / de l'acide / de la graisse chaude / du courant électrique

E Lauge / Säure / heißes Fett / Strom

VI kiềm / axit / mỡ nóng / dòng điện

T liscivia / acido / grasso caldo / corrente elettrica

O 잿물 / 염산 / 뜨거운 지방 / 전류
jaen-mul / yeom-san / tteu-geo-un ji-bang / jeol-lyu

U щелочью / кислотой / кипящим жиром / электрическим током
shcheloch'yu / kislotoy / kipyashchim zhirom / elektricheskim tokom

PL ług / kwas / gorący tłuszcz / prąd elektryczny

AR الغسول \ الحمض \ الدهن الحار \ تيار كهربائي
Al-ghusool / al-himdh / ad-dihn al-haarr / tayyar kahrubaa'ei

PT Lixívia / ácido / gordura quente / corrente eléctrica

K "lye" / asid / gres cho / kouran elektrik

EL καυστική ουσία / οξύ / καυτό λίπος / ηλεκτρικό ρεύμα
kafsteekEE usEEa / oxEE / kaftO IEEpos / eelektreekO revma

HI क्षार मिला पानी / तेजाब / गर्म वसा / विद्युतीय झटका
kShar mila paani / tezaab / garam vasaa / vidyutiya jhatka

Did you inhale the smoke?

ES ¿Respiró humo?

ZH 你有没有吸入浓烟？
nǐ yǒu méi yǒu xī rù nóng yān?

FR Avez-vous inhalé de la fumée?

DE Haben Sie den Rauch eingeatmet?

VI Quý vị có hít phải khói thuốc lá không?

IT Ha inalato il fumo?

KO 연기를 들이마셨습니까?
Yeon-gi-reul deu-ri-ma-syeot-seum-ni-kka?

RU Вы вдыхали дым?
Vy vdykhali dym?

PL Czy nawdychał(a) się Pan(i) dymu?

AR هل استنشقت الدخان؟
Hal istanshaqt ad-dukhaan?

PT Respirou o fumo?

FK Eske ou respire lafimin an?

EL Εισπνεύσατε τον καπνό;
eespnEfsate ton kapnO?

HI क्या आपने धूम्रपान किया था?
Kya aapne dhumrapaan kiya tha?

Did you / do you have breathing difficulties?

ES ¿Tuvo / tiene dificultad para respirar?

ZH 你当时 / 现在有没有呼吸困难？
nǐ dāng shí / xiàn zài yǒu méi yǒu hū xī kùn nán?

FR Avez-vous eu / avez-vous des difficultés respiratoires?

DE Hatten / haben Sie Atembeschwerden?

VI Quý vị có bị / đã bị khó thở không?

IT Ha avuto / ha difficoltà a respirare?

KO 호흡 곤란을 경험하셨습니까 / 경험하시고 계십니까?
Ho-heup gol-la-neul gyeong-heom-ha-syeot-seum-ni-kka / gyeong-heom-ha-si-go gye-sim-ni-kka?

RU У вас было / есть затруднение дыхания?
U vas bylo / est' zatrudnenie dykhaniya?

PL Czy miał(a) / ma Pan(i) trudności z oddychaniem?

AR هل كان عندك \ هل عندك صعوبات فى التنفس؟
Hal kaan "indak / hal "indak su"oobaat fit-tanaffus?

PT Teve / tem dificuldades respiratórias?

FK Eske out e / ou genye difikilte respire?

EL Είχατε / Έχετε δυσκολίες στην αναπνοή;
EEhate / Ehete deeskolEEes steen anapnoEE?

HI क्या आपको सांस लेने में कोई कठिनाई होती थी / है?
Kya aapko saans lene mein koi kaThinayee hoti thi / hai?

19 Dermal Problems, Allergies

Are you allergic to something?

ES	¿Es usted alérgico a algo?
ZH	你对什么东西过敏吗？ nǐ duì shén me dōng xī guò mǐn ma?
FR	Etes-vous allergique à quelque chose?
DE	Sind Sie gegen irgendetwas allergisch?
VI	Quý vị có bị dị ứng với thứ gì không?
IT	Ha qualche allergia?
KO	알레르기가 있으십니까? Al-le-reu-gi-ga i-seu-sim-ni-kka?
RU	У вас есть аллергия к чему-нибудь? U vas est' allergiya k chemu-nibud'?
PL	Czy jest Pan(i) na cokolwiek uczulony(a)?
AR	هل عندك حساسية لشيء من الأشياء؟ Hal "indak hassaasiyyah li-shay' min al-ashyaa'?
PT	É alérgico(a) a alguma coisa?
FK	Eske ou aleji ak okinn bagay?
EL	Είστε αλλεργικοί σε κάτι; EEste alergeekEE se kAtee?
HI	क्या आपको किसी चीज से एलर्जी है? .. Kya aapko kisi cheez se allergy hai?

Have you ever taken penicillin?

¿Lo han tratado alguna vez con penicilina?

以前用过青霉素吗？
yǐ qián yòng guò qīng méi sù ma?

Avez-vous jamais pris de la pénicilline?

Haben Sie schon einmal Penicillin genommen?

Quý vị đã bao giờ uống penicillin chưa?

Ha mai assunto la penicillina?

페니실린을 투약 받으신 적이 있습니까?
Pe-ni-sil-li-neul tu-yak ba-deu-sin jeo-gi it-seum-ni-kka?

Вы когда-нибудь принимали пенициллин?
Vy kogda-nibud' prinimali penitsillin?

Czy przyjmował(a) Pan(i) kiedykolwiek penicylinę?

هل سبق لك أخذ دواء البينيسيلين؟
Hal sabaq lak akhdh dawaa' al-penicilin?

Já alguma vez tomou penicilina?

Eske out e janm pran penisylin?

Έχετε πάρει ποτέ πενικιλίνη;
Ehete pAree potE peneekeelEEnee?

क्या आपने कभी पेंसिलिन ली है?
Kya aapne kabhi pencillin lee hai?

Have you been bitten / stung?

ES ¿Recibió alguna mordedura / picadura?

ZH 你被咬过 / 蜇过吗？
nǐ bèi yǎo guò / zhē guò ma?

FR Avez-vous été mordu(e), piqué(e)?

DE Wurden Sie gebissen / gestochen?

VI Quý vị có bao giờ bị cắn / đốt không?

IT È stato morso / a punto / a?

KO 물리신 적이 있습니까 / 쏘인 적이 있습니까?
Mul-li-sin jeo-gi it-seum-ni-kka / sso-in jeo-gi it-seum-ni-kka?

RU Вас когда-нибудь кусали / жалили?
Vas kogda-nibud' kusali / zhalili?

PL Czy ugryzł / ukąsił Pana (Panią) ?

AR هل اصيب بعضة \ بلدغة؟
Hal usibt bi-"adhdhah / ladghah?

PT Já foi mordido(a) / picado(a) por?

FK Eske yon bèt te janm mode w / pike w?

EL Σας δάγκωσε / τσίμπησε κάτι;
sas dAgose / tsEEbeese kAti?

HI क्या आपको कभी किसी ने काटा / दंश मारा है? ...
Kya aapko kabhi kisi ne kata / dansh mara hai?

tick / spider / (poisonous) snake / bee / wasp / scorpion

S garrapata / araña / víbora (venenosa) / abeja / avispa / escorpión (alacrán)

H 虱子 / 蜘蛛 / 毒蛇 / 蜜蜂 / 大黄蜂 / 蝎子
shī zǐ / zhī zhū / dú shé / mì fēng / dà huáng fēng / xiē zǐ

R tiques / araignée (venimeuse) / serpent / abeille / guêpe / scorpion

E Zecke / Spinne / (Gift)Schlange / Biene / Wespe / Skorpion

T bọ ve / nhện / rắn (độc) / ong / ong bắp cày / bọ cạp

T zecca / ragno / serpente (velenoso) / ape / vespa / scorpione

O 진드기 / 거미 / (독) 뱀 / 벌 / 말벌 / 전갈
jin-deug-i / geo-mi / (dok) baem / beol / mal-beol / jeon-gal

U клещи / пауки / (ядовитые) змеи / пчелы / осы / скорпионы
kleshchi / pauki / (yadovitye) zmei / pchyoly / osy / skorpiony

L kleszcz / pająk / (jadowity) wąż / pszczoła / osa / skorpion

R من قبل قردان (حشرة صغيرة تمص الدم) \ عنكبوت \ ثعبان (سام) \ نحلة \ دبور \ عقرب
Min qibal qirdaan (hasharah sagheerah tamuss ad-damm) / ankaboot / thu"baan (saamm) / nahlah / dabbour / "aqrab

T carraça / aranha / cobra (venenosa) / abelha / vespa / escorpião

K tik / areniye / koulev (ki gen pwazon) / abbey / gep / skorpyon

L τσιμπούρι / αράχνη / (δηλητηριώδες) φίδι / μέλισσα / σφήκα / σκορπιός
tseebUree / arAhnee / (deeleeteereeOdes) fEEdee / mEleesa / sfEEka / skorpeeOs

H चिचड़ा / मकड़ी / (जहरीली) सांप / मक्खी / ततैया / बिच्छू
ChichDa / makDi / (Jaherili) saanp / makkhi / tataiya / biChhu

What symptoms do you have?

ES ¿Qué molestias tiene?

ZH 你有什么不适表现？
nǐ yǒu shén me bù shì biǎo xiàn?

FR Quels symptômes avez-vous ressentis?

DE Welche Symptome haben Sie?

VI Quý vị có những triệu chứng nào?

IT Che sintomi ha?

KO 어떤 증상이 있으십니까?
Eo-tteon jeung-sang-i i-seu-sim-ni-kka?

RU Какие у вас симптомы?
Kakie u vas simptomy?

PL Jakie ma Pan(i) objawy?

AR ما هي الأعراض التي تعاني \ تعانين منها؟
Maa hiya al-a"raadh alati tu"aani / tu"aaneen minha?

PT Que sintomas tem?

FK Ki sintòm ou te genyen?

EL Τι συμπτώματα έχετε;
tee seemptOmata Ehete?

HI आपको कौन–कौन से लक्षण हैं? ...
Aapko kaun-kaun se lakshaN hain?

Did you eat / inhale anything unusual?

¿Inhaló alguna cosa fuera de lo común?

你当时有没有吃下 / 吸入什么异物？
nǐ dāng shí yǒu méi yǒu chī xià / xǐ rù shén me yì wù?

Avez-vous mangé / inhalé quelque chose d'inhabituel?

Haben Sie etwas Ungewöhnliches gegessen / eingeatmet?

Quý vị có ăn / hít phải vật gì bất thường không?

Ha mangiato / inalato qualcosa di insolito?

보통 안먹고 안흡입하는 것을 먹었습니까 / 흡입하셨습니까?
Bo-tong an-meok-go an-heu-bip-ha-neun—geo-seul meo-geot-seum-ni-kka /
heu-bip-ha-syeot-seum-ni-kka?

Вы съели / вдохнули что-нибудь необычное?
Vy s"eli / vdokhnuli chto-nibud' neobychnoe?

Czy jadł / wdychał(a) Pan(i) coś niezwykłego?

كل أكلت \ تنفست شيئاً غير عادٍ؟
Hal akalt / tanaffast shay'an ghayr "aadi?

Comeu / aspirou algo de invulgar?

Eske ou te manje / resoire yon bagay ki anomal?

Φάγατε / Εισπνεύσατε κάτι ασυνήθιστο;
fAgate / eespEfsate kAtee aseenEEtheesto?

क्या आपने कुछ असा धारण खाया / निगला?
Kya aapne kuchh asadharaN khaya / nigla?

Are you using a new kind of soap?

ES ¿Está usando un nuevo tipo de jabón?

ZH 你现在有没有使用新牌子的香皂？
nĭ xiàn zài yŏu méi yŏu shĭ yòng xīn pái zi de xiāng zào?

FR Utilisez-vous un nouveau genre de savon?

DE Verwenden Sie eine neue Seife?

VI Có phải là quý vị đang dùng loại xà bông mới không?

IT Sta utilizzando un nuovo tipo di sapone?

KO 비누를 바꾸셨습니까?
Bi-nu-reul ba-kku-syeot-seum-ni-kka?

RU Вы сейчас пользуетесь новым мылом?
Vy seichas pol'zuetes' novym mylom?

PL Czy używa Pan(i) nowego rodzaju mydła?

AR هل تستعمل \ تستعملين نوعاً جديداً من الصابون؟
Hal tasta"mil / tasta"mileen nau"an jadeedan min as-saaboon?

PT Está a usar um tipo de sabonete novo?

FK Eske ou ap sevi ak yon nouvo kalite savon?

EL Χρησιμοποιείτε κάποιο καινούργιο σαπούνι;
hreeseemopeeEEte kApeeo kenUrgeeo sapUnee?

HI क्या आप नए प्रकार का साबुन प्रयोग कर रहे हैं?
Kya aap naye prakaar ka sabun prayog kar rahe hain?

Do you have pets?

¿Tiene animales en casa?

你养宠物吗？
nǐ yǎng chǒng wù ma?

Avez-vous des animaux domestiques?

Haben Sie Haustiere?

Quý vị có thú nuôi không?

Ha animali?

애완동물이 있으십니까?
Ae-wan-dong-mur-i i-seu-sim-ni-kka?

У вас есть домашние животные?
U vas est' domashnie zhivotnye?

Czy ma Pan(i) zwierzęta domowe?

هل عندك حيوانات منزلية؟
Hal "indak hayawaanaat manziliyyah?

Tem animais de estimação?

Eske ou gen zanimo domestic lakay ou?

Έχετε κατοικίδια ζώα;
Ehete kateekEEdeea zOa?

क्या आपके घर में पालतू जानवर है? ...
Kya aapke ghar mein paltu jaanwar hain?

cats / dogs / birds / rabbits / guinea pigs / hamsters

ES	gatos / perros / pájaros / conejos / cuyos (cobayas) / hámsters
ZH	猫 / 狗 / 鸟 / 兔子 / 豚鼠 / 仓鼠 Mão / gǒu / niǎo / tù zi / tún shǔ / cāng shǔ
FR	chats / chiens / oiseaux / lapins / cobayes / hamsters
DE	Katzen / Hunde / Vögel / Hasen / Meerschweinchen / Hamster
VI	mèo / chó / chim / thỏ / chuột lang / chuột đồng
IT	gatti / cani / uccelli / conigli / porcellini d'india / criceti
KO	고양이 / 개 / 새 / 토끼 / 모르모트 / 햄스터 Go-yang-i / gae / sae / to-kki / mo-reu-mo-teu / haem-seu-teo
RU	кошки / собаки / птицы / кролики / морские свинки / хомяки koshki / sobaki / ptitsy / kroliki / morskie svinki / khomyaki
PL	koty / psy / ptaki / króliki / świnki morskie / chomiki
AR	قطاً \ كلباً \ طيوراً \ ارانباً هنديةً \ جرذان الهامستر Qittan / kalban / tuyooran / araniban hindiyan / jurdhaan al-hamster
PT	gatos / cães / pássaros / coelhos / porquinhos da Índia / hamsters
FK	chat / chyen / zwezo / lapin / kobay / hamster
EL	γάτες / σκύλους / πουλιά / κουνέλια / ινδικά χοιρίδια / χάμστερ gAtes / skEElus / puleeA / kunEleea / eendeekA heerEEdeea / hAmster
HI	बिल्लियां / कुत्ते / पक्षी / खरगोश / गिनी पिग / हैम्सटर billi / kutte / pakShi / KhargoSh / gini pigs / hamsters

Where is the skin rash located?

¿Dónde le salió esa erupción?

皮疹在哪里？
pí zhěn zài nǎ li?

Où était localisée l'éruption cutanée

Wo haben Sie den Hautausschlag?

Các vết nổi mẩn trên da xuất hiện ở đâu?

Dove si trova l'eruzione cutanea?

어디에 피부 발진이 있습니까?
Eo-di-e pi-bu bal-ji-ni it-seum-ni-kka?

В каких местах кожа покрыта сыпью?
V kakikh mestakh kozha pokryta syp'yu?

Gdzie jest umiejscowiona wysypka?

أين الطفح موجود على الجلد؟
Ayn at-tafah maujood "alaa al-jild?

Onde está localizada a erupção cutânea?

Kote iritasyon po a localize?

Πού βρίσκεται το δερματικό εξάνθημα;
pu vrEEskete to dermateekO exAntheema?

त्वचा पर चकत्ता कहां है?
Twacha par Chskatta kahaan hai?

20 Tropical Medicine, Fever

Did you travel do a tropical area / country? Specify travel destination.

ES ¿Viajó a alguna región / país tropical? Indíqueme el lugar de destino

ZH 你有没有到过热带地区 / 国家？具体到过
nǐ yǒu méi yǒu dào guò rè dài dì qū / guó jiā? jù tǐ dào guò

FR Avez-vous voyagé dans une région tropicale / dans un pays tropical? Spécifiez la destination du voyage?

DE Waren Sie in einem tropischen Gebiet / Land? In welchem?

VI Quý vị có đi du lịch tới một quốc gia / vùng nhiệt đới không? Cho biết nơi tới.

IT Ha viaggiato in una zona / un paese tropicale? Specificare la destinazione del viaggio

KO 열대 지역 / 국가로 여행하셨습니까? 여행 목적지를 밝혀주십시오
Yeol-dae ji-yeok / guk-ga-ro yeo-haeng-ha-syeot-seum-ni-kka? Yeo-haeng mok-jeok-ji-reul bal-kyeo-ju-sip-si-o

RU Вы бывали в тропической зоне / стране? Уточните, где именно
Vy byvali v tropicheskoy zone / strane? Utochnite, gde imenno

PL Czy podróżował(a) Pan(i) do tropikalnych miejsc / krajów? Proszę podać konkretne miejsce.

AR هل سافرت إلى منطقة \ دولة إستوائية؟ بين \ بيني مكان السفر.
Hal saafart ilaa mantiqah / Dulah istiwaa'iyyah? Bayyin / bayyinee makaan as-safar.

PT Viajou para uma região / país tropical? Especifique o local de destino da viagem.

FK Eske ou vwayaje al nan yon zon twopikal / payi? Di egzakteman kibo

EL Ταξιδέψατε σε τροπική περιοχή / χώρα; Καθορίστε τον προορισμό του ταξιδιού.
taxeedEpsate se tropeekEE pereeohEE / hOra? kathorEEste ton prooreesmO tu taxeedeeU?

HI क्या आपने उष्णकटिबंधिय ६ ।ीय क्षेत्र / देश की यात्रा की? यात्रा करने वाला स्थान स्पष्ट करें ...
kya aapne uShNkatibandhiya kshetra / desh ki yatra ki? yatra karane wala sthaan spaSt karein

When did you visit and for how long?

¿Cuándo estuvo ahí y por cuánto tiempo?

你什么时候去的，呆了多久？
nǐ shén me shí hòu qù de, dāi le duō jiǔ?

Quand avez-vous visité et combien de temps?

Wann waren Sie dort und wie lange?

Quý vị tới đó khi nào và ở trong bao lâu?

Quando c'è stato e quanto a lungo?

언제 방문하셨고 얼마나 오래?
Eon-je bang-mun-ha-syeot-go eol-ma-na o-rae?

Когда вы там были и как долго находились?
Kogda vy tam byli i kak dolgo nakhodilis'?

Kiedy Pan(i) tam był(a) i na jak długo?

متى قمت بالزيارة ولكم مدة؟
Mattaa qumt biz-ziyaarah wa li-kam muddah?

Quando visitou e durante quanto tempo?

Ki lè ou te al vizite la e pou konbyen tan?

Πότε την επισκεφτήκατε και για πόσο καιρό;
pOte teen epeeskeftEEkate ke geea pOso kerO?

आप कहां गए और कितनी अवधि के लिए?
aap kahan gaye aur kitni avdhi ke liye?

How did you travel?

ES ¿Con quién viajó usted?

ZH 你是怎么去的？
nǐ shi zěn me qù de?

FR Comment avez-vous voyagé?

DE Wie sind Sie gereist?

VI Quý vị đi như thế nào?

IT Come ha viaggiato?

KO 어떻게 여행하셨습니까?
Eo-tteo-ke yeo-haeng-ha-syeot-seum-ni-kka?

RU С кем вы ездили?
S kem vy ezdili?

PL W jaki sposób Pan(i) podróżował(a)?

AR كيف سافرت؟
Kayf saafart?

PT Viajou como?

FK Kijan ou te vwayaje?

EL Πώς ταξιδέψατε;
pos taxeedEpsate?

HI आपने यात्रा कैसे की? ...
aapne yatra kaise ki

alone / with a companion / group

solo / con un acompañante / en grupo

一个人 / 同伴 / 随旅行团
yī gè rén / tóng bàn / suí lǚ xíng tuán

seul(e) / avec un compagnon / en groupe

alleine / zu zweit / in der Gruppe

một mình / đi cùng người khác / đi theo nhóm

solo / a / con un compagno / a / gruppo

혼자 / 다른 한 명하고 / 그룹으로
hon-ja / da-reun han myeong-ha-go / geu-ru-beu-ro

один / с компаньоном / с группой
odin / s kompan'yonom / s gruppoy

sam(a) / z towarzyszem (towarzyszką) / w grupie

لحالك \ مع رفيق \ مع جماعة
Lihaalak / ma" rafeeq / ma" jamaa"ah

só / com um(a) companheiro(a) / em grupo

poukont ou / ak yon moun / ak yon gwoup

μόνος / με συνοδό / ομάδα
mOnos / me seenodO / omAda

अकेले / मित्र के साथ / समूह में
akele / mitra ke saath / samooh mein

Did any health problems occur during your travel?

ES	¿Se presentaron problemas de salud durante el viaje?
ZH	你在旅行过程中得了什么病吗？ nǐ zài lǚ xíng guò chéng zhōng dé le shén me bìng ma?
FR	Avez-vous eu des problèmes de santé au cours de ce voyage?
DE	Sind Beschwerden während der Reise aufgetreten?
VI	Quý vị có gặp vấn đề sức khỏe nào khi đi du lịch không?
IT	Ha avuto problemi di salute durante il viaggio?
KO	여행하는 동안 건강상 문제가 발생했습니까? Yeo-haeng-ha-neun dong-an geon-gang-sang mun-je-ga bal-saeng-haet-seum-ni-kka?
RU	Были ли у вас проблемы со здоровьем во время этой поездки? Byli li u vas problemy so zdorov'em vo vremya etoy poezdki?
PL	Czy podczas podróży zaistniały jakieś problemy zdrowotne?
AR	هل وقعت اية مشاكل صحية أثناء السفر؟ Hal waqa"at ayyi mashaakil sihhiyyah athnaa as-safar?
PT	Teve alguns problemas de saúde durante a sua viagem?
FK	Pandan vwayaj ou eske te gen okinn pwoblè medikal ?
EL	Παρουσιάστηκαν προβλήματα υγείας κατά τη διάρκεια του ταξιδιού; paruseeAsteekan provlEEmata eegEEas katA tee deeArkeea tu taxeedeeU?
HI	क्या आपकी यात्रा के दौरान कोई समस्या हुई? ... kya aapki yatra ke dauraan koi samasya hui?

fever / diarrhea / skin changes / weight loss / constipation

fiebre / diarrea / cambios en la piel / pérdida de peso / estreñimiento

发烧 / 腹泻 / 皮肤变化 / 体重减轻 / 便秘
fā shāo / fù xiè / pí fū biàn huà / tǐ zhòng jiǎn qīng / biàn mì

fièvre / diarrhée / modifications cutanées / perte de poids / constipation

Fieber / Durchfall / Hautveränderungen / Gewichtsverlust / Blähungen

sốt / tiêu chảy / thay đổi về da / giảm cân / táo bón

febbre / diarrea / cambiamenti della pelle / perdita di peso / stipsi

열 / 설사 / 피부 변화 / 체중 감소 / 변비
yeol / seol-sa / pi-bu byeon-hwa / che-jung gam-so / byeon-bi

повышение температуры / понос / изменения кожи / потеря веса / запоры
povyshenie temperatury / ponos / izmeneniya kozhi / poterya vesa / zapory

gorączka / biegunka / zmiany skórne / strata na wadze / zaparcie

الحمى \ الإسهال \ التغيرات في الجلد \ خفض الوزن \ الإمساك
Al-Hummaa / al-is'haal / at-taghyeeraat fil-jild / khafdh il-wazn / al-imsaak

febre / diarreia / alterações da pele / perda de peso / prisão de ventre

lafyev / dyare / chanjman nan po / megri.konstipasyon

πυρετός / διάρροια / δερματικές αλλαγές / απώλεια βάρους / δυσκοιλιότητα
peeretOs / deeAreea / dermateekEs alagEs / apOleea vArus / deeskeeleeOteeta

बुखार / अतिसार / त्वचा में परिवर्तन / वज़न में कमी / कब्ज ....
bukhaar / atisaar / twacha mein parivartan / vazan mein kami / kabz

belching / abdominal pain / blood in urine / urethral discharge

ES eructos / dolor abdominal / sangre en la orina / secreción por la uretra

ZH 打嗝 / 腹痛 / 血尿 / 尿道有分泌物
dǎ gé / fù tòng / xiě niào / niào dào yǒu fēn mì wù

FR des éructations / de la douleur abdominale / du sang dans les urines / des éliminations urétrales

DE Aufstoßen / Bauchschmerzen / Blut im Urin / Ausfluss aus Harnröhre

VI ợ / đau bụng / nước tiểu có máu / niệu đạo có tiết dịch mủ

IT eruttazione / dolori addominali / sangue nelle urine / secrezione uretrale

KO 트림 / 배가 아픔 / 통증 / 소변에 피가 섞임 / 요도 분비물
teu-rim / bae-ga a-peum / tong-jeung / so-byeon-e pi-ga seok-kim / yodo bun-bi-mul

RU отрыжка / боль в животе / кровь в моче / выделения из мочеиспускательного канала
otryzhka / bol' v zhivote / krov' v moche / vydeleniya iz mocheispuskatel'nogo kanala

PL odbijanie się / ból brzucha / krew w moczu / wydzielina z cewki moczowej

AR التجشؤ \ الألم البطني \ الدم في البول \ إفراز إحليلي
At-tajashshu' / al-alam al-batni / ad-damm fil-baul / ifraaz ihleeli

PT Eructações ou arrotos / dor abdominal / sangue na urina / prurido uretral

FK ran gaz / doulè nan vant / san nan pipi / dechaj uretral

EL ρέψιμο / κοιλιακός πόνος / αίμα στα ούρα / ουρηθρικές εκκρίσεις
rEpseemo / keeleeakOs pOnos / Ema sta Ura / ureethreekEs ekrEEsees

HI डकार आना / पेट में दर्द होना / पेशाब में खून आना / मूत्रमार्गीय स्राव ...
dakaar aana / pet mein dard hona / peshab mein khoon aana / mutramargiya sraav

burning sensation during urination / breathing difficulties / sputum

ES ardor al orinar / dificultad para respirar / expectoración (esputo)

ZH 小便时烧灼感 / 呼吸困难 / 多痰
xiǎo biàn shí shāo zhuó gǎn / hū xī kùn nán / duō tán

FR sensation de brûlure au cours de la miction / des difficultés respiratoires / des crachats

DE Brennen beim Wasserlassen / Atemnot / Husten / Auswurf

VI cảm giác bỏng rát khi tiểu tiện / khó thở / có đờm

IT bruciore durante l'urinazione / difficoltà a respirare / espettorato

KO 소변볼 때 쓰린 느낌 / 호흡 곤란 / 침
so-byeon-bol ttae sseu-rin neu-kkim / ho-heup gol-lan / chim

RU жжение при мочеиспускании / затруднение дыхания / мокрота
zhzhenie pri mocheispuskanii / zatrudnenie dykhaniya / mokrota

PL uczucie pieczenia podczas oddawania moczu / trudności w oddychaniu / flegma

AR إحساس إحتراق أثناء التبول \ الصعوبات في التنفس \ البلغم
Ihsaas ihtiraaq athnaa' at-tabawwul / as-su"oobaat fit-tanaffus / al-balgham

PT sensação de ardor durante a micção / dificuldades respiratórias / expectoração

FK sansasyon boule lè ou ap pipi / difikilte respire / kracha

EL αίσθημα καύσου κατά την ούρηση / αναπνευστικές δυσκολίες / πτύελα
Estheema kAfsu katA teen Ureesee / anapnefsteekEs deeskolEEes / ptEEela

HI पेशाब के दौरान ज्वलन संवेदना / सांस लेने में कठिनाई / बलगम
peshaab ke dauran jwalan samvedna / sans lene mein kaThinai / balgam

Do you presently have health problems? Please pecify.

ES ¿Tiene actualmente problemas de salud? Por favor especifique

ZH 你目前有健康问题吗？请具体说明
nǐ mù qián yǒu jiàn kāng wèn tí ma? qǐng jù tǐ shuō míng

FR Avez-vous des problèmes de santé pour le moment? S'il vous plaît veuillez spécifier

DE Haben Sie jetzt Beschwerden? Welche?

VI Quý vị hiện có gặp vấn đề sức khỏe nào không? Xin trình bày rõ.

IT Ha problemi di salute al momento? Specificare, per favore

KO 현재 건강상 문제가 있으십니까? 구체적으로 밝혀주십시오
Hyeon-jae geon-gang-sang mun-je-ga i-seu-sim-ni-kka? Gu-che-jeo-geu-ro bal-kyeo-ju-sip-si-o

RU У вас сейчас есть проблемы со здоровьем? Пожалуйста, уточните.
U vas seychas est' problemy so zdorov'em? Pozhaluysta, utochnite.

PL Czy obecnie ma Pan(i) kłopoty ze zdrowiem? Proszę je bliżej opisać.

AR هل تعاني \ تعانين من مشاكل صحية حالياً؟ الرجاء بيانها.
Hal tu"aani / tu"aaneen min mashaakil sihhiyyah haaliyan? Ar-rajaa' bayaanhaa.

PT Presentemente, tem problemas de saúde? Especifique, por favor.

FK Kounye la eske ou gen okinn pwoblèm lasante ? Tanpri spesifye kisa

EL Έχετε επί του παρόντος προβλήματα υγείας; Παρακαλώ καθορίστε.
Ehete epEE tu parOdos provlEEmata eegEEas? parakalO kathorEEste

HI क्या अभी आपको कोई स्वास्थ्य समस्या है? कृपया स्पष्ट करें ...
kya abhi aapko koi swasthya samasya hai? kripya spaSt karein

If you have diarrhea, how many bowel evacuations occur per day / night?

ES Si tiene diarrea, ¿cuántas evacuaciones tiene cada día / noche?

ZH 你如果有腹泻， 一天 / 一夜有几次？
nǐ rú guǒ yǒu fù xiè, yī tiān / yī yè yǒu jǐ cì?

FR Si vous avez de la diarrhée, combien d'évacuations par jour / par nuit?

DE Wenn Sie Durchfall haben, Anzahl Entleerungen tags / nachts?

VI Nếu quý vị bị tiêu chảy, quý vị đi bao nhiêu lần vào ban ngày / đêm?

IT Se ha la diarrea, quante evacuazioni fa al giorno / notte?

KO 설사를 하신다면, 하루에 / 하루 밤에 몇 번이나 설사를 하십니까?
Seol-sa-reul ha-sin-da-myeon, ha-ru-e / ha-ru ba-me myeot Beo-ni-na seol-sa-reul ha-sim-ni-kka?

RU Если у вас понос, сколько раз вы испражняетесь в течение дня / ночи?
Esli u vas ponos, skol'ko raz vy isprazhnyaetes' v techenie dnya / nochi?

PL Jeśli ma Pan(i) biegunkę, to ile wypróżnień ma miejsce w ciągu dnia / nocy?

AR إذا كان عندك إسهال، كم مرة يحدث إفراغ الغائط فى اليوم \ فى الليل؟
Idhaa kaan "indak is'haal, kam marrah yahduth ifraagh al-ghaa'it fil-youm / fil-leyl?

PT Se tem diarreia, quantas evacuações intestinais ocorrem durante o dia / a noite?

FK Si ou ta gen dyare, konbyen fwa ou al nan watè pa jou / lan nwit ?

EL Εάν έχετε διάρροια, πόσες εκκενώσεις συμβαίνουν κατά την ημέρα / νύχτα;
eAn Ehete deeAreea, pOses ekenOsees seemvEnun katA teen eemEra / nEEhta?

HI यदि आपको अतिसार है, दिन ⁄ रात में कितनी बार दस्त आते हैं? …
yadi aapko atisaar hai, din / raat mein kitni baar dast aate hain?

watery / mushy / bloody / black / pale

ES	acuosas / blandas / con sangre / negras / pálidas
ZH	水样的 / 糊状的 / 带血的 / 黑色的 / 灰白的 shuǐ yàng de / hú zhuàng de / dài xiě de / hēi sè de / huī bái de
FR	aqueuse / mousseuse / sanguinolente / noire / pâle
DE	wässrig / breiig / blutig / schwarz / hell
VI	lỏng / sền sệt / có máu / màu đen / màu xanh xám
IT	acquose / molli / con tracce di sangue / nere / chiare
KO	묽은 / 진 / 피가 섞인 / 검은 / 색이 연한 mul-geun / jin / pi-ga seo-kkin / geo-meun / sae-gi yeon-han
RU	водянистый / кашеобразный / кровянистый / черный / светлый vodyanistyi / kasheobraznyi / krovyanistyi / chernyi / svetlyi
PL	wodnista / papkowata / krwawa / czarna / blada
AR	غائط مائي \ لزج \ دام \ أسود \ شاحب اللون Ghaa'it maa'I / lazij / daami / aswad / shaahib al-loun
PT	aquosas / moles / sanguinolentas / escuras / claras
FK	likid / kouwè pat / gen san / nwa / pal
EL	υδαρή / χυλώδης / αιματώδης / μαύρη / ωχρή eedarEE / heelOdees / ematOdees / mAvree / ohrEE
HI	पानी युक्त / गूदेदार / रक्तयुक्त / काले / पीले paani yukt / goodedaar / raktayukt / kale / pile

Have additional fellow travelers fallen ill? How many?

¿Se enfermaron también compañeros de viaje? ¿Cuántos?

与你一起旅行的人还有人病吗？有几个？
yǔ nǐ yì qǐ lǚ xíng de rén hái yǒu rén bìng ma? yǒu jǐ gè?

D'autres compagnons de voyage sont-ils tombés malades? Combien?

Sind weitere Reiseteilnehmer erkrankt? Wie viele?

Có người nào đi du lịch cùng với quý vị cũng bị ốm không? Bao nhiêu người?

Si sono ammalate altre persone che viaggiavano con Lei? Quante?

같이 여행간 사람 중에도 병이 난 사람이 있습니까? 몇 명입니까?
Ga-chi yeo-haeng-gan sa-ram jung-e-do byeong-i nan sa-ra-mi it-seum-ni-kka?
Myeot myeong-im-ni-kka?

Кто-нибудь из участников поездки заболел? Сколько человек?
Kto-nibud' iz uchastnikov poezdki zabolel! Skol'ko chelovek?

Czy inni uczestnicy wycieczki także się rozchorowali? Ile osób?

هل اصيب من رفاقك الآخرين على السفر بمرض؟ كم فرد؟
Hal useeb min rifaaqak al-aakhareen "alaa as-safar bi-maradh? Kam fard?

Outros companheiros de viagem adoeceram? Quantos deles?

Eske te gen lòt moun ki tap vwayaje vin malad tou? Konbyen ladan yo?

Αρρώστησαν συνταξιδιώτες σας; Πόσοι;
arOsteesan seentaxeedeeOtes sas? pOsee?

क्या आपके अन्य साथी यात्री बीमार हैं? कितने?
kya aapke anya saathi yatri beemaar hain? kitne?

Do you have fever? Since when? How high?

ES ¿Ha tenido fiebre (calentura)? ¿Desde cuándo? ¿Qué tan alta?

ZH 你发烧吗？从什么时候开始？烧到多少度？
nǐ fā shāo ma? cóng shén me shí hòu kāi shǐ? shāo dào duō shǎo dù?

FR Avez-vous de la fièvre? Depuis quand? De quel niveau?

DE Haben Sie Fieber? Seit wann? Wie hoch?

VI Quý vị có bị sốt không? Kể từ khi nào? Nhiệt độ cao bao nhiêu?

IT Ha la febbre? Da quando? Quanto alta?

KO 열이 있으십니까? 언제부터? 열이 얼마나 됩니까?
Yeo-ri i-seu-ni-kka? Eon-je-bu-teo? Yeo-ri eol-ma-na doem-ni-kka?

RU У вас повышена температура? Как долго? Насколько она высокая?
U vas povyshena temperatura? Kak dolgo? Naskol'ko ona vysokaya?

PL Czy ma Pan(i) gorączkę? Od jak dawna? Ile stopni?

AR هل عندك حمى؟ منذ متى؟ كم درجة حرارة الحمى؟
Hal "indak hummaa? Mundhu mattaa? Kam darajat haraarah al-hummaa?

PT Tem febre? Há quanto tempo? Qual é a intensidade?

FK Eske ou gen lafyev? Depi kilè? Kisa tanperati a ye?

EL Έχετε πυρετό; Από πότε; Πόσο υψηλός;
Ehete peeretO? apO pOte? pOso eepseelOs?

HI क्या आपको बुखार है? कबसे? कितना?
kya aapko bukhaar hai? kabse? kitna?

Do you have shaking chills?

¿Ha tenido escalofríos?

你有打寒颤吗？
nǐ yǒu dǎ hán zhàn ma?

Avez-vous des frissons?

Haben Sie Schüttelfrost?

Quý vị có những cơn lạnh run không?

Ha brividi di freddo?

오한이 나서 떨리십니까?
O-ha-ni na-seo tteol-li-sim-ni-kka?

Вас знобит?
Vas znobit?

Czy ma Pan(i) dreszcze?

هل تعاني \ تعانين من رعشات؟
Hal tu"aani / tu"aaneen min ra"shaat?

Tem calafrios acompanhados de tremores?

Eske ou gen frison?

Έχετε ρίγος;
Ehete rEEgos?

क्या आपको कंपाने वाली सर्दी लगती है?
kya aapko kampaane wali sardi lagti hai?

Did you take anti-malarial medication?

ES ¿Tomó algún medicamento contra la malaria (antipalúdicos)?

ZH 你吃过抗疟疾的药吗？
nǐ chī guò kàng nüè jí de yào ma?

FR Avez-vous suivi un traitement antimalarique?

DE Haben Sie eine Malariaprophylaxe genommen?

VI Quý vị có dùng thuốc chống sốt rét không?

IT Ha seguito la profilassi antimalarica?

KO 항 말라리아 약을 드셨습니까?
Hang mal-la-ri-a ya-geul deu-syeot-seum-ni-kka?

RU Вы принимали противомалярийное лекарство?
Vy prinimali protivomalyariynoe lekarstvo?

PL Czy przyjmowała Pani leki na malarię?

AR هل تأخذ / تأخذين أدوية مضادة للملاريا؟
Hal ta"khudh / ta'khudheen adwiyah mudhaaddah lil-malaria?

PT Tomou o medicamento contra a malária?

FK Eske ou te pran medikaman kont malaria?

EL Λάβατε φάρμακα κατά της ελονοσίας;
lavAte fArmaka katA tees elonosEEas?

HI क्या आपने मलेरिया-रोधी दवाई ली थी?
kya aapne maleriya-rodhi dawai li thi?

Lariam / Mephaquin / Nivaquin / Resochin

S Lariam / Mephaquin / Nivaquin / Resochin

H 甲氟喹 / Mephaquin / Nivaquin / Resochin
jiǎ fú kúi / Mephaquin / Nivaquin / Resochin

R Lariam / Mephaquine / Nivaquine / résoquine

E Lariam / Mephaquin / Nivaquin / Resochin

I Lariam / Mephaquin / Nivaquin / Resochin

T Lariam / Mephaquin / Nivaquin / Resochin

O 라리암 / 메파퀸 / 니바퀸 / 레조친
ra-ri-am / me-pa-kuin / ni-ba-kwin / re-jo-chin

U Лариам / мефлохин / Нивахин / резохин
Lariam / meflokhin / Nivakhin / rezokhin

L Lariam / meflochina / Nivaquin / Resochin

R لاريام \ ميفاكين \ نيفاكين \ ريسوخين
Lariam / Mephaquin / Nivaquin / Resochin

T Lariam / Mephaquin / Nivaquin / Resochina

K Lariam / Mephaquin / Nivaquin / Resochin

L Lariam / Mephaquin / Nivaquin / Resochin
Lariam / Mephaquin / Nivaquin / Resochin

I लेरियम / मैफाक्विन / नीवाक्विन / रेसोचिन
Lariam / Mephaquin / Nivaquin / Resochin

Are you still taking this medication? At which dosage?

ES ¿Todavía está tomando ese medicamento? ¿En qué dosis?

ZH 你还在吃这些药吗？ 多大剂量？
nǐ hái zài chī zhè xiē yào ma? duō dà jì liàng?

FR Prenez-vous toujours cette médication? A quelle dose?

DE Nehmen Sie sie noch? Welche Dosierung?

VI Quý vị có còn dùng loại thuốc này không? Theo liều lượng bao nhiêu?

IT Sta ancora prendendo questo farmaco? A quale dosaggio?

KO 이 약을 아직도 드시고 계십니까? 양은 어느 정도?
I ya-geul a-jik-do deu-si-go gye-sim-ni-kka? Yang-eun eo-neu jeong-do?

RU Вы все ещё принимаете это лекарство? В каких дозах?
Vy vse eshchyo prinimaete eto lekarstvo? V kakikh dozakh?

PL Czy ciągle jeszcze przyjmuje Pan(i) ten lek? W jakich dawkach?

AR هل ما زلت تأخذ \ تأخذين هذا الدواء وبأية جرعة؟
Hal maa zilt ta'khudh / ta'khudheen hadhaa ad-dawaa' wa bi-ayyi jur'ah?

PT Ainda está a tomar este medicamento? Qual é a posologia?

FK Eske ou ap pran medikaman sa a toujou? Ki doz?

EL Λαμβάνετε ακόμη αυτό το φάρμακο; Σε ποια δοσολογία;
lamvAnete akOmee aftO to fArmako? se peeA dosologEEa?

HI क्या आप अभी भी यह दवा ले रहे हैं? कितनी खुराक?
kya aap abhi bhi yeh dawa le rahe hain? kitni khuraak?

Did you receive one of the following vaccinations?

S ¿Le aplicaron alguna de las vacunas siguientes?

H 你接种过以下几种疫苗之一吗？
nī jiē zhòng guò yǐ xià jǐ zhǒng yì miáo zhī yī ma?

R Avez-vous reçu une des vaccinations suivantes?

E Haben Sie eine der folgenden Impfungen?

VI Quý vị có được chích ngừa một trong các mũi sau đây không?

T Ha fatto una delle seguenti vaccinazioni?

O 다음 예방주사 중 맞으신 것이 있습니까?
Da-eum ye-bang-ju-sa jung ma-jeu-sin geo-si it-seum-ni-kka?

U Вам делали какие-нибудь из следующих прививок?
Vam delali kakie-nibud' iz sleduyushchikh privivok?

•L Czy otrzymał(a) Pan(i) którąś w następujących szczepionek?

•R هل تلقيت اي من هذه التطعيمات؟
Hal talaqqayt ayyin min hadhihi it-tat"eemaat?

T Recebeu algumas das vacinas seguintes?

K Eske ou te resevwa yon de vaksin swivan yo?

•L Λάβατε κάποιο από τα παρακάτω εμβόλια;
lAvate kApeeo apO ta parakAto emvOleea?

HI क्या आपने निम्नलिखित में से कोई टीका लगवाया?
kya aapne nimnalikhit mein se koi teeka lagwaya?

Typhus / Japanese encephalitis / meningococcal encephalitis

ES Tifus / encefalitis japonesa / encefalitis meningocócica

ZH 斑疹伤寒疫苗 / 日本脑炎 / 脑膜炎 / 球菌脑炎
bān zhěn shāng hán yì miáo / rì běn nǎo yán / nǎo mó yán / qiú jūn nǎo yán

FR Typhus / encéphalite japonaise / encéphalite à méningocoques

DE Typhus / Japanische Enzephalitis / Meningokokken-Enzephalitis

VI Sốt phát ban / viêm não Nhật Bản / viêm màng não

IT Tifo / encefalite giapponese / encefalite meningococcica

KO 발진티푸스 / 일본 뇌염 / 수막구균성 뇌염
bal-jin-ti-pu-seu / il-bon noe-yeom / su-mak-gu-gyun-seong noe-yeom

RU Сыпной тиф / японский энцефалит / менингококковый энцефалит
Sypnoy tif / yaponskiy entsefalit / meningokokkovyi entsefalit

PL Przeciw durowi plamistemu / przeciw Japońskiemu zapaleniu mózgu / przeciw
meningokokowemu zapaleniu mózgu

AR تطعيم التايفوس \ إلتهاب الدماغ الياباني \ إلتهاب الدماغ والسحايا
Tat"eem at-taifous / iltihaab ad-dimaagh al-yaabaani / iltihaab ad-dimaagh was-
sihaayaa

PT Tifo / encefalite japonesa / encefalite meningocócica

FK Fyev tifoyed / Ensefelit Japonè / mininjit

EL τύφος / ιαπωνική εγκεφαλίτιδα / μηνιγγιτιδοκοκκική εγκεφαλίτιδα
tEEfos / eeaponeekEE egefalEEteeda / meeneegeeteedokokeekEE egefalEEteeda

HI टाइफस / जापानी एनसेफलीटीस / मेनिंगोकोकल एनसेफलीटीस ...
Typhus / Japanese encephalitis / meningococcal encephalitis

Did you already have one of the following diseases?

¿Ya ha tenido alguna de las siguientes enfermedades?

你得过以下疾病之一吗？
nǐ dé guò yǐ xià jí bìng zhī yī ma?

Avez-vous déjà eu une des maladies suivantes?

Haben Sie bereits eine der folgenden Erkrankungen gehabt?

Quý vị có từng mắc một trong các căn bệnh sau đây không?

Ha già avuto una delle seguenti malattie?

다음 질환 중 이미 앓은 적이 있는 것이 있습니까?
Da-eum jil-hwan jung i-mi a-reun jeo-gi in-neun geo-si It-seum-ni-kka?

Вы ранее болели какой-нибудь из следующих болезней?
Vy ranee boleli kakoy-nibud' iz sleduyushchikh bolezney?

Czy przechodził(a) Pan(i) już którąś w następujących chorób?

هل سبق أن اصبت بأية من الأمراض التالية؟
Hal sabaq an usibt bi-ayyin min al-amraadh it-taaliyah?

Já teve alguma das doenças seguintes?

Eske ou deja gen yon nan maladi sa yo?

Είχατε ήδη μία από τις ακόλουθες νόσους;
EEhate EEdee mEEa apO tees akOluthes nOsus?

क्या आपको पहले से निम्नलिखित में से कोई बीमारी थी? ...
kya aapko pehle se nimnlikhit mei se koi beemari thi?

malaria / amoebae / filariae / bilharziosis / worms

ES malaria (paludismo) / amebas / filarias / bilharziosis / lombrices

ZH 疟疾 / 阿米巴病 / 丝虫病 / 血吸虫病 / 蠕虫病
nüè jí / ā mǐ bā bìng / sī chóng bìng / xuè xī chóng bìng / rú chóng bìng

FR malaria / amibes / filaires / bilharziose / des vers

DE Malaria / Amöben / Filarien / Bilharziose / Wurmerkrankungen

VI sốt rét / amíp / bệnh giun chỉ / bệnh sán / giun sán

IT malaria / amoeba / filaria / bilharziosi / vermi

KO 말라리아 / 아메바 / 심장충 / 발하지오시스 / 기생충
mal-la-ri-a / a-me-ba / sim-jang-chung / bal-ha-ji-o-si-seu / gi-saeng-chung

RU малярия / амебеоз / филяриоз / бильгарциоз / глисты
malyariya / amebeoz / filyarioz / bil'gartsioz / glisty

PL malarię / zakażenie amebowe / filariozę / przywrzycę / robaczycę

AR الملاريا \ إلتهاب بالأميبات \ الإلتهاب بالخيطات \ البيلهارتسيوسيس \ الدود
Al-Malariya / iltihaab bil-ameebaayaat / al-iltihaab bil-khuyaytaat / al-bilhartsiosis / ad-dood

PT malária / amebas / filariae / bilharziose / lombrigas

FK malaria / "amoebae" / "filariae " / "bilharziosis" / ve (parazit)

EL ελονοσία / αμοιβάδες / φιλάρια / σχιστοσωμίαση / σκώληκες
elonosEEa / ameevAdes / feelAreea / sheestosomEEasee / skOleekes

HI मलेरिया / अमीबा / फिलारिया / बिलहरजिओसिस / कीड़े ...
malaria / amoebae / filariae / bilharziosis / kiRe

jaundice / typhus / tuberculosis / genital diseases

ES ictericia / tifus / tuberculosis / enfermedades genitales

ZH 黄疸 / 斑疹伤寒 / 结核 / 性病
huáng dǎn / bān zhěn shāng hán / jiē hé / xìng bìng

FR ictère / typhus / tuberculose / maladies génitales

DE Gelbsucht / Typhus / Tuberkulose / Geschlechtskrankheiten

VI bệnh vàng da / sốt phát ban / bệnh lao / bệnh liên quan tới bộ phận sinh dục

IT itterizia / tifo / tubercolosi / malattie genitali

KO 황달 / 발진티푸스 / 결핵 / 생식기 질환
hwang-dal / bal-jin-ti-pu-seu / gyeol-haek / saeng-sik-gi jil-hwan

RU желтуха / сыпной тиф / туберкулёз / заболевания половых органов
zheltukha / sypnoy tif / tuberkulyoz / zabolevaniya polovykh organov

PL żółtaczkę / dur plamisty / gruźlicę / choroby organów płciowych

AR اليرقان \ حمى التايفوس \ السل \ الأمراض التناسلية
Al-yarqaan / hummaa at-taifous / as-sull / al-amraadh at-tanaasuliyyah

PT icterícia / tifo / tuberculose / doenças genitais

FK lajondis / tifoyed / tibekiloz / infexsyon jenital

EL ίκτερος / τύφος / φυματίωση / ασθένειες των γεννητικών οργάνων
EEkteros / tEEfos / feematEEosee / asthEnee-es ton geneteekOn orgAnon

HI पीलिया / टाइफस / तपेदिक / जननांगिक बीमारी
pilia / typhus / tapedik / jannangik beemari

Did you have close contact with animals? Animal bite / sting?

ES ¿Ha tenido contacto con animales? ¿Lo han mordido / picado?

ZH 你有没有与动物密切接触过？被动物咬 / 蜇过吗？
nǐ yǒu méi yǒu yǔ dòng wù mì qiè jiē chù guò? bèi dòng wù yǎo / zhē guò ma?

FR Avez-vous eu des contacts étroits avec des animaux / des morsures / des piqûres?

DE Hatten Sie engen Kontakt zu Tieren? Tierbiss / Stich?

VI Quý vị có tiếp xúc gần gũi với thú vật không? Bị thú vật cắn / đốt?

IT Ha avuto contatti stretti con animali? Morsi / punture di animali?

KO 동물들을 가까이 하신 적이 있으십니까? 동물한테 물렸나요 / 쏘였나요?
Dong-mul-deu-reul ga-kka-i ha-sin jeo-gi i-seu-sim-ni-kka? Dong-mul-han-te mul-lyeon-na-yo / sso-yeon-na-yo?

RU У вас был близкий контакт с животными? Укус животного / насекомого?
U vas byl blizkiy kontakt s zhivotnymi? Ukus zhivotnogo / nasekomogo?

PL Czy miał(a) Pan(i) bliski kontakt ze zwierzętami? Czy ugryzło / ukąsiło Pana (Panią) zwierzę ?

AR هل كنت متعرضاً \ متعرضة للحيوانات؟ عضات او لدغات حيوان؟
Hal kunta / kunti muta"arridh / muta"arridhah lil-haywaanaat? "adhdhaaat au ladghaat haywaan?

PT Teve contacto com animais? Foi mordido(a) / picado(a)?

FK Eske ou gen kontak ak zanimo? Yon zanimo mode w / pike w?

EL Είχατε στενή επαφή με ζώα; Δάγκωμα / Τσίμπημα ζώου;
EEhate stenEE epafEE me zOa? dAgoma / tsEEbeema zOu?

HI क्या आप पशुओं के नज़दीकी संपर्क में रहे हैं? पशु ने काटा / डंक मारा? ...
kya aap pashuon ke nsjdeeki sampark mein rahe hain? pashu ne kaata / dank maara?

dogs / cats / birds / snake / scorpion / insect

S perros / gatos / pájaros / serpiente / escorpión (alacrán) / insecto

H 狗 / 猫 / 鸟 / 蛇 / 蝎子 / 昆虫
gǒu / māo / niǎo / shé / xiē zi / kūn chóng

R chiens / chats / oiseaux / serpents / scorpion / insecte

E Hunde / Katzen / Vögel / Schlange / Skorpion / Insekt

V chó / mèo / chim / rắn / bọ cạp / côn trùng

T cani / gatti / uccelli / serpente / scorpione / insetto

O 개 / 고양이 / 새 / 뱀 / 전갈 / 곤충
gae / go-yang-i / sae / baem / jeon-gal / gon-chung

U собаки / кошки / птицы / змея / скорпион / насекомое
sobaki / koshki / ptitsy / zmeya / skorpion / nasekomoe

L psy / koty / ptaki / wąż / skorpion / owad

R الكلاب \ القطط \ الطيور \ التعابين \ العقارب \ الحشرات
Al-kilaab / al-qitat / at-tuyoor / ath-tha"aabeen / al-"aqaarib / al-hasharaat

T cães / gatos / pássaros / cobra / escorpião / insecto

K chyen / chat / zwezo / koulev / skorpyon / bigay

L σκύλοι / γάτες / πουλιά / φίδι / σκορπιός / έντομο
skEElee / gAtes / puleeA / fEEdee / skorpeeOs / Edomo

H कुत्ते / बिल्लियाँ / चिड़ियाँ / सांप / बिच्छू / कीड़े–मकोड़े
kutte / billiyan / chiRiya / saanp / bichCHu / kiDe makoDe

21 Pediatrics

Is this your son / daughter? How old is he / she?

ES ¿Es su hijo / hija? ¿Qué edad tiene él (m) / ella (f)?

ZH 这是你的儿子 / 女儿吗？他 / 她多大了？
zhè shì nǐ de ér zi / nǚ ér ma? tā / tā duō dà le?

FR Est-ce votre fils / fille? Quel âge a-t-il / elle?

DE Ist das Ihr Sohn / Ihre Tochter? Wie alt ist er / sie?

VI Đây có phải là con quý vị không? Năm nay em bao nhiêu tuổi?

IT È Suo figlio / Sua figlia? Quanti anni ha?

KO 이 사람이 아들 / 딸 입니까? 몇 살입니까?
I sa-ra-mi a-deul / ttal im-ni-kka? Myeot sa-rim-ni-kka?

RU Это ваш сын / ваша дочь? Сколько ему / ей лет?
Eto vash syn / vasha doch'? Skol'ko emu / ey let?

PL Czy to jest Pana(i) syn / córka? Ile on(a) ma lat?

AR هل هذا إبنك \ هذه بنتك؟ كم عمره \ عمرها؟
Hal hadha ibnak / hadhihi bintak? Kam "umroh / "umrhaa?

PT Esta criança é seu filho / sua filha? Que idade tem ele / ela?

FK Eske sa a se pitit gason w / fi w? Ki laj li genyen ?

EL Είναι ο γιος / η κόρη σας; Πόσο χρονών είναι αυτός / αυτή;
EEne o geeOs / ee kOree sas; pOso hronOn EEne aftOs / aftEE;

HI क्या यह आपका बेटा / बेटी है? इसकी उम्र क्या है?
Kya yeh aapka beta / beti hai? Iski Umra kya hai?

Who is your pediatrician?

S ¿Quién es su pediatra?

H 你的儿科医生是谁？
nǐ de ér kē yī shēng shì shuí?

R Quel est votre pédiatre?

E Wer ist Ihr Kinderarzt?

VI Bác sĩ khoa nhi của con quý vị là ai?

T Chi è il pediatra?

O 소아과 의사의 이름이 뭡니까?
So-a-gwa ui-sa-ui i-reu-mi mwom-ni-kka?

U Кто ваш педиатр?
Kto vash pediatr?

L Kto jest Pana(i) pediatrą?

R من طبيب أطفالك؟
Man tabeeb atfaalak?

T Quem é o(a) seu(sua) médico(a) pediatra?

K Ki es ki pedyat ou?

L Ποιος είναι ο παιδίατρός σας;
peeOs EEne o pedEEatrOs sas?

NI आपका चिकित्सक कौन है?
Apka chikitsak kaun hai?

What is wrong with your child? About which health issue is it complaining about?

ES ¿Qué le pasa al niño (m) / la niña (f)? ¿De qué problema o molestia se queja?

ZH 你的孩子哪里不舒服？是哪一方面的健康问题？
nǐ de hái zǐ nǎ li bù shū fú? shì nǎ yī fāng miàn de jiàn kāng wèn tí?

FR Quest-ce qui ne va pas avec votre enfant? De quel problème de santé se plaint-il?

DE Was fehlt Ihrem Kind? Über welche Beschwerden klagt es?

VI Con quý vị gặp vấn đề gì? Con quý vị có bệnh tật gì?

IT Cosa ha Suo figlio / a? Di cosa si lamenta?

KO 아이가 어디가 아픕니까? 어떤 건강 상의 문제를 아이가 호소합니까?
A-i-ga eo-di-ga a-peum-ni-kka? Eo-tteon geon-gang sang-ui mun-je-reul a-i-ga ho-so-ham-ni-kka?

RU Что случилось с вашим ребенком? На что он жалуется?
Chto sluchilos s vashim rebenkom? Na chto on zhaluetsya?

PL Co Pana(i) dziecku dolega? Na jaki problem ze zdrowiem on(a) się skarży?

AR ما هى المشكلة عند طفلك؟ ما هى القضية الصحية التى يشتكى طفلك منها؟
Maa hiya al-mushkilah "ind atfaalak? Maa hia al-qadhiyyah as-sihhiyah ilati yishtiki tiflak minhaa?

PT O que é que o(a) seu(sua) filho(a) tem? De que problema de saúde é que ele(ela) se queixa?

FK Kisa pitit ou genyen? De ki pwoblèm sante ke lap plenyen ?

EL Τι έχει το παιδί σας; Για πιο θέμα υγείας παραπονιέται;
tee Ehee to pedEE sas? geea peeo thEma eegEEas paraponeeEte?

HI आपके बच्चे को क्या हुआ है? इसे किस स्वास्थ्य मुद्दे के बारे में शिकायत है? ...
Aapke bachche ko kya hua hai? ise kis swasthya mudde ke baare mein shikayat hai?

Health Issue 431

fever / cough / common cold / pain / breathing difficulties / lack of appetite

ES fiebre / tos / resfriado / dolor / dificultad para respirar / falta de apetito

ZH 发烧 / 咳嗽 / 普通感冒 / 痛 / 呼吸困难 / 食欲减退
fā shāo / ké sou / pǔ tōng gǎn mào / tòng hū xī kùn nán / shí yù jiān tuì

FR fièvre / toux / rhume banal / douleur / difficultés respiratoires / perte d'appétit

DE Fieber / Husten / Schnupfen / Schmerzen / Atemnot / Appetitlosigkeit

VI sốt / ho / cảm lạnh thông thường / đau / khó thở / không chịu ăn

IT febbre / tosse / raffreddore comune / dolori / difficoltà di respirazione / mancanza di appetito

KO 열 / 기침 / 일반 감기 / 통증 / 호흡 곤란 / 입맛 없음
yeol / gi-chim / il-ban gam-gi / tong-jeung / ho-heup gol-lan / im-mat eop-seum

RU повышенная температура тела / кашель / простуда / боль / затруднение дыхания / отсутствие аппетита
povyshennaya temperatura tela / kashel' / prostuda / bol' / zatrudnenie dykhaniya / otsutstvie appetita

PL gorączkę / kaszel / przeziębienie / ból / trudności z oddychaniem / brak apetytu

AR الحمّى \ السعال \ الزكام العادي \ الألم \ الصعوبات في التنفس \ قلة الشهية للأكل
Al-hummaa / as-su"aal / az-zukaam al-"aadi / al-alam / as-su"oubaat fit-tanaffus / qillat ash-shahyah lil-'akl

PT febre / tosse / constipação / dor / dificuldades respiratórias / falta de apetite

FK lafyèv / touse / la grip / doulèdifikilte respire / mank apeti

EL πυρετός / βήχας / κοινό κρυολόγημα / πόνος / αναπνευστικές δυσκολίες / έλλειψη όρεξης
peeretOs / vEEhas / keenO kreeolOgeema / pOnos / anapnefsteekEs deeskolEEes / Eleepsee Orexees

HI बुखार / खांसी / सामान्य सर्दी / दर्द / सांस लेने में कठिनाई / भूख न लगना ....
bukhaar / khaansi / samanya sardi / dard / saans lene mein kathinaayi / bhookh na lagna

heat / cold / diarrhea / nausea / vomiting / abdominal pain / head aches / itching

ES
calor / frío / diarrea / náusea / vómito / dolor de estómago / dolor de cabeza / comezón (picazón)

ZH
感觉热 / 冷 / 腹泻 / 恶心 / 呕吐 / 肚子痛 / 头痛 / 痒
gǎn jué rè / lěng / fù xiè / ě xīn / ǒu tù / dù zǐ tòng / tóu tòng / yǎng

FR
chaud / froid / diarrhée / nausée / vomissement / douleur abdominale / céphalées / démangeaisons

DE
Hitze / Kälte / Durchfall / Übelkeit / Erbrechen / Bauchweh / Kopfweh / Juckreiz

VI
nóng / lạnh / tiêu chảy / buồn nôn / ói mửa / đau bụng / đau đầu / ngứa

IT
caldo / freddo / diarrea / nausea / vomito / dolori addominali / mal di testa / prurito

KO
더움 / 추움 / 설사 / 구토증 / 토함 / 복통 / 두통 / 가려움
deo-um / chu-um / seol-sa / gu-to-jeung / to-ham / bok-tong / dutong / ga-ryeo-um

RU
жарко / холодно / понос / тошнота / рвота / боль в животе / головные боли / зуд
zharko / kholodno / ponos / toshnota / rvota / bol' v zhivote / golovnye boli / zud

PL
gorąco / zimno / bigunkę / mdłości / wymioty / ból brzucha / bóle głowy / swędzenie

AR
الحرارة / البرد / الإسهال / شعور الغثيان / التقيّؤ / ألم بطني / الصداعات / الحكّ
Al-haraarah / al-bard / al-is'haal / shu"oor al-ghithyaan / at-taqayyu' / alam batni / as-sudaa"aat / al-hakk

PT
calor / frio / diarreia / náusea / vómitos / dor abdominal / dores de cabeça / comichão

FK
chalè / fredi / noze / vomisman / doulè nan vant / mal tèt / grate

EL
ζέστη / κρύο / διάρροια / ναυτία / εμετός / κοιλιακός πόνος / πονοκέφαλοι / φαγούρα
zEstee / krEEo / deeAreea / naftEEa / emetOs / keeleeakOs pOnos / ponokEfalee / fagUra

HI
गर्मी / सर्दी / अतिसार / मतली / उल्टी / पेट में दर्द / सिरदर्द / खुजली
garmi / sardi / atisaar / matli / ulti / pet mein dard / sirdard / khujli

Have you noticed any behavioral changes in your child?

¿Ha notado cambios en su comportamiento?

孩子的行为有什么异常吗？
hái zǐ de xíng wéi yǒu shén me yì cháng ma?

Avez-vous remarqué un changement de comportement chez votre enfant?

Haben Sie Änderungen im Verhalten Ihres Kindes bemerkt?

Quý vị có thấy con quý vị có thay đổi gì về hành vi không?

Ha notato cambiamenti nel comportamento di Suo / a figlio / a?

아이의 행동이 달라진 것을 느끼셨습니까?
A-i-ui haeng-dong-i dal-la-jin geo-seul neu-kki-syeot-seum-ni-kka?

Заметили ли вы какие-нибудь изменения в поведении вашего ребенка?
Zametili li vy kakie-nibud' izmeneniya v povedenii vashego rebenka?

Czy zauważył(a) Pan(i) jakieś zmiany w zachowaniu swojego dziecka?

هل لاحظت أية تغييرات سلوكية في طفلك؟
Hal laahadht ayy taghyeeraat sulookiyah fi tiflak?

Notou algumas mudanças no comportamento do(a) seu(sua) filho(a)?

Eske ou remake okinn changman nan atitid pitit ou?

Παρατηρήσατε οποιεσδήποτε αλλαγές στη συμπεριφορά του παιδιού σας;
parateerEEsate opee-esdEEpote alagEs stee seebereeforA tu pedeeU sas?

क्या आपने अपने बच्चे के व्यवहार में कोई परिवर्तन नोट किया है?...
Kya aapne apne bachche ke vyavhaar mein koi parivartan note kiya hai?

lethargic / no desire to play / cries frequently

ES	aletargado / no quiere jugar / llora mucho
ZH	没精神 / 不想玩 / 好哭 méi jīng shén / bù xiǎng wán / hǎo kū
FR	léthargie / aucun désir de jouer / pleure fréquemment
DE	lethargisch / keine Spielfreude / weint viel
VI	kêu la đau đớn / không muốn chơi / khóc nhiều
IT	apatico / a / non ha voglia di giocare / piange frequentemente
KO	나름해함 / 놀고 싶은 생각이 없음 / 자주 운다 na-reun-hae-ham / nol-go si-peun saeng-ga-gi eop-seum / ja-ju un-da
RU	сонливость / отсутствие интереса к играм / частый плач sonlivost' / otsutstvie interesa k igram / chastyi plach
PL	ospałość / brak ochoty do zabawy / często płacze
AR	خامل / لا رغبة فى اللعب / كثرة البكاء Khaamil / laa raghbah fil-la"ab / kathrat al-bukaa'
PT	letárgico / sem vontade de brincar / chora com frequência
FK	pa domi byen / li pa vle jouwe / kriye anpil
EL	ληθαργικό / δεν έχει διάθεση να παίξει / κλαίει συχνά leethargeekO / den Exee deeAthesee na pExee / klEee seehnA
HI	सुस्त / खेलने के प्रति अनिच्छा / अक्सर रोना ... sust / khelne ke prati aniCha / aksar rona

cramps / cough / decreased appetite

cólicos / tos / pérdida del apetito

痙攣 / 咳嗽 / 食欲減退
jìng luán / ké sou / shí yù jiǎn tuì

crampes / toux / perte d'appétit

Krämpfe / Husten / wenig Appetit

chứng vọp bẻ / ho / chán ăn

crampi / tosse / meno appetito

급격한 복통 / 기침 / 식욕저하
geup-gyeo-kan bok-tong / gi-chim / si-gyok-jeo-ha

спастические боли / кашель / сниженный аппетит
spasticheskie boli / kashel' / snizhennyi appetit

skurcze / kaszel / brak apetytu

التشنجات / السعال / النقص فى الشهية
At-tashannujaat / as-su"aal / an-naqs fish-shahyah

cólicas / tosse / menos apetite

la karmp / touse / apeti li diminye (koupe)

κράμπες / βήχας / μειωμένη όρεξη
krAbes / vEEhas / meeomEnee Orexee

ऐंठन / खांसी / भूख न लगना
ainThan / khaansi / bhookh na lagna

For how long has your child been already ill? Days / weeks / months / years

ES ¿Cuánto tiempo hace que el niño está enfermo? Días / semanas / meses / años

ZH 孩子病了多久了？几天／几周／几个月／几年
hái zi bìng le duō jiǔ le? jǐ tiān / jǐ zhōu / jǐ ge yuè / jǐ nián

FR Depuis combien de temps votre enfant est-il réellement malade? Jours / semaines / mois / années

DE Wie lange ist es schon krank? Tage / Wochen / Monate / Jahre

VI Con quý vị đã đau bệnh trong bao lâu? Ngày / tuần / tháng / năm

IT Da quanto tempo sta male Suo / a figlio / a? Giorni / settimane / mesi / anni

KO 벌써 아픈 지가 얼마나 되었습니까? 일 / 주 / 달 / 년
Beol-sseo a-peun ji-ga eol-ma-na doe-eot-seum-ni-kka? il / ju / dal / nyeon

RU Как долго уже ваш ребенок болен? Дней / недель / месяцев / лет?
Kak dolgo uzhe vash rebenok bolen? Dney / nedel' / mesyatsev / let?

PL Od jak dawna już dziecko choruje? Dni / tygodni / miesięcy / lat

AR لكم مدة كان طفلك مريضاً؟ أيام \ أسابيع \ شهور \ سنوات
li-kam muddah kan tiflak mareedh? Ayyaah / asaabee" / shuhoor / sanawaat

PT Há quanto tempo é que o(a) seu(sua) filho(a) tem estado doente? dias / semanas / meses / anos

FK Pandan konbyen tan ke pitit ou malad? Jou / semen / plizye mwa / plizye ane

EL Για πόσο καιρό ήταν το παιδί σας ήδη άρρωστο; Ημέρες / Εβδομάδες / Μήνες / Χρόνια
geea pOso kerO EEtan to pedEE sas EEdee Arosto? eemEres / evdomAdes / mEEnes / hrOneea

HI आपका बच्चा कितने समय पहले से बीमार है? दिन／हफ्ते／महीने／वर्ष
Aapka bachcha kitne samay pahle se bimaar hai? Din / hafte / mahine / varSh

Has your child experienced the same health problems in the past?

¿Ya había tenido el niño estos mismos problemas?

孩子以前得过这样的病吗？
hái zǐ zǐ yǐ qián dé guò zhè yàng de bìng ma?

Votre enfant a-t-il déjà eu les mêmes problèmes de santé dans le passé?

Hatte es in der Vergangenheit die gleichen Beschwerden?

Trước đây, con quý vị có bao giờ gặp các vấn đề sức khỏe tương tự như vậy chưa?

Suo / a figlio / a ha avuto gli stessi problemi di salute in passato?

과거에도 아이가 동일한 건강 문제를 경험한 적이 있었습니까?
Gwa-geo-e-do a-i-ga dong-il-han geon-gang mun-je-reul gyeong-heom-han jeo-gi it-sot-seum-ni-kka?

У вашего ребенка уже были подобные проблемы в прошлом?
U vashego rebenka uzhe byli podobnye problemy v proshlom?

Czy Pana(i) dziecko miało już wcześniej te same kłopoty ze zdrowiem?

هل عانى طفلك من نفس المشاكل الصحية فى الماضى؟
Hal "aanaa tiflak min nafs il-mashaakil as-sihhiyyah fil-madhee?

O(a) seu(sua) filho(a) já sofreu os mesmos problemas de saúde anteriormente?

Eske pitit ou te gen menm pwoblèm lasante nan le pase ?

Είχε το παιδί σας τα ίδια προβλήματα υγείας στο παρελθόν;
EEhe to pedEE sas ta EEdeea provlEEmata egEEas sto parelthOn?

क्या आपके बच्चे ने पहले भी इसी तरह की स्वास्थ्य समस्या का अनुभव किया था?
Kya aapke bachche ne pahle bhi isi tarah ki swasthya samasya ka anubhav kiya tha?

Do you breast-feed? What do you feed your child?

ES ¿Le está dando el pecho? ¿Qué le da de comer?

ZH 是母乳喂养吗？你喂孩子什么？
shì mǔ rǔ wèi yǎng ma? nǐ wèi hái zǐ shén me?

FR Le nourrissez-vous au sein? Que lui donnez-vous à manger?

DE Stillen Sie? Mit was füttern Sie es?

VI Quý vị có cho con bú sữa mẹ không? Quý vị cho em ăn gì?

IT Lei allatta? Che cibo dà a Suo / a figlio / a?

KO 모유를 먹이십니까? 아이한테 어떤 것을 먹이십니까?
Mo-yu-reul meo-gi-sim-ni-kka? A-i-han-te eo-tteon geo-seul meo-gi-sim-ni-kka?

RU Вы кормите грудью? Чем вы кормите вашего ребенка?
Vy kormite grud'yu? Chem vy kormite vashego rebenka?

PL Czy Pani karmi piersią? Czym Pani karmi dziecko?

AR هل ترضّعين من الصدر؟ بماذا تغذّين طفلك؟
Hal tiradhdhi"een min as-sadr? Bi-madhaa tighadhdheen tiflak?

PT Amamenta o(a) seu(sua) filho(a)? Alimenta-o(a) com o quê??

FK Eske ou bay tete? Kisa ou bay pitit ou manje ?

EL Θηλάζετε; Τι ταΐζεται το παιδί σας;
theelAzete? tee taEEzete to pedEE sas?

HI क्या आप स्तन–पान कराती हैं? आप अपने बच्चे को खाने में क्या देती हैं?
Kya aap stan-paan karaati hain? Aap apne bachche ko khane mein kya deti hain?

milk powder / cow's milk / cereals with cream

S leche en polvo / leche de vaca / cereal con crema

H 奶粉 / 牛奶 / 麦片加奶
nǎi fěn / niú nǎi / mài piàn jiā nǎi

R lait en poudre / lait de vache / céréales avec de la crème

E Milchpulver / Kuhmilch / Getreide mit Sahne

VI sữa bột / sữa bò / ngũ cốc với kem

T latte in polvere / latte vaccino / cereali con la panna

O 분유 / 우유 / 크림과 먹는 씨리얼
bun-yu / u-yu / keu-rim-gwa meong-neun ssi-ri-eol

RU молочной смесью / коровьем молоком / хлопьями со сливками
molochnoy smes'yu / korov'yem molokom / khlop'yami so slivkami

PL mlekiem w proszku / krowim mlekiem / płatkami zbożowymi ze śmietanką

AR مسحوق حليب \ حليب البقرة \ الحبوب بالقشطة
Mas'hooq haleeb / haleeb al-baqarah / al-huboob bil-qashtah

PT leite em pó / leite de vaca / cereal (papa) com leite

K lèt an poud / lèt bef / sereyal ak krem fre

EL γάλα σε σκόνη / αγελαδινό γάλα / δημητριακά με κρέμα
gAla se skOnee / ageladenO gAla / deemeetreeakA me krEma

HI दूध पाउडर / गाय का दूध / क्रीम के साथ अनाज ...
dhoodh powder / gaaye ka dhoodh / cream ke saath anaaj

vegetables / meat / ready-to-eat meals

ES	verduras / carne / alimento preparado

| ZH | 蔬菜 / 肉 / 速食品 |
| | shū cài / ròu / sù shí pǐn |

| FR | légumes / viande / repas tout préparés |

| DE | Gemüse / Fleisch / Fertiggerichte |

| VI | rau / thịt / đồ ăn liền |

| IT | verdure / carne / pasti preconfezionati |

| KO | 야채 / 고기 / 판매되는 바로 먹게 준비된 식사 |
| | ya-chae / go-gi / pan-mae-doe-neun ba-ro meog-ge jun-bi-doen sik-sa |

| RU | овощами / мясом / готовой к употреблению пищей |
| | ovoshchami / myasom / gotovoy k upotrebleniyu pishchey |

| PL | warzywami / mięsem / posiłkami gotowymi do spożycia |

| AR | الخضار \ اللحم \ وجبات طعام جاهزة للأكل |
| | Al-khudhaar / al-lahm / wajbaat ta"aam jaahizah lil-'akl |

| PT | legumes / carne / refeições prontas a comer |

| FK | legim / vyan / manje ki tou pare pou manje |

| EL | λαχανικά / κρέας / έτοιμα γεύματα |
| | lahaneekA / krEas / Eteema gEvmata |

| HI | सब्जियां / मांस / खाने के लिए तैयार भोजन |
| | sabjiyan / maans / khaane ke liye taiyaar bhojan |

Has your child received all the necessary vaccinations?

S ¿Le han aplicado todas las vacunas necesarias?

H 你得孩子接种过所有必要的疫苗吗？
nǐ de hái zǐ jiē zhòng guò suǒ yǒu bì yào de yì miáo ma?

R Votre enfant a-t-il reçu toutes les vaccinations nécessaires?

E Sind die Impfungen Ihres Kindes vollständig?

I Con quý vị có được tiêm tất cả các mũi chích ngừa cần thiết không?

T Suo / a figlio / a ha fatto tutte le vaccinazioni necessarie?

O 아이가 필요한 예방주사를 모두 맞았습니까?
A-i-ga pi-ryo-han ye-bang-ju-sa-reul mo-du ma-jat-seum-ni-kka?

U Ваш ребенок получил все необходимые прививки?
Vash rebenok poluchil vse neobkhodimye privivki?

L Czy dziecko otrzymało wszystkie niezbędne szczepionki?

R هل تلقى طفلك كلّ التطعيمات اللازمة؟
Hal talaqqaa tiflak kull it-tat"eemaat al-laazimah?

T O(a) seu(sua) filho(a) recebeu todas as vacinas necessárias?

K Eske pitit ou a resevwa tout vaksin ki nèsesè ?

L Έκανε το παιδί σας όλα τα απαραίτητα εμβόλια;
Ekane to pedEE sas Ola ta aparEteeta emvOleea?

क्या आपके बच्चे को सभी जरूरी टीके लगे हैं?
Kya aapke bachche ko sabhi jarooree teeke lage hain?

In which grade is your child?

ES ¿En qué grado escolar está el niño (m) / la niña (f)?

ZH 你孩子上几年级？
nǐ hái zǐ shàng jǐ nián jí?

FR Dans quelle classe est votre enfant?

DE In welcher Klasse ist es?

VI Con quý vị học lớp mấy?

IT In che classe sta Suo / a figlio / a?

KO 아이가 몇 학년입니까?
A-i-ga myeot hang-nyeon-im-ni-kka?

RU В каком классе ваш ребенок?
V kakom klasse vash rebenok?

PL W ktorej klasie jest Pana(i) dziecko?

AR في اي سنة دراسية طفلك؟
Fi ayy sanah diraasiyah tiflak?

PT Em que classe está o(a) seu(sua) filho(a)?

FK Nan ki klas pitit ou ye?

EL Σε ποια τάξη είναι το παιδί σας;
se peea tAxee EEne to pedEE sas?

HI आपका बच्चा कौन—से ग्रेड में है?
Aapka bachcha kaun se grade mein hai?

Is your child attending a special school?

¿Asiste a una escuela especial?

你的孩子上特殊学校吗？
nǐ de hái zǐ shàng tè shū xué xiào ma?

Votre enfant est-il dans une école spéciale?

Geht Ihr Kind auf eine besondere Schule?

Con quý vị có theo học tại một trường học đặc biệt không?

Suo / a figlio / a frequenta una scuola speciale?

아이가 특수학교에 다닙니까?
A-i-ga teuk-su-hak-gyo-e da-nim-ni-kka?

Ваш ребенок посещает специальную школу?
Vash rebenok poseshchaet spetsial'nuyu shkolu?

Czy Pana(i) dziecko uczęszcza do specjalnej szkoły?

هل يحضر طفلك مدرسة خاصّة؟
Hal yahdhur tiflak madrasah khaasah?

O(a) seu(sua) filho(a) frequenta uma escola especial?

Eske li nan yon lekòl espesyal?

Παρακολουθεί το παιδί σας ειδικό σχολείο;
parakoluthEE to pedEE sas eedeekO sholEEo?

क्या आपका बच्चा किसी विशेष स्कूल में जा रहा है?
Kya aapka bachcha kisi vishesh school mein ja raha hai?

How much does he / she weigh? How tall is he / she?

ES	¿Cuánto pesa? ¿Cuánto mide?
ZH	他 / 她体重是多少？身高是多少？ tā / tā tǐ zhòng shì duō shǎo? shēn gāo shì duō shǎo?
FR	Combien pèse-t-il / elle? Quelle est sa taille?
DE	Wie viel wiegt er / sie? Wie groß ist er / sie?
VI	Em cân nặng bao nhiêu? Em cao bao nhiêu?
IT	Quanto pesa? Quanto è alto / a?
KO	아이의 체중은? 아이의 키는? A-i-ui che-jung-eun? A-i-ui ki-neun?
RU	Какой у него / неё вес? Какой у него / неё рост? Kakoy u nego / neyo ves? Kakoy u nego / neyo rost?
PL	Ile on / ona waży? Ile on / ona ma wzrostu?
AR	كم وزنه \ وزنها؟ كم طوله \ طولها؟ Kam waznoh / waznhaa? Kam tooloh / toolhaa?
PT	Quanto é que ele / ela pesa? Qual é a sua altura?
FK	Konbyen ke li peze? Ki wote pitit ou a?
EL	Πόσο ζυγίζει αυτός / αυτή; Τι ύψος έχει αυτός / αυτή; pOso zeegEEzee aftOs / aftEE? tee EEpsos Ehee aftOs / aftEE?
HI	उसका वज़न कितना है? उसकी लंबाई कितनी है? Uska vazan kitna hai? Uski lambaayi kitnee hai?

Is he / she losing / gaining weight? How much?

¿Ha estado bajando / subiendo de peso? ¿Qué tanto?

他 / 她的体重有没有减少 / 增加？是多少？
tā / tā de tǐ zhòng yǒu méi yǒu jiǎn shāo / zēng jiā? shì duō shǎo?

Perd-t-il / elle du poids ou en gagne-t-il / elle? Combien?

Nimmt er / sie an Gewicht zu / ab? Wieviel?

Em có giảm / tăng cân không? Giảm / tăng bao nhiêu cân?

Sta aumentando / diminuendo di peso? Quanto?

아이의 체중이 감소 / 증가 되었습니까? 얼마나?
A-i-ui che-jung-i gam-so / jeung-ga doe-eot-seum-ni-kka? Eol-ma-na?

Он / она теряет / набирает вес? Как много?
On / ona teryaet / nabiraet ves? Kak mnogo?

Czy on / ona traci / zyskuje na wadze? Ile?

هل يزيد او ينزل وازنه \ وزنها؟ كم من الوزن؟
Hal yazeed au yanzil waznoh / waznhaa? Kam min al-wazn?

Tem perdido / aumentado peso? Quanto?

Eske li ap megri / gwosi? Konbyen ?

Αυτός / Αυτή χάνει / παίρνει βάρος; Πόσο;
aftOs / aftEE hAnee / pErnee vAros? pOso?

क्या उसका वज़न घट / बढ़ रहा है? कितना?
Kya uska vazan baDh / ghat raha hai? Kitna?

For how long did he / she have fever / vomit / have diarrhea?

ES ¿Cuánto tiempo lleva con fiebre / vómito / diarrea?

ZH 他 / 她发烧 / 呕吐 / 腹泻多久了？
tā / tā fā shāo / ǒu tù / fù xiè duō jiǔ le?

FR Depuis combien de temps a-t-il / elle de la fièvre / vomi / de la diarrhée?

DE Wie lange hatte er / sie Fieber / erbrochen / Durchfall?

VI Em đã bị sốt / ói mửa / tiêu chảy trong bao lâu?

IT Per quanto tempo ha avuto la febbre / ha vomitato / ha avuto la diarrea?

KO 아이가 열 / 토 / 설사한 지가 얼마나 됐습니까?
A-i-ga yeol / to / seol-sa-han ji-ga eol-ma-na doet-seum-ni-kka?

RU Как долго у него / неё была повышена температура тела / рвота / понос?
Kak dolgo u nego / neyo byla povyshena temperatura tela / rvota / ponos?

PL Od jak dawna ma on / ona gorączkę / wymioty / biegunkę?

AR لكم مدة عانى \ عانت من الحمى \ التقيؤ \ الإسهال؟
Li-kam muddah "aanaa / "aanat min al-hummaa / at-taqayyu' / al-is'haal?

PT Durante quanto tempo é que ele / ela teve febre / vómitos / diarreia?

FK Pandan konbyen tan ke li gen lafyèv la / vomi / gen dyare?

EL Για πόσο καιρό είχε αυτός / αυτή πυρετό / εμετό / διάρροια;
geea pOso kerO eehe aftOs / aftEE peeretO / emetO / deeAreea?

HI उसे कितने समय से बुखार / उल्टी / अतिसार है?
Usey kitne samay se bukhaar / ulti / atisaar hai?

For how long did he / she experience wheezing / pain?

¿Cuánto tiempo ha tenido respiración ruidosa / dolor?

他 / 她气喘 / 疼痛多久了？
tā / tā qì chuǎn / téng tòng duō jiǔ le?

Depuis combien de temps a-t-il / elle une respiration d'asthmatique / de la douleur?

Wie lange hatte er / sie keuchende Atmung / Schmerzen?

Em có hiện tượng thở khò khè / đau trong bao lâu?

Per quanto tempo ha avuto rantoli / dolore?

숨 쉴 때 쌕쌕 소리가 난 지 / 통증이 있은 지 얼마나 됐습니까?
Sum swil ttae ssaek-ssaek so-ri-ga nan ji / tong-jeung-i i-seun ji eol-ma-na dwaet-seum-ni-kka?

Как долго у него / неё было свистящее дыхание / боль?
Kak dolgo u nego / neyo bylo svistyashchee dykhanie / bol'?

Od jak dawna ma świszczący oddech / odczuwa ból?

لكم مدة عاني \ عانت من الأزيز في التنفس \ الألم؟
Li-kam muddah "aanaa / "aanat min al-azeed fit-tanaffus / al-alam?

Durante quanto tempo é que ele / ela teve pieira / sentiu dor?

Pandan konbyen tan ke l ap soufri ak sifleman an / doulè a?

Για πόσο καιρό είχε συριγμό / πόνο;
geea pOso kerO EEhe seereegmO / pOno?

उसे कितने समय से घरघराहट / दर्द महसूस होता है?
usey kitne samay se ghargharahat / dard mehsoos hota hai?

Does he / she only vomit during / after a meal?

ES ¿Vomita solamente durante / después de las comidas?

ZH 他 / 她是不是只在吃饭时 / 饭后呕吐？
tā / tā shì bù shì zhǐ zài chī fàn shí / fàn hòu ǒu tù?

FR A-t-il / elle vomi au cours ou après un repas?

DE Erbricht er / sie immer / nur beim / nach dem Essen?

VI Có phải em chỉ ói mửa trong khi / sau khi ăn không?

IT Vomita solo durante / dopo i pasti?

KO 식사 중 / 후에만 토합니까?
Sik-sa jung / hu-e-man to-ham-ni-kka?

RU Он / она рвет только во время / после еды?
On / ona rvet tol'ko vo vremya / posle edy?

PL Czy on / ona wymiotuje tylko w czasie jedzenia / po jedzeniu?

AR هل يتقيأ \ تتقيأ فقط أثناء تناول وجبات الطعام او بعده ؟
Hal taqayya' / titqayya' faqat athnaa' au tanaawul wajbaat at-ta"aam au ba"doh?

PT Ele / ela só vomita durante / depois de uma refeição?

FK Eske li vomi pandan / apre li manje?

EL Κάνει αυτός / αυτή εμετό μόνο κατά τη διάρκεια / μετά από ένα γεύμα;
kAnee aftOs / aftEE emetO mOno katA tee deeArkeea / metA apO Ena gEvma?

HI क्या वह केवल भोजन के दौरान / बाद में उल्टी करता / करती है?
Kya vah keval bhojan ke dauraan / baad mein ulti karta / karti hai?

How often did he / she have bowel movement within the last 24 hours?

S ¿Cuántas veces ha evacuado en las últimas 24 horas?

H 在过去的24小时内，他 / 她多久大便一次？
zài guò qù de 24 xiǎo shí nèi, tā / tā duō jiǔ dà biàn yī cì?

R Combien de fois a-t-il / elle été à la selle au cours des dernières 24 heures?

E Wie oft hatte er / sie Stuhlgang in den letzten 24 Stunden?

VI Trong 24 giờ qua, em đã đi cầu bao nhiêu lần?

T Quante volte è andato / a di corpo nelle ultime 24 ore?

O 지난 24 시간 동안 아이가 대변을 몇 번 봤습니까?
Ji-nan i-sip-sa-si-gan dong-an a-i-ga dae-byeo-neul myeot beon bwat-seum-ni-kka?

U Сколько актов дефекации было у него / неё за последние сутки?
Skol'ko aktov defekatsii bylo u nego / neyo za poslednie sutki?

L Jak często miał(a) wypróżnienia w ciągu ostatnich 24 godzin?

R كم مرّة تغوط \ تغوطت ضمن الساعات الـ24 الأخيرة؟
Kam marrah taghawwat / taghawwatat dhimn as-saa"aat al-arba"h wa-"ishreen al-akheerah?

T Com que frequência é que ele / ela teve um movimento intestinal durante as últimas 24 horas?

K Konbyen fwa ke li te al nan watè nan denye 24 hètan yo?

L Πόσο συχνά ενεργήθηκε αυτός / αυτή εντός των τελευταίων 24 ωρών;
pOso seehnA energEEtheeke aftOs / aftEE edOs ton teleftEon EEkosee tesAron orOn?

H उसे पिछले 24 घंटों में कितनी बार दस्त हुआ?
Use piChle 24 ghanton mein kitni baar dast hua?

Is the stool watery / mucous / bloody?

ES ¿El excremento es líquido / mucoso / con sangre?

ZH 大便是稀水样／粘液样／带血的吗？
dà biàn shì xī shuǐ yàng / nián yè yàng / dài xiě de ma?

FR Est-ce que les selles étaient aqueuses / muqueuses / sanguinolentes

DE Ist der Stuhl wässrig / schleimig / blutig?

VI Phân có lỏng / nhầy / có máu không?

IT Le feci sono acquose / contengono muco / sangue?

KO 대변이 묽었습니까 / 끈적했습니까 / 피가 섞여 있었습니까?
Dae-byeo-ni mul-geot-seum-ni-kka / kkeun-jeok-haet-seum-ni-kka / pi-ga seok-kyeo i-seot-seum-ni-kka?

RU Кал водянистый / слизистый / кровавый?
Kal vodyanistyi / slizistyi / krovavyi?

PL Czy stolec był wodnisty / śluzowaty / krwawy?

AR هل الغائط مائي \ لزج \ دامٍ؟
Hal al-ghaa'it maa'ee / lazij / daami?

PT As fezes são muito aquosas / com mucosidade / sanguinolentas?

FK Eske watè a te dlo anpil / gen pi / san?

EL Είναι τα κόπρανα υδαρά / βλεννώδη / αιματηρά;
EEne ta kOprana eedarA / vlenOdee / emateerA?

HI क्या मल पानीयुक्त / कफयुक्त / रक्तयुक्त है?
Kya mal paniyukta / kuffyukta / raktyukta hai?

What did you give him / her to eat?

¿Qué le dio usted de comer?

你给他 / 她吃了什么？
nǐ gěi tā / tā chī le shén me?

Qu'est-ce que vous lui avez donné à manger?

Was haben Sie ihm / ihr zu Essen gegeben?

Quý vị đã cho em ăn gì?

Cosa gli / le ha dato da mangiare?

아이한테 어떤 음식을 주었습니까?
A-i-han-te eo-tteon eum-si-geul ju-eot-seum-ni-kka?

Чем вы его / её кормили?
Chem vy ego / eyo kormili?

Co mu / jej Pan(i) podawał(a) do jedzenia?

ماذا أعطيته / اعطيتها للأكل؟
Maadha a"ateytoh / a"ateyt'haa lil-akl?

O que é que lhe deu de comer?

Kisa ou bal manje?

Τι του / της δώσατε να φάει;
tee tu / tees dOsate na fAee?

आपने उसे खाने के लिए क्या दिया? ...क्यूक्यू पी
Aapne use khaane ke liye kya diya?

When was the last time he / she urinated?

ES ¿Cuándo orinó el niño (m) / la niña (f) por última vez?

ZH 他 / 她最后一次小便是什么时候？
tā / tā zuì hòu yī cì xiǎo biàn shì shén me shí hòu?

FR Quand a-t-il / elle uriné pour la dernière fois?

DE Wann hat er / sie das letzte Mal Wasser gelassen?

VI Lần em tiểu tiện gần đây nhất là khi nào?

IT Quando ha urinato l'ultima volta?

KO 아이가 마지막으로 소변을 본 게 언제 입니까?
A-i-ga ma-ji-ma-geu-ro so-byeo-neul bon ge eon-je im-ni-kka?

RU Когда он / она последний раз мочился / мочилась?
Kogda on / ona poslednii raz mochilsya / mochilas'?

PL Kiedy on / ona ostatni raz oddał(a) mocz?

AR متى كان آخر مرّة تبول \ تبوّلت؟
Mattaa kaan aakhir marrah tabawwal / tabawwalat?

PT Quando é que ele / ela urinou pela última vez?

FK Ki denye fwa ke li pipi?

EL Πότε ήταν η τελευταία φορά που ούρησε;
pOte EEtan ee teleftEa forA pu Ureese?

HI उसने अंतिम बार पेशाब कब किया?
Usne antim baar peshaab kab kiya?

Is anyone else ill?

ES ¿Hay alguien más enfermo en

ZH 还有什么人生病吗？
hái yǒu shén me rén shēng bìng ma?

FR Y a-t-il quelqu'un d'autre qui soit malade?

DE Ist sonst noch jemand krank?

VI Có còn ai khác bị đau bệnh không?

IT Qualcun altro sta male?

KO 아픈 사람이 또 있습니까?
A-peun sa-ra-mi tto it-seum-ni-kka?

RU Кто-нибудь ещё болен?
Kto-nibud' eshchyo bolen?

PL Czy ktoś jeszcze jest chory?

AR هل هناك أي شخص آخر مريض؟
Hal hunaak ayy shakhs aakhar mareedh?

PT Está mais alguém doente?

FK Eske gen lòt moun ki malad?

EL Είναι κάποιος άλλος άρρωστος;
EEne kApeeos Alos Arostos?

HI क्या कोई और बीमार है? ....
kya koi aur bimaar hai?

at home / in kindergarten / in school / day-care center

ES	la casa / el jardín de niños / la escuela / la guardería?
ZH	在家里 / 幼儿园 / 学校 / 托儿所 zài jiā lǐ / yòu ér yuán / xué xiào / tuō er suǒ
FR	à la maison / au jardin d'enfant / à l'école / au centre journalier de soin
DE	zu Hause / im Kindergarten / in der Schule / Kindertagesstätte
VI	ở nhà / ở lớp mẫu giáo / ở trường học / trung tâm giữ trẻ ban ngày
IT	a casa / all'asilo / a scuola / all'asilo nido
KO	집에 / 유치원에 / 학교에 / 유아원 ji-be / yu-chi-wo-ne / hak-gyo-e / yu-a-won
RU	дома / в детском саду / в школе / в яслях doma / v detskom sadu / v shkole / v yaslyakh
PL	w domu / w przedszkolu / w szkole
AR	فى البيت \ فى روضة الأطفال \ فى المدرسة \ عند مركز الرعاية النهارية Fil-beyt / fi roudhat il-atfaal / fil-madrasah / "ind markaz ar-ri"aayat in-nahaariyah
PT	em casa / na escola infantil / na escola / no infantário
FK	lakay / nan jadin danfan / lekol la / gadri
EL	στο σπίτι / στο νηπιαγωγείο / στο σχολείο / στο παιδικό σταθμό sto stEEte / sto neepeeagogEEo / sto sholEEo / sto pedeekO stathmO
HI	घर में / किंडरगार्टेन में / स्कूल में / दिन परिचर्या केंद्र ghar mein / kindergarten mein / school mein / din paricharya kendra

Has he / she been complaining about a head ache / stiff neck?

ES ¿Se ha quejado de dolor de cabeza / tensión en el cuello?

ZH 他／她有没有说过头痛／脖子发紧？
tā / tā yǒu méi yǒu shuō guò tóu tòng / bó zi fā jǐn?

FR S'est-il / elle plaint(e) de maux de tête / de raideur de la nuque?

DE Hat er / sie über Kopfschmerzen / steifen Nacken geklagt?

VI Em có kêu bị đau đầu / cứng cổ không?

IT Dice di avere mal di testa / torcicollo?

KO 아이가 두통이나 목이 뻐근하다는 호소를 해왔습니까?
A-i-ga du-tong-i-na mo-gi ppeo-geun-ha-da-neun ho-so-reul hae-wat-seum-ni-kka?

RU Были ли у него / неё жалобы на головную боль / напряжённость затылочных мышц?
Byli li u nego / neyo zhaloby na golovnuyu bol' / napryazhennost' zatylochnykh myshts?

PL Czy on / ona skarży się na ból głowy / sztywną szyję?

AR هل كان يشتكي / كانت تشتكي من الصداع \ الرقبة المتصلّبة؟
Hal kaan yishtiki / kaanat tishtiki min as-sudaa" / ar-ruqbat il-mutasallibah?

PT Ele / ela tem-se queixado de dor de cabeça / dor no pescoço?

FK Eske li tap plenyin ke kè l ap fè l mal / kou l rèd?

EL Παραπονιέται αυτός / αυτή για πονοκέφαλο / αυχενική δυσκαμψία;
paraponeeEte aftOs / aftEE geea ponokEEfalo / afheneekEE deeskampsEEa?

HI क्या वह सिरदर्द / गले में खराश की शिकायत कर रहा / रही है?
Kya vah sirdard / gale me kharash ki shikayat kar raha / rahi hai?

Did the wheezing occur suddenly / gradually?

ES ¿El ruido al respirar empezó de repente / poco a poco?

ZH 喘气是突然出现的 / 慢慢出现的？
chuǎn qì shì tū rán chū xiàn de / màn màn chū xiàn de?

FR Est-ce que le sifflement de la respiration est arrivé busquement / graduellement?

DE Hat die keuchende Atmung plötzlich / allmählich begonnen?

VI Hiện tượng thở khò khè có xảy ra đột ngột / dần dần không?

IT I rantoli si sono verificati improvvisamente / gradualmente?

KO 숨 쉴 때 쌕쌕 하는 소리가 갑자기 / 점차로 시작됐습니까?
Sum swil ttae ssaek-ssaek ha-neun so-ri-ga gap-ja-gi / jeom-cha-ro si-jak-dwaet-seum-ni-kka?

RU Свистящее дыхание появилось внезапно / постепенно?
Svistyashchee dykhanie poyavilos' vnezapno / postepenno?

PL Czy ten świszczący oddech pojawił się nagle / stopniowo?

AR هل وقع الأزيز بالفجأة \ بشكل تدريجي؟
Hal waqa" al-azeez bil-faj'ah / bi-shekl tadreeji?

PT A pieira ocorreu de repente / gradualmente?

FK Eske sifleman an komanse sibitman / yon bagay gradyel?

EL Συνέβη ο συριγμός ξαφνικά / σταδιακά;
seenEvee o seereegmOs xafneekA / stadeeakA?

HI क्या घरघराहट अचानक / ε ीरे– ε ीरे हुई थी?
Kya ghargharahat achanak / dheere-dheere hui thi?

Is he / she taking medication for this condition?

¿Está tomando medicamentos para este problema?

他 / 她现在吃什么药治疗呢？
tā / tā xiàn zài chī shén me yào zhì liáo ne?

a-t-il / elle pris des médicaments pour cet état?

Nimmt er / sie Medikamente dagegen?

Em có đang dùng thuốc để chữa bệnh này không?

Sta prendendo farmaci per questo disturbo?

아이가 이 증상에 대한 약을 먹고 있습니까?
A-i-ga i jeung-sang-e dae-han ya-geul meok-go it-seum-ni-kka?

Он / она принимает лекарства от этого?
On / ona prinimaet lekarstva ot etogo?

Czy on / ona przyjmuje z tego względu jakieś leki?

هل يأخذ \ تأخذ دواءاً لهذا المرض؟
Hal ya'khudh / ta'khudh dawaa'an li-hadhal-maradh?

Ele / ela está a tomar algum medicamento para este problema?

Eske lap pran medikaman pou kondisyon sa?

Λαμβάνει αυτός / αυτή φάρμακα για αυτήν την πάθηση;
lamvAnee aftOs / aftEE fArmaka geea aftEEn teen pAtheesee?

क्या वह इस दशा के लिए दवा ले रहा / रही है?
Kya vah is dasha ke liye davaa le raha / rahi hai?

What triggers the wheezing?

ES ¿Con qué se pone ruidosa la respiración?

ZH 是什么引发了喘气？
shì shén me yǐn fā le chuǎn qì?

FR Quel est le facteur déclenchant du sifflement?

DE Was löst die keuchende Atmung aus?

VI Vì sao lại có hiện tượng thở khò khè?

IT Cosa provoca i rantoli?

KO 어떤 때에 숨 쉴 때 쌕쌕 소리가 납니까?
Eo-tteon ttae-e sum swil ttae ssaek-ssaek so-ri-ga nam-ni-kka?

RU Что вызывает свистяще дыхание?
Chto vyzyvaet svistyashche dykhanie?

PL Co wywołuje ten świszczący oddech?

AR ما هو الشيء الذي يسبب الازيز؟
Ma huwa ash-shey' 'iladhee yesabbib al-azeez?

PT O que é que provoca a pieira?

FK Kisa ki koze sifleman an komanse?

EL Τι προκαλεί το συριγμό;
tee prokalEE to seereegmO?

HI घरघराहट का क्या कारण था? ...
Ghargharahat ka kya kaaraN tha?

Common cold / cold air / dust / pets

Enfriamiento / polvo del aire / animales domésticos

普通感冒 / 冷空气 / 灰尘 / 宠物
pǔ tōng gǎn mào / lěng kōng qì / huī chén / chǒng wù

Rhume banal / air froid / poussières / animaux domestiques

Erkältung / kalte Luft / Staub / Haustiere

Cảm lạnh thông thường / không khí lạnh / bụi / thú nuôi

Raffreddore comune / aria fredda / polvere / animali domestici

일반 감기 / 차가운 공기 / 먼지 / 애완 동물
il-ban gam-gi / cha-ga-un gong-gi / meon-ji / ae-wan dong-mul

Простуда / холодный воздух / пыль / домашние животные
Prostuda / kholodnyi vozdukh / pyl' / domashnie zhivotnye

Przeziębienie / zimne powietrze / kurz / zwierzęta domowe

الزكام العادي \ الهواء البارد \ الغبار \ الحيوانات الأليفة
Az-zukkaam al-"aadi / al-hawaa' al-baarid / al-ghubaar / al-haywaanaat al-'aleefah

Constipação / ar frio / pó / animais de estimação

Lagrip / tan fret / pousye / ninpòt ki zanimo domestic

κοινό κρυολόγημα / κρύος αέρας / σκόνη / κατοικίδια
keenO kreeolOgeema / krEEos aEras / skOnee / kateekEEdeea

सामान्य जुकाम / नज़ला / गड़बड़ / चिड़चिड़ापन ...
samanya jhukam / nazla / gaDbaD / chiDchiDapan

pollen / physical activity / anger

ES polen / actividad física / enojo

ZH 花粉 / 运动 / 生气
huā fěn / yùn dòng / shēng qì

FR pollen / activité physique / irritabilité

DE Pollen / körperliche Betätigung / Ärger

VI phấn hoa / vận động cơ thể / giận dữ

IT polline / attività fisica / rabbia

KO 꽃가루 / 육체적 활동 / 분노
kkot-ga-ru / yuk-che-jeok hwal-dong / bun-no

RU пыльца / физическая активность / гнев
pyl'tsa / fizicheskaya aktivnost' / gnev

PL pyłek kwiatowy / aktywność fizyczna / gniew

AR غبار الطلع / النشاط الجسماني \ الغضب
Ghubar at-tala" / an-nashaat al-jismaani / al-ghadhab

PT pólen / actividade física / ira

FK pollen / aktivite fizik / kolè

EL γύρη / σωματική δραστηριότητα / θυμός
gEEree / somateekEE drasteereeOteeta / theemOs

HI रजयुक्त / शारीरिक गतिविधि ६ T / क्रो ६ T
rajyukta / sharirik gatividhi / krodh

Is he / she experiencing coughing / allergies / an eczema / skin rashes / itching skin?

S ¿Ha tenido tos / alergias / eccema / erupciones / comezón (picazón)?

H 他 / 她是否有咳嗽 / 过敏 / 湿疹 / 皮肤出疹 / 皮肤搔痒?
tā / tā shì fǒu yǒu ké sou / guò mǐn / shī zhěn / pí fū chū zhěn / pí fū são yǎng?

R A-t-il / elle toussé / présenté une allergie / un eczéma / une éruption cutanée / des démangeaisons?

E Hat er / sie Husten / Allergien / ein Ekzem, Hautausschlag / juckende Haut?

I Em có đang bị ho / dị ứng / chàm bội nhiễm / nổi mẩn trên da / ngứa da không?

T Ha tosse / allergie / un eczema / eruzioni cutanee / prurito alla pelle?

O 아이가 기침 / 알레르기 / 습진 / 피부 발진 / 가려운 피부를 경험하고 있습니까?
A-i-ga gi-chim / al-le-reu-gi / seup-jin / pi-bu bal-jin / ga-ryeo-un pi-bu-reul gyeong-heom-ha-go it-seum-ni-kka?

U Есть ли у него / неё сейчас кашель / аллергия / экзема / кожная сыпь / кожный зуд?
Est' li u nego / neyo seychas kashel' / allergiya / ekzema / kozhnaya syp' / kozhnyi zud?

L Czy on / ona ma kaszel / uczulenia / egzemę / wysypki skórne / świąd skóry?

R هل يعاني \ تعاني من السعال \ الحساسيات \ أكزيما \ الطفح الجلدي \ الحك في الجلد؟
Hal yu"aani / tu"aani min as-su"aal / al-hassaasiyaat / ikzeema / at-tafah al-jildi / al-hakk fil-jild?

T Ele / ela tem tido tosse / alergias / um eczema / erupções cutâneas / comichão na pele?

K Eske lap touse / aleji / egzema / iritasyon po / po l ap grate l?

L Παθαίνει αυτός / αυτή βήχα / αλλεργίες / εκζήμα / δερματικά εξανθήματα / φαγούρα στο δέρμα;
pathEnee aftOs / aftEE vEEha / alergEEes / ekzEEma / dermateekA exanthEEmata / fagUra sto dErma;

HI क्या वह खांसी / एलर्जी / खुजली / त्वचा छिलना / खारिश का अनुभव कर रहा / रही है?
Kya vah khaansi / alergy / khujli / twacha Chilna / kharish ka anubhav kar raha / rahi hai?

Has he / she swallowed something small?

ES	¿Se tragó algún objeto pequeño?
ZH	他 / 她有没有吞咽什么小东西？ tā / tā yǒu méi yǒu tūn yàn shén me xiǎo dōng xi?
FR	a-t-il / elle avalé un petit objet?
DE	Hat er / sie etwas Kleines verschluckt?
VI	Em có nuốt phải một vật gì nhỏ không?
IT	Ha inghiottito qualcosa di piccole dimensioni?
KO	작은 물체를 삼켰습니까? Ja-geun mul-che-reul sam-kyeot-seum-ni-kka?
RU	Он / она проглотил / проглотила что-нибудь маленькое? On / ona proglotil / proglotila chto-nibud' malen'koe?
PL	Czy on / ona połknął(a) jakąś małą rzecz?
AR	هل ابتلع \ إبتلعت شيئاً صغيراً؟ Hal ibtala"a / ibtala"at shey' sagheer?
PT	Ele / ela engoliu algum objecto pequeno?
FK	Eske li janm vale yon bagay ki piti?
EL	Κατάπιε αυτός / αυτή κάτι μικρό; katApee-e aftOs / aftEE kAtee meekrO?
HI	क्या उसने कोई छोटी चीज निगल ली है? ... Kya usne koi Choti cheez nigal li hai?

coin / piece of jewelry / pearl / peanut

moneda / alhaja / perla / cacahuete (maní)

硬币 / 小首饰 / 珠子 / 花生米
yìng bì / xiǎo shǒu shì / zhū zǐ / huā shēng mǐ

une pièce de monnaie / un bijou / une perle / une arachide

Münze / Schmuckstück / Perle / Erdnuss

đồng xu / đồ trang sức / hạt ngọc trai / đậu phộng

moneta / gioiello / buccia / arachide

동전 / 보석 / 진주 / 땅콩
dong-jeon / bo-seok / jin-ju / ttang-kong

монету / ювелирное изделие / жемчужину / арахис
monetu / yuvelirnoe izdelie / zhemchuzhinu / arakhis

monetę / klejnot / perłę / orzeszek ziemny?

عملة معدنية \ قطعة من المجوهرات \ لؤلؤة حبة فول سوداني
"Umlah ma"daniyah / qit"ah min al-mujauharaat / lu'lu'ah / habbat fool soudaani

moeda / jóia / casca / amendoim

monin / yon moso bijou / po / pistach

κέρμα / κομμάτι κοσμήματος / μαργαριτάρι / φιστίκι
kEmra / komAtee kosmEEmatos / margareetAree / feestEEkee

सिक्का / ज़ेवर का हिस्सा / मोती / मटर
sikka / zevar ka hissa / moti / matar

22 Pain

Do you presently have pain? Where is the pain located?

ES ¿Tiene actualmente algún dolor? ¿Dónde lo siente?

ZH 你现在痛吗？哪里痛呢？
nǐ xiàn zài tòng ma? nǎ lǐ tòng ne?

FR Avez-vous mal en ce moment? Où est localisée la douleur?

DE Haben Sie jetzt gerade Schmerzen? Wo (noch)?

VI Quý vị hiện có bị đau gì không? Quý vị bị đau ở đâu?

IT Prova dolore in questo momento? Dove è localizzato il dolore?

KO 현재 통증이 있으십니까? 어디에 통증이 있습니까?
Hyeon-jae tong-jeung-i i-seu-sim-ni-kka? Eo-di-e tong-jeung-i it-seum-ni-kka?

RU Вы сейчас испытываете боль? Где эта боль находится?
Vy seychas ispytyvaete bol'? Gde eta bol' nakhoditsya?

PL Czy oczuwa Pan(i) ból? Gdzie Pana (Panią) boli?

AR هل عندك ألم في الوقت الحاضر؟ أين مكان الألم؟
Hal "indak alam fil-waqt il-haadhir? Ayna makaan al-alam?

PT Neste momento sente alguma dor? Onde é que a dor está localizada?

FK Eske ou gen doulè kounye la? Kote doulè a ye ?

EL Έχετε πόνο επί του παρόντος; Πού βρίσκεται ο πόνος;
Ehete pOno epEE tu parOdos? pu vrEEskete o pOnos?

HI क्या आपको अभी दर्द है? दर्द कहां पर है?
Kya aapko abhi dard hai? Dard kahaan par hai?

Have you experienced any type of pain before? Where was the pain located? When?

S ¿Había tenido algún tipo de dolor antes? ¿Dónde lo sentía entonces? ¿Cuándo?

H 你以前有过何种痛吗？哪里痛？什么时候？
nǐ yǐ qián yǒu guò hé zhǒng tòng ma? nǎ li tòng? shén me shí hòu?

R Avez-vous déjà eu n'importe quel type de douleur auparavant? Où était-t-elle localisée? Quand?

E Hatten Sie früher irgendwelche Schmerzen? Wo? Wann?

VI Trước đây quý vị đã bao giờ bị đau chưa? Quý vị đã bị đau ở đâu? Khi nào?

T Ha mai avuto un qualunque tipo di dolore in precedenza? Dove era localizzato il dolore? Quando?

O 이전에 통증을 경험하신 적 있습니까? 어디에 통증이 있었습니까? 언제?
I-jeon-e tong-jeung-eul gyeong-heom-ha-sin jeok it-seum-ni-kka? Eo-di-e tong-jeung-i i-seot-seum-ni-kka? Eo-nje?

U Ранее вы испытывали какую-нибудь боль? Где эта боль находилась? Когда?
Ranee vy ispytyvali kakuyu-nibud' bol'? Gde eta bol' nakhodilas'? Kogda?

L Czy odczuwał(a) Pan(i) już wcześniej jakiś ból? Gdzie on był umiejscowiony? Kiedy?

R هَلْ سبق لك أن عانيت بنوع من الألم قبل ذلك؟ أين مكان الألم؟ متى وقع الألم؟
Hal sabaq lak an "aanayt bi-nou" min al-alam qabla dhaalik? Ayna al-alam? Mattaa waqa" al-alam?

Já sentiu algum tipo de dor? Onde é que a dor estava localizada? Quando?

K Eske ou te gen ninpòt ki kalite doulè avan? Kote doulè a te ye? Ki lè?

L Είχατε οποιοδήποτε είδος πόνου πριν; Πού βρισκόταν ο πόνος; Πότε;
EEhate opeeodEEpote EEdos pOnu preen? pu vreeskOtan o pOnos?

HI क्या आपने पहले भी किसी प्रकार के दर्द महसूस किया है? दर्द कहां पर था? कब?
Kya aapne pahle bhi kisi prakaar ke dard mehsoos kiya Hai? Dard kahaan par tha? Kab?

For how long do / did you have this pain?

ES ¿Cuánto tiempo le ha durado / le duró el dolor?

ZH 现在 / 以前痛了多久？
xiàn zài / yǐ qián tòng le duō jiǔ?

FR Depuis combien de temps avez-vous / eu cette douleur?

DE Wie lange haben / hatten Sie diese Schmerzen?

VI Quý vị bị / đã bị đau như thế này trong bao lâu?

IT Da quanto tempo ha / per quanto tempo ha avuto questo dolore?

KO 이 통증은 얼마나 갑 / 갔습니까?
I tong-jeung-eun eol-ma-na gap-ni-kka / ga-seum-ni-kka?

RU Как долго вы испытываете / испытывали эту боль?
Kak dolgo vy ispytyvaete / ispytyvali etu bol'?

PL Od jak dawna Pan(i) go odczuwa / odczuwał(a)?

AR لكم مدة يكون \ كان عندك هذا الألم؟
Li-kam muddah yakoon \ kaan "indak hadhaa al-alam?

PT Há quanto tempo tem / teve esta dor?

FK Panda konbyen tan ou gen / te gen doulè sa ?

EL Για πόσο έχετε / είχατε αυτόν τον πόνο;
geea pOso Ehete / EEhate aftOn ton pOno?

HI आपको यह दर्द कितने समय तक रहता है / रहा? ...
Aapko yeh dard kitne samay tak rahta hai / raha?

... hours / ... days ... weeks / ... years

... horas / ... días / ... semanas / ... años

几小时 / 几天 / 几周 / 几年
jǐ xiǎo shí / jǐ tiān / jǐ zhōu / jǐ nián

... heures / ... jours / ... semaines / ... années

... Stunden / ... Tage / ... Wochen / ... Jahre

... giờ / ... ngày ... tuần / ... năm

... ore / ... giorni / ... settimane / ... anni

... 시간 / ... 일 / ... 주 / ... 년
... si-gan / ... il / ... ju / ... nyeon

... часов / ... дней / ... недель / ... лет
... chasov / ... dney ... nedel' / ... let

... godzin / ... dni / ... tygodni / ... lat

... ساعة \ ... يوم \ ... \ اسبوع \ ... سنة
... saa"ah / ... youm / ... usboo" / ... sanah

... horas / ... dias / ... semanas / ... anos

... hètan / ... jou / ... semen / ... ane

...
... Ores / ... eemEres ... evdomAdes / ... hrOneea

... घंटे / ... दिन ... सप्ताह / ... वर्ष
... ghante / ... din ... saptaah / ... varSh

When does the pain occur?

ES	¿A qué hora aparece el dolor?
ZH	什么时候痛？ shén me shí hòu tòng?
FR	Quand la douleur survient-elle?
DE	Wann tritt der Schmerz auf?
VI	Quý vị bắt đầu đau từ khi nào?
IT	Quando si verifica il dolore?
KO	언제 통증이 생깁니까? Eon-je tong-jeung-i saeng-gim-ni-kka?
RU	Когда возникает эта боль? Kogda voznikaet eta bol'?
PL	Kiedy ten ból się pojawia?
AR	متى يقع الألم؟ Mattaa yaqa" al-alam?
PT	Quando é que a dor ocorre?
FK	Ki lè doulè a pran w?
EL	Πότε συμβαίνει ο πόνος; pOte seemvEnee o pOnos?
HI	दर्द कब होता है? ... Dard kab hota hai?

irregularly / in the morning / evening / at night / at daytime / before (after) meals

a cualquier hora / por la mañana / tarde / en la noche / en el día / antes (después) de comer

不规则 / 在早上 / 晚饭后 / 夜间 / 白天 / 饭前(饭后)
bù guī zé / zài zǎo shàng / wǎn fàn hòu / yè jiān / bái tiān / fàn qián (fàn hòu)

Irrégulièrement / le matin / le soir / la nuit / le jour / avant (après) les repas

(un)regelmäßig / morgens / abends / nachts / tagsüber / vor (nach) dem Essen

không thường xuyên / vào buổi sáng / buổi tối / buổi đêm / vào ban ngày / trước (sau) khi ăn

irregolarmente / la mattina / la sera / la notte / durante il giorno / prima (dopo) i pasti

대중없이 / 아침에 / 저녁에 / 밤에 / 낮에 / 식사 전(후)
dae-jung-eop-si / a-chi-me / jeo-nyeo-ge / ba-me / na-je / sik-sa jeon(hu)

нерегулярно / утром / вечером / ночью / днём / до (после) еды
neregulyarno / utrom / vecherom / noch'yu / dnyom / do (posle) edy

nieregulamie / rano / wieczorem / w nocy / w ciągu dnia / przed (po) posiłku

لا يقع في وقت معين \ في الصباح \ في المساء \ في الليل \ في النهار \ قبل (بعد) وجبات الطعام
La yaqa" fi waqt mu"ayyan / fis-sabaah / fil-masaa / fil-leyl / fin-nahaar / qabl (ba"d) wajbaat at-ta"aam

irregularmente / de manhã / de tarde / à noite / durante o dia / antes (depois) das refeições

Pa regilye / nan matin / aswe / pandan lan nwit la / lajounin / avan (apre) ou fin manje

ακανόνιστα / το πρωί / το απόγευμα / τη νύχτα / την ημέρα / πριν (μετά) τα γεύματα
akanOneesta / to proEE / to apOgevma / tee nEEhta / teen eemEra / preen (metA) ta gEvmata

अनियमित रूप से / सुबह / शाम / रात में / दिन में / खाना खाने से पहले (बाद) ...
A-niyamit roop se / subah / shaam / raat mein / din mein / khana khane se pahle (baad)

during meals / while walking / lying / moving / after physical exertion

ES	al comer / al caminar / al acostarse / al moverse / al hacer un esfuerzo

ZH 吃饭时 / 行走时 / 躺倒时 / 活动身子时 / 体育锻炼之后
chī fàn shí / xíng zǒu shí / tǎng dǎo shí / huó dòng shēn zǐ shí / tǐ yù duàn liàn zhī hòu

FR au cours des repas / en marchant / en étant couché / en mouvement / au cours d'un exercice physique

DE während des Essens / Gehens / Liegens / Bewegens / nach körperlicher Betätigung

VI trong khi ăn / khi đi bộ / nằm / cử động / sau khi vận động mạnh

IT durante i pasti / quando cammino / sono steso / a / / quando mi muovo / dopo aver fatto sforzi fisici

KO 식사 중에 / 걸을 때 / 누워있을 때 / 움직일 때 / 육체적으로 힘을 많이 쓴 후
sik-sa-jung-e / geo-reul ttae / nu-wo-i-seul ttae / um-ji-gil ttae / yuk-che-jeo-geu-ro hi-meul ma-ni ssen hu

RU во время еды / при ходьбе / в лежачем положении / при движении / после физического напряжения
vo vremya edy / pri khod'be / v lezhachem polozhenii / pri dvizhenii / posle fizicheskogo napryazheniya

PL podczas jedzenia / podczas chodzenia / leżenia / poruszania się / po wysiłku fizycznym

AR أثناء وجبات الطعام \ عند المشي \ عند الكذب \ عند التحرك \ بعد المشقة
Athnaa' wajbaat at-ta"aam / "ind al-mashiy / "ind al-kadhib / "ind at-taharruk / ba"d al-mashaqqah

PT durante as refeições / enquanto caminha / enquanto está deitado / enquanto se movimenta / depois de esforços físicos

FK pandan ou ap manje / pandant ou ap mache / kouche / apre ou fin bay kou w anpil mouvman

EL κατά τη διάρκεια των γευμάτων / ενώ περπατάτε / ξαπλώνετε / κινείστε / μετά από σωματικό κόπο
katA tee deeArkeea ton gevmAton / enO perpatAte / xaplOnete / keenEEste / metA apO somateekO kOpo

HI खाना खाने के दौरान / चलते समय / लेटे हुए / घूमते हुए / शारीरिक परिश्रम के बाद
khaana khaane ke dauraan / chalte samay / lete hue / ghoomte hue / shaaririk pariShram ke baad

Did the pain occur suddenly?

¿El dolor empezó de repente?

是突然痛的吗？
shì tū rán tòng de ma?

Cette douleur survient-elle brusquement?

Kam der Schmerz ganz plötzlich?

Cơn đau có khởi phát đột ngột không?

Il dolore si è verificato improvvisamente?

이 통증은 갑자기 생겼습니까?
I tong-jeung-eun gap-ja-gi saeng-gyeot-seum-ni-kka?

Эта боль появилась внезапно?
Eta bol' poyavilas' vnezapno?

Czy ten ból pojawił się nagle?

هل وقع الألم فجأة؟
Hal waqa" al-alam faj'atan?

A dor ocorreu de repente?

Eske doulè a parèt sou ou sibitman?

Συνέβη ο πόνος ξαφνικά;
seenEvee o pOnos xafneekA?

क्या दर्द अचानक हुआ?
Kya dard achaanak hua?

Does the pain recur / stay the same?

ES ¿El dolor se repite / se mantiene igual?

ZH 是反复发作痛 / 还是一直不变？
shì fǎn fù fā zuò tòng / hái shì yì zhí bù biàn?

FR Est-ce que cette douleur revient / ou est permanente?

DE Tritt der Schmerz wiederholt auf / ist er gleichbleibend?

VI Cơn đau có tái phát / vẫn như vậy không?

IT Il dolore ritorna / rimane lo stesso?

KO 이 통증은 없어졌다 다시 생겼다 합니까 / 이 통증은 항상 같습니까?
I tong-jeung-eun eop-seo-jyeot-da da-si saeng-gyeot-da-ham-ni-kka / i tong-jeung-eun hang-sang gat-seum-ni-kka?

RU Эта боль возникает снова / остается такой же?
Eta bol' voznikaet snova / ostaetsya takoy zhe?

PL Czy ten ból powraca / jest stale taki sam?

AR هل يتكرر الألم \ يبقى كما هو؟
Hal yitkarrir al-alam / yibqaa kamaa huwa?

PT A dor é reincidente / fica na mesma?

FK Eske doulè a reparè / rete mem jan an?

EL Υποτροπιάζει / Παραμένει ίδιος ο πόνος;
eepotropeeAzee / paramEnee EEdeeos o pOnos?

HI क्या दर्द दोबारा हुआ / उसी तरह बना रहा?
Kya dard dobaara hua / usi tarah banaa raha?

For how long does the pain last?

S ¿Cuánto tiempo dura el dolor?

H 痛了多久？
tòng le duō jiǔ?

R Combien de temps dure la douleur?

E Wie lange hält der Schmerz an?

VI Cơn đau kéo dài trong bao lâu?

T Quanto dura il dolore?

O 이 통증은 얼마나 오래 갑니까?
I tong-jeung-eun eol-ma-na o-rae gam-ni-kka?

U Как долго длится боль?
Kak dolgo dlitsya bol'?

.L Jak długo ten ból już trwa?

.R كم مدة يدوم الألم؟
Kam muddah yadoum al-alam?

T Durante quanto tempo é que a dor dura?

K Pandan konbyen tan doulè a ret sou ou?

L Για πόσο καιρό διαρκεί ο πόνος;
geea pOso kerO deearkEE o pOnos?

II दर्द कितनी देर तक रहा? ...
Dard kitni der tak raha?

always present / minutes / hours / days / comes and goes

ES	no se quita / minutos / horas / días / va y viene
ZH	一直痛／几分钟／几小时／几天／断断续续的痛 yì zhí tòng / jǐ fēn zhōng / jǐ xiǎo shí / jǐ tiān / duàn duàn xù xù de tòng
FR	elle est toujours présente / minutes / heures / jours / vient et s'en va
DE	ständig / Minuten / Stunden / Tage / er kommt und geht
VI	luôn cảm thấy đau / phút / giờ / ngày / hết rồi lại thấy đau
IT	sempre presente / minuti / ore / giorni / va e viene
KO	항상 있다 / 몇 분 / 몇 시간 / 수일 / 있다가 없다가 한다 hang-sang it-da / myeot bun / myeot si-gan / su-il / it-da-ga eop-da-ga han-da
RU	всегда присутствует / минуты / часы / дни / проходящая vsegda prisutstvuet / minuty / chasy / dni / prokhodyashchaya
PL	stale obecny / minuty / godziny / dni / mija i powraca
AR	موجود بشكل دائم \ يدوم عدة دقائق \ يدوم ساعات \ يدوم أيام \ يجيء ويذهب Maujoud bi-shekl daa'im / yadoum "iddati daqaa'iq / yadoim saa"aat / yadoum ayyam / yijee wa yadh-hab
PT	sempre presente / minutos / horas / dias / vai e vem
FK	toujou la / minit / plize hètan / plize jou / ale vini
EL	πάντα υπάρχει / λεπτά / ώρες / ημέρες / έρχεται και φεύγει pAnda eepArhee / leptA / Ores / eemEres / Erhete ke fEvgee
HI	हमेशा मौजूद / मिनट / घंटे / दिन / आता जाता रहा hamesha maujood / minute / ghante / din / aata jaata rahaa

How severe is the pain?

ES ¿Qué tan fuerte es el dolor?

ZH 痛的严重程度怎样？
tòng de yán zhòng chéng dù zěn yàng?

FR Quelle est l'intensité de la douleur?

DE Wie stark ist der Schmerz?

VI Quý vị thấy đau tới mức nào?

IT Quanto è forte il dolore?

KO 통증이 어느 정도입니까?
Tong-jeung-i eo-neu jeong-do-im-ni-kka?

RU Насколько боль сильная?
Naskol'ko bol' sil'naya?

PL Jak silny jest ten ból?

AR كيف شدة الألم؟
Kayf shiddat al-alam?

PT Qual é a intensidade da dor?

FK Ki nivo doulè a?

EL Πόσο σοβαρός είναι ο πόνος;
pOso sovarOs EEne o pOnos?

HI दर्द कितना तीव्र था? ...
Dard kita teevra tha?

pain scale from 0 to 10: 0 = no pain, 10 = unbearable pain

ES escala del dolor de 0 a 10: 0 = ningún dolor, 10 = dolor insoportable

ZH 痛的严重度从0到10：0是不痛，10是最痛
tòng de yán zhòng dù cóng 0 dào 10: 0 shì bù tòng, 10 shì zuì tòng

FR échelle de la douleur de 0 à 10: 0= pas de douleur, 10 = douleur insupportable

DE Schmerzskala von 0 bis 10: 0=kein Schmerz, 10= unerträglicher Schmerz

VI mức độ đau từ 0 tới 10: 0 = không đau, 10 = đau tới mức không chịu được

IT in una scala da 0 a 10: 0 = niente dolore, 10 = dolore insopportabile

KO 에서 10까지 통증을 표시한다면, 0=무통증, 10=참을 수 없는 통증
yeung-e-seo sip-kka-ji tong-jeung-eul pyo-si-han-da-myeon, yeung=mu-tong-jeung, sip=cha-meul su eom-neun tong-jeung

RU шкала боли от ноля (0) до десяти (10): ноль - нет боли, десять – невыносимая боль
shkala boli ot nolya (0) do desyati (10): nol' - net boli, desyat' - nevynosimaya bol'

PL w skali bólu od 0 do 10: 0= nie ma bólu, 10= ból jest nie do zniesienia

AR حسب المقياس من ٠ إلى ١٠ حيث ١٠ . يساوي لا ألم و ١٠ = ألم لا يُطاق
Hasab al-miqyaas min 0 ilaa 10 haithoo

PT Escala da dor de 0 a 10: 0 = sem dor, 10 = dor insuportável

FK nivo to doulè a de 0 a 10: 0= pa gen doulè; 10 = gen anpil doulè

EL κλίμακα πόνου από 0 έως 10: 0 = καθόλου πόνος, 10 = αφόρητος πόνος
klEEmaka pOnu apO meedEn EEos dEka: meedEn EEson kathOlu pOnos, dEka EEson afOreetos pOnos

HI दर्द मापी 0 से 10: 0 ऱ कोई दर्द नहीं, 10 ऱअसहनीय दर्द
Dard maapi 0 se 10: 0 = Koi dard nahi, 10=A-sahniya dard

Have you had this type of pain before?

ES ¿Ya había tenido antes este tipo de dolor?

ZH 你以前有过类似的痛吗？
nǐ yǐ qián yǒu guò lèi sì de tòng ma?

FR Avez-vous déjà eu ce type de douleur auparavant?

DE Hatten Sie diese Art von Schmerzen früher schon einmal?

VI Quý vị đã bao giờ bị đau như thế này chưa?

IT Ha mai avuto questo tipo di dolore in passato?

KO 이런 통증이 이전에도 있었습니까?
I-reon tong-jeung-i i-jeon-e-do i-seot-seum-ni-kka?

RU У вас была такая боль ранее?
U vas byla takaya bol' ranee?

PL Czy doznawał(a) Pan(i) już wcześniej tego rodzaju bólu?

AR هل سبق لك التعرض لمثل هذا الألم من قبل؟
Hal sabaq lak at-ta"arrudh li-mithl hadhaa al-alam min qabl?

PT Já alguma vez sentiu este tipo de dor?

FK Eske ou te jan gen kalite doulè sa a deja?

EL Είχατε αυτό το είδος πόνου πριν;
EEhate aftO to EEdos pOnu preen?

HI क्या आपको इस तरह का दर्द पहले भी हुआ था?
Kya aapko is tarah ka dard pahle bhi hua tha?

Did you receive treatment for this condition? Was the treatment successful?

ES	¿Le dieron tratamiento para ese problema? ¿Resultó útil el tratamiento?
ZH	你以前为这个痛接受过治疗吗？效果怎么样？ nǐ yǐ qián wèi zhè gè tòng jiē shòu guò zhì liáo ma? xiào guǒ zěn me yàng?
FR	Avez-vous reçu un traitement pour cet état? Le traitement a-t-il été efficace?
DE	Wurden Sie dagegen behandelt? Erfolgreich?
VI	Quý vị có được điều trị cho căn bệnh đó không? Biện pháp điều trị có hiệu quả không?
IT	È stato / a curato / a per questo disturbo? La cura ha avuto successo?
KO	이 증상에 대해 치료를 받았습니까? 치료가 성공적이었습니까? I jeung-sang-e dae-hae chi-ryo-reul ba-dat-seum-ni-kka? Chi-ryo-ga seong-gong-jeo-gi-eot-seum-ni-kka?
RU	Вам назначали лечение по этому поводу? Было ли лечение успешным? Vam naznachali lechenie po etomu povodu? Bylo li lechenie uspeshnym?
PL	Czy był(a) Pan(i) leczony(a) na tę chorobę? Czy to leczenie było skuteczne?
AR	هل تلقّيت علاجاً لهذا الوضع؟ هل كان العلاج ناجحاً؟ Hal talaqqayt "ilaaj li-haadha al-wadha"? Hal kaan al-"ilaaj naajih?
PT	Recebeu tratamento para esta condição? O tratamento foi bem sucedido?
FK	Eske ou te resevwa tretman pou kondisyon sa? Eske tretman an te gen sikse ?
EL	Λάβατε θεραπεία για αυτήν την πάθηση; Ήταν επιτυχής η θεραπεία; lAvate therapEEa geea aftEEn teen pAtheesee? EEtan epeeteehEEs ee therapEEa?
HI	क्या आपने इस दशा के लिए कोई इलाज करवाया? क्या इलाज सफल रहा था? Kya aapne is dasha ke liye koi ilaaj karvaya? Kya ilaaj safal raha tha?

How does the pain feel?

¿Cómo se siente el dolor?

感觉是什么样的痛？
gǎn jué shì shén me yàng de tòng?

Comment ressentez-vous la douleur?

Wie fühlt sich der Schmerz an?

Tình trạng đau hiện như thế nào?

Come descriverebbe il dolore?

어떤 식으로 아픈 지 설명해주시겠습니까?
Eo-tteon si-geu-ro a-peun ji seol-myeong-hae-ju-si-get-seum-ni-kka?

Какая это боль?
Kakaya eto bol'?

Jaki to jest ból ?

كيف شعور الألم؟
Kayf shu"oor al-alam?

Que tipo de dor sente?

Ki jan ou santi doulè a ?

Πώς νιώθετε τον πόνο;
pos neeOthete ton pOno?

दर्द कैसा है? ...
Dard kaisa hai?

sharp / pounding / burning / stabbing / cramping / shooting

ES cortante / palpitante / quemante / punzante / calambre / lancinante

ZH 尖痛 / 跳痛 / 火烧样痛 / 刺痛 / 绞痛 / 据痛
jiān tòng / tiào tòng / huǒ shāo yàng tòng / cì tòng / jiǎo tòng / jù tòng

FR aiguë / martèlement / brûlure / lancinante / crampe / élancement

DE reißend / pochend / brennend / stechend / krampfartig / ziehend

VI đau buốt / đau điếng người / nóng rát / đau nhói / đau thắt / nhói buốt

IT acuto / martellante / bruciante / lancinante / a crampi / a fitte

KO 날카로운 / 두들기듯 / 쓰림 / 아리는 / 경련성의 / 콕콕 쑤시는
nal-ka-ro-un / du-dul gi-deut / sseu-rim / a-ri-neun / gyeong-lyeon-seong-ui / kuk-kuk ssu-si-neun

RU острая / пульсирующая / жгучая / колющая / спастическая / стреляющая
ostraya / pul'siruyushchaya / zhguchaya / kolyushchaya / spasticheskaya / strelyayushchaya

PL ostry / pulsujący / piekący / kłujący / skurczowy / przeszywający

AR حاد \ ضارب \ محترق \ طاعن \ متشنج \ نابض
Haadd / dhaarib / muhtariq / taa"in / mutashannij / naabidh

PT aguda / latejante / ardente / penetrante / cólicas / muito forte

FK tranchant / egu / boulè / pesan / kramp / lanse

EL οξύς / συνθλιπτικός / καυστικός / διαξιφιστικός / συσφικτικός / σουβλιές
oxEEs / seenthleepteekOs / kafstikOs / deeaxeefeesteekOs / seesfeekteekOs / suvleeEs

HI बहुत तेज / तोड़ देने वाला / ज्वलनशील / कटु / मरोड़ देने वाला / मारने वाला
bahut tez / toD dene wala / jwalansheel / katu / maroD dene vala / maarne wala

Does the pain always occur in the same body region? Where?

¿Siente el dolor siempre en la misma parte del cuerpo? ¿Dónde?

一直是一个地方痛吗？是哪里？
yì zhí shì yī gè dì fāng tòng ma? shì nǎ lǐ?

La douleur revient-elle toujours au même endroit du corps? Où?

Tritt der Schmerz immer im gleichen Körperteil auf? Wo?

Quý vị có luôn thấy đau ở cùng một vùng trên cơ thể không? Ở chỗ nào?

Il dolore si verifica sempre nella stessa zona del corpo? Dove?

이 통증은 항상 같은 신체 부위에 생깁니까? 어디 입니까?
I tong-jeung-eun hang-sang ga-tun sin-che bu-wi-e saeng-gim-ni-kka? Eo-di im-ni-kka?

Боль всегда возникает в одном и том же месте? Где?
Bol' vsegda voznikaet v odnom i tom zhe meste? Gde?

Czy ten ból zawsze pojawia się w tej samej okolicy? Gdzie?

هل يقع الألم دائماً في نفس منطقة الجسم؟ أين يقع؟
Hal yaqa" al-alam daa'iman fi nafs mantiqat il-jism? Ayna yaqa"?

A dor ocorre sempre na mesma parte do corpo? Onde?

Eske doulè a toujou parèt nan mem kote a nan ko w ? Ki bo ?

Συμβαίνει ο πόνος πάντα στην ίδια περιοχή του σώματος; Πού;
seemvEnee o pOnos pAnda steen EEdeea pereeohEE tu sOmatos? pu?

क्या दर्द हमेशा शरीर के एक ही भाग में होता है? कहां?
Kya dard hamesha Shareer ke ek hi bhaag mein hota hai? Kahaan?

Does the pain radiate in a particular direction? Which direction?

ES ¿Se irradia el dolor en una dirección en especial? ¿Hacia dónde?

ZH 疼痛向哪里放射吗？向哪里呢？
téng tòng xiàng nǎ lǐ fàng shè ma? xiàng nǎ lǐ ne?

FR La douleur irradie-t-elle dans une direction particulière? Quelle direction?

DE Strahlt der Schmerz aus? Wohin?

VI Cơn đau có lan tỏa theo hướng nào đó không? Hướng nào?

IT Il dolore si irradia in una particolare direzione? In che direzione?

KO 이 통증이 일정한 방향으로 퍼집니까? 어떤 방향입니까?
I tong-jeung-i il-jeong-han bang-hyang-eu-ro peo-jim-ni-kka? Eo-tteon bang-hyang-im-ni-kka?

RU Эта боль отражается в каком-то определенном направлении? Куда именно?
Eta bol' otrazhaetsya v kakom-to opredelennom napravlenii? Kuda imenno?

PL Czy ból ten promieniuje w jakimś szczególnym kierunku? W jakim kierunku?

AR هل ينتشر الألم في إتجاه معيّن؟ أي الإتّجاه؟
Hal yantashir al-alam fi ittijaah mu"ayyan? Ayyi ittijaah?

PT A dor irradia numa direcção especial? Em que direcção?

FK Eske doulè a mache nan yon direksyon an patikilye? Nan ki direksyon?

EL Διαχέεται ο πόνος προς κάποια συγκεκριμένη κατεύθυνση; Ποια κατεύθυνση;
deeahEete o pOnos pros kApeea seegekreemEnee katEftheensee? peeA katEftheensee?

HI क्या दर्द किसी निश्चित दिशा में बढ़ता है? कौनसी दिशा में?
Kya dard kisi nishchit disha mein baDhta hai? Kaunsi disha mein?

Where do you feel pain at the moment?

¿Dónde siente el dolor en este momento?

你现在哪里痛？
nǐ xiàn zài nǎ lǐ tòng?

Où ressentez-vous la douleur, en ce moment?

Wo tut es Ihnen jetzt weh?

Hiện giờ quý vị cảm thấy đau ở đâu?

In questo momento dove prova dolore?

지금 어디에 통증이 있으십니까?
Ji-geum eo-di-e tong-jeung-i i-seu-sim-ni-kka?

Где у вас сейчас болит?
Gde u vas seychas bolit?

Gdzie odczuwa Pan(i) ból w tej chwili?

أين تشعر \ تشعرين بالألم في الوقت الحاضر؟
Ayna tish"ur / tish"ureen bil-alam fil-waqt al-haadhir?

Neste momento onde é que sente a dor?

Kote ou santi doulè a kounye la?

Πού νιώθετε τον πόνο αυτήν τη στιγμή;
pu neeOthete ton pOno aftEEn tee steegmEE?

आप इस समय कहां पर दर्द महसूस कर रहे हैं?
Aap is samay kahaan par dard mehsoos kar rahe hain?

What alleviates the pain?

ES · ¿Con qué se alivia el dolor?

ZH · 怎么样能使疼痛减轻？
zěn me yàng néng shǐ téng tòng jiǎn qīng?

FR · Qu'est-ce qui soulage la douleur?

DE · Was hilft gegen die Schmerzen?

VI · Điều gì giúp làm giảm đau?

IT · Cosa allevia il dolore?

KO · 어떻게 하면 통증이 경감됩니까?
Eo-tteo-ke ha-myeon tong-jeung-i gyeong-gam-doem-ni-kka?

RU · Что облегчает эту боль?
Chto oblegchaet etu bol'?

PL · Co ból łagodzi?

AR · ما هو الذي يخفّف الألم؟
Maa huwa aladhi yikhaffif al-alam?

PT · O que é que alivia a dor?

FK · Kisa ki ba ou soulajman pou doulè a?

EL · Τι ανακουφίζει τον πόνο;
tee anakufEEzee ton pOno?

HI · दर्द किससे कम होता है? ...
Dard kisse kam hota hai?

change of body position / heat / cold / physical rest / medications (specify) / nothing

cambio de posición / calor / frío / reposo / medicamentos (especifique) / con nada

改变体位／热敷／冷敷／休息／药物（哪一种）／没办法减轻
gǎi biàn tǐ wèi / rè fū / lěng fū / xiū xi / yào wù (nǎ yī zhǒng) / méi bàn fā jiǎn qīng

Changement de position du corps / le chaud / le froid / le repos / des médicaments (spécifiez lesquels) / rien

Position verändern / Wärme / Kälte / Schonung / Medikamente (welche?) / nichts

thay đổi tư thế cơ thể / nóng / lạnh / nghỉ ngơi / dùng thuốc (trình bày rõ) / không có gì cả

cambiare posizione del corpo / calore / freddo / riposo / medicine(specificare) / nulla

몸의 자세를 변화시킴 / 따뜻하게 함 / 차게 함 / 육체 휴식 / 약 (구체적으로) / 아무 것도 없다
mom-ui ja-se-reul byeon-hwa-si-kim / tta-tteu-ta-ge ham / cha-ge ham / yuk-che hyu-sik / yak (gu-che-jeo-geuro) / a-mu geot-do eop-da

изменение положения тела / тепло / холод / отдых / лекарства (уточните) / ничто
izmenenie polozheniya tela / teplo / kholod / otdykh / lekarstva (utochnite) / nichto

zmiana pozycji ciała / ciepło / zimno / odpoczynek fizyczny / leki (proszę uściślić) / nic

تغير موقع الجسم \ الحرارة \ البرد \ الإستراحة الجسمانية \ الأدوية (بين \ بيني نوعها) \ لا شيء
Taghyeer mauqa" al-jism / al-haraarah / al-bard / al-istiraahah al-jismaaniyah / al-adwiyyah (bayyin / bayyinee nau"ihaa) / laa shey'

mudar a posição do corpo/calor/frio/descanso físico / medicamentos (especifique) / nada

Chanje pozisyon kou w / chale / fredi / repo / medikaman (di ki les) / anyen

αλλαγή στάσης σώματος / θερμότητα / κρύο / σωματική ξεκούραση / φάρμακα (καθορίστε) / τίποτα
alagEE stAsees sOmatos / thermOteeta / krEEo / somateekEE xekUrasee / fArmaka (kathorEEste) / tEEpota

शरीर की स्थिति में बदलाव / गर्मी / सर्दी / शारीरिक आराम / दवा (स्पष्ट करें) में परिवर्तन / किसी से नहीं
Sharir ki sThiti mein badlaav / garmi / sardi / sharirik aaraam / davaa (spaSht karein) mein parivartan / kisi se nahi

23 Examination

I am going to examine you now

ES Ahora voy a examinarlo

ZH 我来给你检查一下
wǒ lái gěi nǐ jiǎn chá yī xià

FR Je vais vous examiner maintenant

DE Ich möchte Sie / dich jetzt untersuchen

VI Bây giờ tôi sẽ khám cho quý vị

IT Ora La visito

KO 이제 진단을 하겠습니다
I-je jin-da-neul ha-get-seum-ni-da

RU Я хочу осмотреть вас
Ya khochu osmotret' vas

PL Teraz Pana / Panią zbadam

AR سأقوم بفحصك الآن
Sa'aqoom bi-fahsak al-aan

PT Vou examiná-lo(a) agora

FK Kounye la mwen pral fè yon egzamin pou ou

EL Θα σας εξετάσω τώρα
tha sas exetAso tOra

HI मैं अब आपकी जाँच करने जा रहा हूं
mein ab aapki jaanch karne jaa raha hun

Please remove your pants / dress / top clothing

Por favor quítese el pantalón / vestido / la ropa de arriba

请脱去裤子 / 外套 / 上衣
qǐng tuō qù kù zǐ / wài tào / shàng yī

Veuillez, s'il vous plaît, enlever votre pantalon / votre robe / le dessus

Bitte die Hose / den Rock / das Oberteil ausziehen

Xin cởi bỏ quần / váy / áo ra

Per favore si tolga i pantaloni / il vestito / gli indumenti della parte superiore

바지 / 드레스 / 웃옷을 벗으십시오
Ba-ji / deu-re-seu / ut-o-seul beo-seu-sip-si-o

Пожалуйста, снимите ваши брюки / платье / верхнюю одежду
Pozhaluysta, snimite vashi bryuki / plat'ye / verkhnyuyu odezhdu

Proszę zdjąć spodnie / sukienkę / górną część garderoby

الرجاء فك البناطيل \ الفستان \ الملابس الخارجية
Ar-rajaa' fakk al-banaateel / al-fustaan / al-malaabis al-khaarijiyah

Por favor, tire as calças / vestido / roupa de cima

Tanpri retire pantaloon w / rad ou / rat ki anle yo

Παρακαλώ βγάλτε το παντελόνι / φόρεμα / μπλούζα σας
parakalO vgAlte to padelOnee / fOrema / blUza sas

कृपया अपनी पैंट / कपड़े / ऊपर के कपड़े उतारें
kripya apnai pants / kapRe / upper ke kapRe utarein

Please put your clothes back on

ES Por favor vuelva a vestirse

ZH 请穿回衣服
qǐng chuān huí yī fú

FR S'il vous plaît, remettez vos vêtements

DE Bitte wieder anziehen

VI Quý vị có thể mặc lại quần áo

IT Per favore si rivesta

KO 옷을 다시 입으십시오
O-seul da-si i-beu-sip-si-o

RU Пожалуйста, оденьтесь
Pozhaluysta, oden'tes'

PL Proszę się ubrać

AR الرجاء ارتداء الملابس
Ar-rajaa' irtidaa' al-malaabis

PT Por favor, volte a vestir a roupa

FK Tanpri abiye w anko

EL Παρακαλώ φορέστε ξανά τα ρούχα σας
parakalO forEste xanA ta rUha sas

HI कृपया अपने कपड़े पहन लें
kripya apne kapRe pehene lein

Please lie down / stand up

ES Por favor acuéstese / póngase de pie

ZH 请躺下 / 站起来
qǐng tǎng xià / zhàn qǐ lái

FR S'il vous plaît, couchez-vous / levez-vous

DE Bitte hinlegen / aufstehen

VI Xin nằm xuống / đứng lên

IT Si stenda / si alzi, per favore

KO 누우십시오 / 일어서십시오
Nu-u-sip-si-o / i-reo-seo-sip-si-o

RU Пожалуйста, лягте / встаньте
Pozhaluysta, lyagte / vstan'te

PL Proszę się położyć / wstać

AR الرجاء انبطح \ انبطحي \ قم \ قمي
Ar-rajaa' inbatih / inbatihee / qum / qumee

PT Deite-se / levante-se, por favor

HT Tanpri kouche / kanpe

EL Παρακαλώ ξαπλώστε / σηκωθείτε όρθιοι
parakalO xaplOste / seekothEEte Orthee-ee

HI कृपया लेट जाएं / खड़े हो जाएं
kripya let jaayein / khaRe ho jaayein

Please repeat

ES	Por favor repita
ZH	请再来一次 qǐng zài lái yī cì
FR	Veuillez répéter, s'il vous plaît
DE	Noch einmal bitte
VI	Xin vui lòng nhắc lại
IT	Ripeta, per favore
KO	반복하십시오 Ban-bok-ha-sip-si-o
RU	Пожалуйста, повторите Pozhaluysta, povtorite
PL	Proszę powtórzyć
AR	الرجاء كرر \ كرري Ar-rajaa' karrir / karriree
PT	Repita, por favor
FK	Tanpre repete l anko
EL	Παρακαλώ επαναλάβετε parakalO epanalAvete
HI	कृपया दोहराएं kripya dohrein

Does it hurt if I press here / let go here?

¿Le duele si aprieto aquí / si suelto aquí?

我压 / 松开这里时你感觉痛吗？
wǒ yā / sōng kāi zhè lǐ shí nǐ gǎn jué tòng ma?

Est-ce que cela fait mal si je pousse ici / si je lâche ici?

Tut es weh, wenn ich hier drücke / loslasse?

Quý vị có thấy đau không khi tôi ấn vào đây / di tay tới đây?

Le fa male se spingo qui / lascio qui?

여기를 누르면 / 여기에서 손을 떼면 아픕니까?
Yeo-gi-reul nu-reu-myeon / yeo-gi-e-seo so-neul tte-myeon a-peum-ni-kka?

Здесь болит, когда я давлю / отпускаю?
Zdes' bolit, kogda ya davlyu / otpuskayu?

Czy boli gdy tu uciskam / zwalniam ucisk?

هل تشعر \ تشعرين بالألم إذا ضغطت هنا \ ازلت الضغط هنا؟
Hal tish"ur / tish"ureen bil-alam idhaa dhaghattu hinaa / azalt idh-dhaghat huna?

Dói-lhe quando faço pressão aqui / deixo de fazer pressão aqui?

Eske li fè w mal lè mwen peze la a / lage la a ?

Πονάει εάν πιέσω εδώ / αφήσω εδώ;
ponAee eAn peeEso edO / afEEso edO?

क्या दर्द होता है यदि मैं यहां दबाऊं / यहां जाने दूं?
kya dard hota hai yadi main yahan dabaaun / yaha jane dun?

Please follow what I am doing

ES · Por favor haga lo mismo que yo

ZH · 请跟着我的动作做
qǐng gēn zhè wǒ de dòng zuò zuò

FR · S'il vous plaît, veuillez suivre ce que je fais

DE · Bitte das machen, was ich mache

VI · Xin làm theo những gì tôi đang làm

IT · Per favore, segua ciò che faccio

KO · 제가 하는 대로 따라 해보십시오
Je-ga ha-neun dae-ro tta-ra hae-bo-sip-si-o

RU · Пожалуйста, повторяйте за мной
Pozhaluysta, povtoryayte za mnoy

PL · Proszę uważać na to, co robię

AR · لطفاً تابع \ تابعى مع الذى افعله
Lutfan taabi" / taabi"ee ma" aladhi af"aloh

PT · Por favor, siga o que eu estou a fazer

FK · Tanpri swiv sa map fè a

EL · Παρακαλώ ακολουθήστε αυτό που κάνω
parakalO akolouthEEste aftO pu kAno

HI · कृपया अनुशरण करें जो मैं कर रहा हूँ
kripya anusharaN karein jo main kar raha hun

Please move

Por favor mueva

请移动
qǐng yí dòng

S'il vous plaît, changez de place

Bitte bewegen

Xin cử động

Per favore, muova

을 / 를 움직이십시오
eul / reul um-ji-gi-sip-si-o

Пожалуйста, подвигайте
Pozhaluysta, podvigayte

Proszę się poruszyć

الرجاء تحرك \ تحركي
Ar-rajaa' taharrak / taharrakee

Por favor, mova-se

Tanpri deplase (fe movman ak)

Παρακαλώ κινηθείτε
parakalO keeneethEEte

कृपया चलें ...
kripya chalein

I want to take your temperature / blood pressure / pulse

ES Quiero medirle la temperatura / la presión / el pulso

ZH 我想给你量一下体温 / 血压 / 脉搏
wǒ xiǎng gěi nǐ liáng yī xià tǐ wēn / xuè yā / mài bó

FR J'ai l'intention de prendre votre température / votre pression sanguine / votre pouls

DE Ich möchte Ihre / n Temperatur / Blutdruck / Puls messen

VI Tôi muốn đo nhiệt độ / huyết áp / mạch của quý vị

IT Voglio misurarLe la temperatura / la pressione / il polso

KO 체온 / 혈압 / 맥박을 재겠습니다
Che-on / hyeo-rap / maek-ba-geul jae-get-seum-ni-da

RU Я хочу измерить вашу температуру / артериальное давление / пульс
Ya khochu izmerit' vashu temperaturu / arterial'noe davlenie / pul's

PL Chcę zmierzyć Pani(i) temperaturę / ciśnienie krwi / tętno

AR انا اريد أن اقيس درجة حرارتك \ ضغط دمك \ نبضتك
Ana ureed an aqees daraja haraaratak / dhaght dammak / nabdhatak

PT Quero tirar a sua temperatura / medir a sua tensão arterial / contar as suas pulsações

FK Mwen vle pran tanperati w / tansyon w / to batman kè w

EL Θέλω να πάρω τη θερμοκρασία / αρτηριακή πίεση / παλμούς σας
thElo na pAro tee thermokrasEEa / arteereeakEE pEEesee / palmUs sas

HI मैं आपका तापमान / रक्तचाप / नब्ज़ देखना चाहता हूं
mein aapka taapmaan / raktchaap / nabz dekhna chahta hun

Please open your mouth / stick out your tongue / say "Ahh"

Por favor abra la boca / saque la lengua / diga "Aaah"

请张开口 / 伸出舌头 / 说"啊"
qǐng zhāng kāi kǒu / shēn chū shé tóu shuō "ā"

Veuillez ouvrir la bouche, s'il vous plaît / sortez la langue / dites "Ahh"

Bitte den Mund öffnen / die Zunge zeigen / "ah" sagen

Vui lòng há miệng / thè lưỡi ra / nói "Ahh"

La prego di aprire la bocca / tirare fuori la lingua / dica "Ahh"

입을 벌려 주십시오 / 혀를 내밀어 주십시오 / "아" 하십시오
I-beul beol-lyeo ju-sip-si-o / hyeo-reul nae-mi-reo ju-sip-si-o / "a" ha-sip-si-o

Пожалуйста, откройте рот / высуньте язык / скажите «А»
Pozhaluysta, otkroyte rot / vysun'te yazyk / skazhite «A»

Proszę otworzyć usta / pokazać język / powiedzieć „Aaa"

الرجاء فتح الفم \ إخراج اللسان \ النطق بـ"اه"
Ar-rajaa' fat'h al-famm / ikhraaj al-lisaan / an-nutq bi-"aah"

Por favor, abra boca / deite a língua de fora / diga "Ah"

Tanpri louvri bouch ou / met lang ou deyo / di "Ahh"

Παρακαλώ ανοίξτε το στόμα σας / βγάλτε τη γλώσσα σας / πείτε «Ααα»
parakalO anEExte to stOma sas / vgAlte tee glOssa sas / pEEte aaa

कृपया अपना मुंह खोलें / अपनी जीभ बाहर निकालें / "आह" कहें
kripya apna muhn kholein / apni jeebh baahar nikalein / "ahh" kahein

Please open / close your eyes

ES Por favor abra / cierre los ojos

ZH 请睁开眼 / 闭上眼
qǐng zhēng kāi yǎn / bì shàng yǎn

FR Veuillez, s'il vous plaît, ouvrir / fermer les yeux

DE Bitte die Augen öffnen / schließen

VI Vui lòng mở mắt / nhắm mắt

IT La prego di aprire / chiudere gli occhi

KO 눈을 떠 / 감아 주십시오
Nu-neul tteo / ga-ma ju-sip-si-o

RU Пожалуйста, откройте / закройте глаза
Pozhaluysta, otkroyte / zakroyte glaza

PL Proszę otworzyć / zamknąć oczy

AR الرجاء فتح \ غلق العينين
Ar-rajaa' fat'h / ghalq al-"aynayn

PT Por favor, abra / feche os olhos

FK Tanpri louvri / femin zye w

EL Παρακαλώ ανοίξτε / κλείστε τα μάτια σας
parakalO anEExte / klEEste ta mAteea sas

HI कृपया अपनी आंखें खोलें / बंद करें
kripya apni ankhein kholein / band karein

Please look up / down / towards the side

Mire por favor para arriba / abajo / hacia un lado

请向上看 / 向下 / 向侧面看
qǐng xiàng shàng kàn / xiàng xià / xiàng cè miàn kàn

Veuillez, s'il vous plaît, regarder vers le haut / vers le bas / sur le côté

Bitte nach oben / unten / auf die Seite schauen

Vui lòng nhìn lên / xuống / sang bên cạnh

La prego di guardare in alto / in basso / di lato

위로 / 아래로 / 옆으로 보십시오
Wi-ro / a-rae-ro / yeo-peu-ro bo-sip-si-o

Пожалуйста, посмотрите вверх / вниз / в сторону
Pozhaluysta, posmotrite vverkh / vniz / v storonu

Proszę spojrzeć w górę / w dół / w bok

الرجاء انظر \ انظري فوق \ تحت \ إلى الجانب
Ar-rajaa' undhur / undhuree fauq / taht / ilaa al-jaanib

Por favor, olhe para cima / para baixo / para o lado

Tanpri gade anlè / anba / sou kote

Παρακαλώ κοιτάξτε επάνω / κάτω / προς το πλάι
parakalO keetAxte epAno / kAto / pros to plAee

कृपया ऊपर / नीचे / एक तरफ देखें
kripya oopar / neeche / ek taraf dekhein

Please look right / left / towards here / towards the light

ES
Por favor mire a la derecha / a la izquierda / hacia acá / hacia la luz

ZH
请看右边 / 左边 / 这里 / 灯光
qǐng kàn yòu biān / zuǒ biān / zhè lǐ / dēng guāng

FR
Veuillez, s'il vous plaît, regarder à droite / à gauche / vers moi / vers la lumière

DE
Bitte nach rechts / links / hierhin / zum Licht schauen

VI
Vui lòng nhìn về phía bên phải / bên trái / hướng về đây / hướng về phía có ánh sáng

IT
La prego di guardare a destra / a sinistra / verso di me / verso la luce

KO
오른쪽으로 / 왼쪽으로 / 이쪽으로 / 빛 쪽으로 보십시오
O-reun-jjo-geu-ro / oen-jjo-geu-ro / i-jjo-geu-ro / bit jjo-geu-ro bo-sip-si-o

RU
Пожалуйста, посмотрите направо / налево / сюда / на свет
Pozhaluysta, posmotrite napravo / nalevo / syuda / na svet

PL
Proszę spojrzeć w prawo / w lewo / w tę stronę / w stronę światła

AR
الرجاء انظر \ انظري لليمين \ لليسار \ إلى هذا الطرف \ إلى الضوء
Ar-rajaa' undhur / undhuree lil-yameen / lil-yasaar / ilaa hadha at-taraf / ilaa adh-dhoo'

PT
Por favor, olhe para a direita / esquerda / para aqui / para a luz

FK
Tanpri gad a dwat / a goch / zon isit la / nan direksyon limye a

EL
Παρακαλώ κοιτάξτε δεξιά / αριστερά / προς τα εδώ / προς το φως
parakalO keetAxte dexeeA / areesterA / pros ta edO / pros to fos

HI
कृपया दाएं/ बाएं/ इस तरफ/ उस तरफ प्रकाश की ओर देखें
kripya dayein / bayein / is taraf / us taraf prakash ki or dekhein

Please follow my finger

Por favor siga mi dedo con la vista

请顺着我的手指看
qǐng shùn zhè wǒ de shǒu zhǐ kàn

Veuillez, s'il vous plaît, suivre mon doigt

Bitte meinem Finger folgen

Vui lòng nhìn theo ngón tay của tôi

Segua il mio dito, per favore

제 손가락을 눈으로 따라 가십시오
Je son-ga-ra-geul nu-neu-ro tta-ra ga-sip-si-o

Пожалуйста, следите за моим пальцем
Pozhaluysta, sledite za moim pal'tsem

Proszę patrzeć na mój palec

الرجاء تابع \ تابعي اصبعي
Ar-rajaa' tabi" / tabi"ee usbu"ee

Por favor siga o meu dedo

Tanpri swiv dwet mwen

Παρακαλώ ακολουθήστε το δάχτυλό μου
parakalO akoluthEEste to dAhteelO mou

कृपया मेरी अंगुली का अनुशरण करें
kripya meri anguli ka anushraN karein

How many fingers do you see?

ES ¿Cuántos dedos ve?

ZH 你能看到几个手指？
nǐ néng kàn dào jǐ gè shǒu zhǐ?

FR Combien de doigts voyez-vous?

DE Wie viele Finger sehen Sie?

VI Quý vị nhìn thấy bao nhiêu ngón tay?

IT Quante dita vede?

KO 손가락이 몇 개 보입니까?
Son-ga-ra-gi myeot gae bo-im-ni-kka?

RU Сколько пальцев вы видите?
Skol'ko pal'tsev vy vidite?

PL Ile palców Pan(i) widzi?

AR كم اصبع تراه \ ترينه؟
Kam usbu" taraahu / taraeenoh?

PT Quantos dedos vê?

FK Konbyen dwet ke ou we?

EL Πόσα δάχτυλα βλέπετε;
pOsa dAhteela vlEpete?

HI आपको कितनी अंगुलियां दिखाई देती हैं?
aapko kitni angulian dekhaee deti hain

Can you read this? Please read the letters

¿Puede leer esto? Por favor léame las letras

你能看清这些吗？清读这些字
nǐ néng kàn qīng zhè xiē ma? qīng dú zhè xiē zì

Savez-vous lire ceci? Veuillez, s'il vous plaît, lire les lettres

Können Sie das lesen? Lesen Sie die Buchstaben

Quý vị có thể đọc được phần này không? Vui lòng đọc các chữ cái

Riesce a leggere qui? Legga le lettere, per favore

이것을 읽을 수 있습니까? 글자를 읽어 보십시오
I-geo-seul il-geul su it-seum-ni-kka? Geul-ja-reul il-geo bo-sip-si-o

Вы можете прочитать это? Пожалуйста, назовите буквы
Vy mozhete prochitat' eto? Pozhaluysta, nazovite bukvy

Czy jest Pan(i) w stanie to przeczytać? Proszę przeczytać litery

هل تستطيع \ تستطيعين قراءة هذا؟ لطفاً اقرأ \ أقرأي الحروف
Hal tastatee" / tastatee"een qiraa'at hadhaa? Lutfan iqra' / iqra'ee / il-huroof

Pode ler isto? Leia as letras, por favor

Eske ou ka li sa a? Tanpri li lèt yo

Το διαβάζετε αυτό; Παρακαλώ διαβάστε τα γράμματα
to deeavAzete aft0? parakalO deeavAste ta grAmata

क्या आप इसे पढ सकते हैं? कृपया वर्णों को पढें
kya aap ise paDh sakte hain? kripya vaRnon ko paDhein

I will now examine you by auscultation

ES	Ahora le voy a auscultar
ZH	我现在给你做听诊检查 wǒ xiàn zài gěi nǐ zuò tīng zhěn jiǎn chá
FR	Je vais maintenant vous ausculter
DE	Ich werde Sie jetzt abhören
VI	Bây giờ, tôi sẽ khám cho quý vị bằng ống nghe
IT	Ora La devo auscultare
KO	이제 청진기로 진단을 하겠습니다 I-je cheong-jin-gi-ro jin-da-neul ha-get-seum-ni-da
RU	Я теперь вас послушаю Ya teper' vas poslushayu
PL	Zbadam Pana (Panią) teraz osłuchowo
AR	سأقوم الآن بفحصك من خلال الإنصات Sa'aqoom al-aan bi-fahsak min khilal il-insaat
PT	Agora, vou examiná-lo(a) por auscultação
FK	Kounye la mwen pral fè yon egzamin pa okiltasyon
EL	Τώρα θα σας εξετάσω με ακρόαση tOra tha sas exetAso me akrOasee
HI	मैं अब आपकी जांच परिश्रवण द्वारा करूंगा mein ab aapki janch pariShravan dwara karoonga

Please hold you breath

Por favor aguante la respiración

请闭住呼吸
qǐng bì zhù hū xī

Veuillez, s'il vous plaît, retenir votre respiration

Halten Sie bitte den Atem an

Vui lòng nín thở

Trattenga il respiro, per favore

숨을 멎으십시오
Su-meul meo-jeu-sip-si-o

Пожалуйста, задержите дыхание
Pozhaluysta, zaderzhite dykhanie

Proszę wstrzymać oddech

الرجاء احبس \ احبسي الأنفاس
Ar-rajaa' ihbis / ihbisee al-anfaas

Por favor, contenha a respiração

Tanpri kanbe souf ou

Παρακαλώ κρατήστε την αναπνοή σας
parakalO kratEEste teen anapnoEE sas

कृपया अपनी सांस रोकें
kripya apni saans rokein

cough / (deeply) inhale / exhale

ES tosa / inhale (profundamente) / exhale

ZH 咳嗽 / （深）吸气 / 呼气
ké sou / (shēn) xī qì / hū qì

FR toussez / inspirez (fort) / expirez

DE husten / (tief) einatmen / ausatmen

VI ho / hít vào (sâu) / thở ra

IT tossisca / inspiri (profondamente) / espiri

KO 기침하십시오 / (깊이) 숨을 들이 쉬십시오 / 숨을 내뱉으십시오
Gi-chim-ha-sip-si-o / (gi-pi) su-meul deu-ri swi-sip-si-o / su-Meul nae-bae-teu-sip-si-o

RU покашляйте / (глубоко) вдохните / выдохните
pokashlyaite / (gluboko) vdokhnite / vydokhnite

PL zakaszleć / wziąć (głęboki) oddech / wydech

AR اسعل \ اسعلي \ استنشق \ استنشقي (عميقاً) \ اخرج \ اخرجي النفس
ls"al / is"alee / istanshiq / istanshiqee ("ameeqan) / akhrij / akhrijee an-nafas

PT tussa / inale (a fundo) / exale

FK touse / pran yon gwo souf / lage souf ou

EL βήξτε / εισπνεύστε (βαθιά) / εκπνεύστε
vEExte / eespnEfste (vatheeA) / ekpnEfste

HI खांसे / (जोर से) खींचें / छोड़ें
khanse / (jor se) kheenchein / ChoDein

I must now do a rectal examination

:S Tengo que hacerle un examen rectal

H 我现在必须给你做肛门检查
wǒ xiàn zài bì xū gěi nǐ zuò gāng mén jiǎn chá

R Je dois maintenant faire un examen rectal

E Ich muss Sie rektal untersuchen

VI Bây giờ tôi phải làm khám trực tràng

T Ora devo effettuare un esame rettale

O 직장 검사를 하겠습니다
Jik-jang geom-sa-reul ha-get-seum-ni-da

U Сейчас я должен провести ректальный осмотр
Seychas ya dolzhen provesti rektal'nyi osmotr

L Muszę teraz dokonać badania odbytu

R يجب الآن أن اقوم بفحص الدبر
Yajib al-aan an aqoom bi-fahs ad-dubur

T Agora, vou fazer um exame ao recto

K Kounye la fòk mwen fè yon egzamin ren

L Τώρα πρέπει να κάνω εξέταση ορθού
tOra prEpee na kAno exEtasee orthU

H अब मुझे आपकी गुदा संबंधी जांच करनी है
ab mujhe aapki guda sambandhi jaanch karni hai

I must insert a rectal / urethral catheter

ES Tengo que introducir una sonda rectal / uretral

ZH 我必须给你放肛导管 / 导尿管
wǒ bì xū gěi nǐ fàng gāng dǎo guǎn / dǎo niào guǎn

FR Je dois insérer un cathéter rectal / urétral

DE Ich muss einen Darm- / Blasenkatheter einführen

VI Tôi phải đưa vào một ống thông qua trực tràng / niệu đạo

IT Ora devo inserire un catetere rettale / uretrale

KO 직장에 / 요도에 카테터를 삽입해야 합니다
Jik-jang-e / yo-do-e ka-te-teo-reul sa-bi-pae-ya ham-ni-da

RU Я должен ввести ректальный / мочевой катетер
Ya dolzhen vvesti rektal'nyi / mochevoy kateter

PL Muszę wprowadzić cewnik do odbytnicy / do cewki moczowej

AR يجب عليّ إدخال مسبار مستقيمي \ إحليلي
Yajib "alayyi idkhaal misbaar mustaqimi / ihleeli

PT Vou introduzir um cateter rectal / uretral

FK Fòk mwen mete yon katatè ren / uretral

EL Πρέπει να εισάγω ορθικό / ουρηθρικό καθετήρα
prEpee na eesAgo ortheekO / ureethreekO kathetEEra

HI मैं गुदासंबंधी ६ ९ी / मूत्रसंबंधी ६ ९ी नलिका डालूंगा
mein gudasambandhi / mutrasambandhi nalika daloonga

I must examine your pelvic area

Tengo que examinar la región pélvica

我必须给你做骨盆部位检查
wǒ bì xū gěi nǐ zuò gǔ pén bù wèi jiǎn chá

Je dois examiner la région de votre bassin

Ich muss Ihren Unterleib untersuchen

Tôi phải khám vùng xương chậu của quý vị

Le devo esaminare l'area pelvica

골반 부위를 검사해야 합니다
Gol-ban bu-wi-reul geom-sa-hae-ya ham-ni-da

Я должен провести гинекологический осмотр
Ya dolzhen provesti ginekologicheskiy osmotr

Muszę dokonać badania miednicowego

يجب أن افحص المنطقة الحوضية عندك
Yajib an afhas al-mantiqah al-haudhiyyah "indak

Tenho que examinar a sua zona pélvica

Fòk mwen fè yon egzamin nan zon basin w

Πρέπει να εξετάσω την περιοχή της πυέλου σας
prEpee na exetAso teen pereeohEE tees peeElu sas

मुझे आपके नितंब के आसपास जांच करनी है
mujhe aapke nitamb ke aaspass jaanch karni hai

I will now feel your breasts

ES Ahora voy a palparle los pechos

ZH 我现在给你做乳房检查
wǒ xiàn zài gěi nǐ zuò rǔ fáng jiǎn chá

FR Je vais maintenant examiner vos seins

DE Ich werde jetzt Ihre Brüste abtasten

VI Bây giờ tôi sẽ chạm vào vú của quý vị

IT Ora devo palparle il seno

KO 이제 유방을 만져 보겠습니다
I-je yu-bang-eul man-jyeo bo-get-seum-ni-da

RU Сейчас я обследую вашу грудь
Seychas ya obsleduyu vashu grud'

PL Zbadam teraz Pani piersi

AR يجب أن احسس ثديك الآن
Yajib an uhassis thadyik al-'aan

PT Agora vou fazer a palpação da mama

FK Kounye la mwen pral manyen tete w

EL Τώρα θα ψηλαφίσω το στήθος σας
tOra tha pseelafEEso to stEEthos sas

HI अब मैं आपके स्तनों को छूऊंगा
ab mein aapke stanon ko Chuunga

Do you feel this?

S ¿Siente esto?

H 你能感到这个吗？
nǐ néng gǎn dào zhè gè ma?

R Sentez-vous ceci?

E Spüren Sie / spürst du das?

VI Quý vị có cảm thấy gì không?

T Sente questo?

O 이것이 느껴지십니까?
I-geo-si neu-kkyeo-ji-sim-ni-kka?

RU Вы это чувствуете?
Vy eto chuvstvuete?

PL Czy Pan(i) to czuje?

AR هل تشعر \ تشعرين بهذا؟
Hal tash"ur / tash"ureen bi-hadhaa?

T Sente isto?

K Eske ou santi sa a?

EL Το νιώθετε αυτό;
to neeOthete aftO?

HI क्या आप इसे महसूस करती हैं
kya aap ise mahsoos karti hain

How does this feel? Sharp / dull / hot / cold

ES ¿Cómo lo siente? Agudo / romo / caliente / frío

ZH 有什么感觉？是尖锐 / 钝的 / 热的 / 冷的
yǒu shén me gǎn jué？shì jiān ruì / dùn de / rè de / lěng de

FR Comment sentez-vous ceci? Tranchant / lourd / chaud / froid

DE Wie fühlt es sich an? spitz / stumpf / heiß / kalt

VI Cảm giác này như thế nào? Đau buốt / không có cảm giác / nóng / lạnh

IT Come lo sente? Aguzzo / smussato / caldo / freddo

KO 이것은 느낌이 어떻습니까? 날카로운 / 둔한 / 뜨거운 / 차가운
I-geo-seun neu-kki-mi eo-tteo-sseum-ni-kka? Nal-ka-ro-un / dun-han / tteu-geo-un / cha-ga-un

RU Какое это ощущение? Острое / тупое / теплое / холодное
Kakoe eto oshchushchenie? Ostroe / tupoe / teploe / kholodnoe

PL Jak Pan(i) to odczuwa? Ostry / tępy / gorący / zimny

AR كيف يشعر هذا؟ حاد \ كليل \ حار \ بارد
Kayf yash"ur hadha? Haadd / kaliil / haarr / baarid

PT O que é que sente? Uma sensação aguda / sem intensidade / quente / fria

FK Kijan ou santi sa a? Egu / pa egu / cho / fret

EL Πώς το νιώθετε αυτό; Οξύ / Αμβλύ / Θερμό / Κρύο
pos to neeOthete aftO? oxEE / amvlEE / thermO / krEEo

HI यह कैसा लगता है? सख्त / ढीला / गर्म / ठंडा
yeh kaisa lagta hai? sakht / Dheela / garm / Thanda

Press my fingers

Apriete mis dedos

压我的手指
yā wǒ de shǒu zhǐ

Pressez mes doigts

Drücken Sie meine Finger

Ấn các ngón tay của tôi

Prema le mie dita

제 손가락을 꼭 쥐십시오
Je son-ga-ra-geul kkok jwi-sip-si-o

Сожмите мои пальцы
Sozhmite moi pal'tsy

Proszę ścisnąć moje palce

اضغط \ اضغطي على اصابعي
Idhghat / idhghatee "alaa asaabi"ee

Faça pressão sobre os meus dedos

Peze dwet mwen

Πιέστε τα δάχτυλά μου
peeEste ta dAhteelA mu

च्तमे उल पिदहमते
esjh vaxqfy;ka nck,a

I need a sample for the laboratory

ES Necesito una muestra para análisis

ZH 我需要一个样本送实验室检查
wǒ xū yào yī gè yàng běn sòng shí yàn shì jiǎn chá

FR Je vais prendre un échantillon pour le laboratoire

DE Ich brauche eine Probe für das Labor

VI Tôi cần lấy mẫu xét nghiệm

IT Ho bisogno di un campione da mandare al laboratorio

KO 시험실 검사를 할 표본이 필요합니다
Si-heom-sil geom-sa-reul hal pyo-bo-ni pi-ryo-ham-ni-da

RU Для лабораторного анализа мне нужна проба
Dlya laboratornogo analiza mne nuzhna proba

PL Potrzebna mi jest dla laboratorium próbka

AR يجب أن أخذ عينة من للمخبر
Yajib an akhudh "ayyinah min lil-makhbar

PT Preciso de uma amostra para análise laboratorial

FK Mwen bezwin yon echantiyon pou laboratwa a

EL Χρειάζομαι δείγμα για το εργαστήριο
hreeAzome dEEgma geea to ergastEEreeo

HI मुझे प्रयोगशाला के लिए नमूने की जरूरत है ...
muJhe prayogshala ke liye namune ki jaroorat hai

of your blood / urine / stool

S de sangre / orina / heces (excremento)

H 血样 / 尿样 / 大便
xiě yàng / niào yàng / dà biàn

R de votre sang / d'urine / des selles

E von Ihrem Blut / Urin / Stuhl

T mẫu máu / nước tiểu / phân của quý vị

T di sangue / di urina / delle feci

O 혈액 표본 / 소변 표본 / 대변 표본
Hyeo-raek pyo-bon / so-byeon pyo-bon / dae-byeon pyo-bon

U вашей крови / мочи / вашего кала
vashey krovi / mochi / vashego kala

L Pana(i) krwi / moczu / stolca

R من دمك \ بولك \ غائطك
Dammak / baulak / ghaa'itak

T de sangue / de urina / de fezes

K san w / urin / lasel

L του αίματος / των ούρων / των κοπράνων σας
tu Ematos / ton Uron / ton koprAnon sas

I आपके खून / पेशाब / मल
aapke khoon / peshab / mal

We must examine your spinal fluid

ES	Tenemos que estudiar su líquido raquídeo
ZH	我们必须给你做一个脑脊液检查 wǒ mén bì xū gěi nǐ zuò yī gè nǎo jǐ yè jiǎn chá
FR	Nous devons examiner votre liquide cérébro-spinal
DE	Wir müssen Ihre Rückenmarksflüssigkeit untersuchen
VI	Chúng tôi phải khám tủy sống của quý vị
IT	Dobbiamo esaminare il Suo liquido cerebrospinale
KO	척수액을 검사해야 합니다 Cheok-su-ae-geul geom-sa-hae-ya ham-ni-da
RU	Нам нужно исследовать вашу спинномозговую жидкость Nam nuzhno issledovat' vashu spinnomozgovuyu zhidkost'
PL	Musimy zbadać Pana(i) płyn mózgowo-rdzeniowy
AR	يجب أن نفحص السائل الشوكي عندك Yajib an afhas as-saa'il ash-shouki "indak
PT	Temos que examinar o seu líquido raquidiano
FK	Kounye la fòk nou fè egzamin likid kolon vetebral ou
EL	Πρέπει να εξετάσουμε το σπονδυλικό υγρό σας prEpee na exetAsume to spondeeleekO eegrO sas
HI	हमें आपकी रीढ़ की हड्डी के तरल की जांच करनी है hamein aapki reeDh ki haddi ke taral ki janch karni hai

We will now take an x-ray picture

S Vamos a tomar una radiografía

H 我们现在给你照X光片
wǒ mén xiàn zài gěi nǐ zhào X guāng piān

R Nous allons maintenant prendre un cliché radiographique

•E Wir machen eine Röntgenaufnahme

/I Bây giờ chúng tôi sẽ chụp X-quang

T Ora Le faremo una radiografia

O 이제 엑스레이를 찍을 겁니다
I-je ek-seu-re-i-reul jji-geul geom-ni-da

U Сейчас мы сделаем рентгеновский снимок
Seychas my sdelaem rentgenovskiy snimok

"L Zrobimy teraz zdjęcie rentgenowskie

R الآن سنأخذ صورة أشعة
Al-aan sana'khudh soorah ashi""ah

T Agora, vamos tirar uma radiografia

K Kounye la a nou pral fè yon radyografi

L Τώρα θα πάρουμε ακτίνα X
tOra the pArume aktEEna hee

-ll अब हम आपका एक्स—रे लेंगे
ab ham aapka x-ray lenge

We will now do a heart catheterization

ES Vamos a hacer un cateterismo cardíaco

ZH 我们现在给你放心导管
wǒ mén xiàn zài gěi nǐ fàng xīn dǎo guǎn

FR Nous allons maintenant effectuer un cathétérisme cardiaque

DE Wir machen eine Herzkatheteruntersuchung

VI Bây giờ chúng tôi sẽ đặt một ống thông vào tim

IT Ora Le faremo un angiogramma coronarico

KO 이제 심장 카테테르법을 실시할 겁니다
I-je sim-jang ka-te-te-reu-beo-beul sil-si-hal geom-ni-da

RU Сейчас мы выполним катетеризацию сердца
Seychas my vypolnim kateterizatsiyu serdtsa

PL Przeprowadzimy teraz cewnikowanie serca

AR نقوم الآن بعملية قسطرة القلب
Naqoom al-aan bi-"amaliyyah qastarat il-qalb

PT Agora, vamos fazer um cateterismo cardíaco

FK Kounye la nou pral fè yon katteterism kè w

EL Τώρα θα κάνουμε καθετηριασμό καρδίας
tOra the kAnume katheteereeasmO kardeeAs

HI अब हम हृदय नलिका की जांच करेंगे
ab ham hridya nalika ki jaanch karenge

We will now do a computer tomography scan

Vamos a hacer una tomografía por computadora

我们现在给你做CT扫描
wǒ mén xiàn zài gěi nǐ zuò CT sǎo miáo

Nous allons prendre un cliché tomodensitométrique

Wir machen eine Computertomographie

Bây giờ chúng tôi sẽ chụp X-quang bằng máy tính

Ora Le faremo una TAC

CT (전산 단층 조영술) 촬영을 할 겁니다
CT (jeon-san dan-cheung jo-yeong-sul) chwa-ryeong-eul hal geom-ni-da

Сейчас мы выполним компьютерную томографию
Seychas my vypolnim komp'yuternuyu tomografiyu

Przeprowadzimy teraz badania tomografii komputerowej

نقوم الآن بتصوير سطوحي بالكمبيوتر
Naqoom al-aan bi-tasweer sutoohi bil-computer

Agora, vamos fazer uma tomografia computorizada

Kounye la nou pral fè yon radyografi tomografi kompitè

Τώρα θα κάνουμε αξονική τομογραφία
tOra the kAnume axoneekEE tomografEEa

अब हम कंप्यूटर टॉमोग्राफी स्कैन करेंगे
ab ham computer tomography scan karenge

We will now do an ultrasound examination

ES	Vamos a hacer un estudio de ultrasonido
ZH	我们现在给你做超声波检查 wǒ mén xiàn zài gěi nǐ zuò chāo shēng bō jiǎn chá
FR	Nous allons pratiquer une échographie
DE	Wir machen eine Ultraschalluntersuchung
VI	Bây giờ chúng tôi sẽ làm khám siêu âm
IT	Ora Le faremo un'ecografia
KO	초음파 검사를 할 겁니다 Cho-eum-pa geom-sa-reul hal geom-ni-da
RU	Сейчас мы выполним ультразвуковое обследование Seychas my vypolnim ul'trazvukovoe obsledovanie
PL	Wykonamy teraz badanie ultrasonograficzne
AR	نقوم الآن بفحص فوق السمعية Naqoom al-aan bi-fahs fauq as-sam"iyah
PT	Agora, vamos fazer uma ecografia ou ultra-som
FK	Kounye la nou pral fè yon egzamin ultrason
EL	Τώρα θα κάνουμε εξέταση με υπερήχους tOra the kAnume exEEtasee me eeperEEhus
HI	अब हम आपकी अल्ट्रासाउंड जांच करेंगे ab ham aapki ultrasound jaanch karenge

We will now perform an electroencephalogram (recordings of brain waves)

ES Vamos a hacer ahora un electroencefalograma (registro de las ondas cerebrales)

ZH 我们现在给你做脑电图
wǒ mén xiàn zài gěi nǐ zuò nǎo diàn tú

FR Nous allons maintenant réaliser un électroencéphalogramme (enregistrement des ondes du cerveau)

DE Wir machen ein EEG (Messung der Hirnströme)

VI Bây giờ chúng tôi sẽ làm điện não đồ (bản ghi chép dao động của sóng não)

IT Ora Le faremo un elettroencefalogramma (registrazione delle onde celebrali)

KO 뇌파 검사를 할 겁니다(뇌파 기록)
Noe-pa geom-sa-reul hal geom-ni-da(noe-pa gi-rok)

RU Сейчас мы сделаем электроэнцефалограмму (запись мозговых волн)
Seychas my sdelaem elektrontsefalogrammu (zapis' mozgovykh voln)

PL Przeprowadzimy teraz elektroencefalogram (zapis fal mózgowych)

AR نقوم الآن بفحص تخطيط الموجات الدماغية (تسجيلٌ لموجات الدماغ)
Naqoom al-aan bi-fahs takhteet al-moujaat ad-dimaaghiyyah (tasjeel li-moujaat ad-dimaagh)

PT Agora, vamos tirar um electroencefalograma (registos das ondas cerebrais)

FK Kounye la nou pral fè yon elektwoericefalogram (yon anrekistreman sinyal elektrik sevo w)

EL Τώρα θα εκτελέσουμε ηλεκτροεγκεφαλογράφημα (καταγραφή των εγκεφαλικών κυμάτων)
tOra tha ektelEEsume eelektroegefalogrAfeema (katagrafEE ton egefaleekOn keemAton)

HI अब हम आपकी इलेक्ट्रोएनसेफलोग्राम (मस्तिष्क तरंगों की रिकार्डिंग)
ab ham aapki electroencephalogram (mastiSk tarangon ki recordings)

We will now do an NMR (imaging of the body's interior)

ES Haremos ahora una resonancia magnética (imagen del interior del cuerpo)

ZH 我们现在给你做一个NMR（体内成像）
wǒ mén xiàn zài gěi nǐ zuò yī gè NMR (tǐ nèi chéng xiàng)

FR Nous allons maintenant réaliser une IRM (une image de l'intérieur de votre corps)

DE Wir machen ein NMR (Aufnahme des Körperinneren)

VI Bây giờ chúng tôi sẽ chụp theo dạng cộng hưởng từ hạt nhân (chụp hình các bộ phận bên trong cơ thể)

IT Ora Le faremo una RMN (immagini dell'interno del corpo)

KO NMR (핵 자기 공명 진단장치) 검사를 할 겁니다(신체 내부 촬영)
NMR (haek ja-gi gong-myeong jin-dan-jang-chi) geom-sa-reul hal geom-ni-da(sin-che nae-bu chwa-ryeong)

RU Сейчас мы выполним ЯМР (визуализацию внутренностей тела)
Seychas my vypolnim YaMR (vizualizatsiyu vnutrennostey tela)

PL Przeprowadzimy teraz badanie NMR (obrazowanie wnętrz organizmu)

AR نقوم الآن بفحص ان ام آر (تصوير داخل الجسم)
Naqoom al-aan bi-fahs NMR (tasweer daakhil al-jism)

PT Agora vamos fazer uma RNM (imagem do interior do corpo)

FK Kounye la nou pral fè yon NMR (radyografi andan ko a)

EL Τώρα θα κάνουμε τομογραφία πυρηνικού μαγνητικού συντονισμού (απεικόνιση του εσωτερικού του σώματος)
tOra tha kAnume tomografEEa peereeneekU magneeteekU seedoneesmU (apeekOneesee tu esotereekU tu sOmatos)

HI अब हम एनएमआर (शरीर की आंतरिक तस्वीर) करेंगे
ab ham NMR karenge (sharir ki antarik tasveer)

We will now perform a mammography

S Vamos a realizar una mamografía

H 我们现在给你做乳房照影
wǒ mén xiàn zài gěi nǐ zuò rǔ fáng zhào yīng

R Nous allons maintenant réaliser une mammographie

E Wir machen eine Mammographie

I Bây giờ chúng tôi sẽ chụp khám ung thư vú

T Ora Le faremo una mammografia

O 유방 뢴트겐 조영법을 하겠습니다
Yu-bang Roen-teu-gen jo-yeong-beo-beul ha-get-seum-ni-da

U Сейчас мы выполним маммографию
Seychas my vypolnim mammografiyu

L Przeprowadzimy teraz badanie mammograficzne

R نقوم الآن بفحص الثدي
Naqoom al-aan bi-fahs ath-thadi

T Agora vamos fazer uma mamografia

K Kounye la nou pral fè yon mamografi

L Τώρα θα κάνουμε μαστογραφία
tOra the kAnume mastografEa

II अब हम आपकी मेमोग्राफी करेंगे
ab ham aapki mammography karengein

We will now record a ECG (evaluation of heart function)

ES Vamos a obtener un electrocardiograma (para estudiar la función del corazón)

ZH 我们现在给你做心电图
wǒ mén xiàn zài gěi nǐ zuò xīn diàn tú

FR Nous allons maintenant réaliser un ECG (évaluation de la fonction du coeur)

DE Wir machen jetzt ein EKG (Messung der Herzfunktion)

VI Bây giờ chúng tôi sẽ ghi lại điện tâm đồ (đánh giá chức năng hoạt động của tim

IT Ora Le faremo un elettrocardiogramma (valutazione del funzionamento del cuore)

KO 심전도 검사를 하겠습니다(심장 기능 평가)
Sim-jeon-do geom-sa-reul ha-get-seum-ni-da(sim-jang gi-neung pyeong-ga)

RU Сейчас мы выполним ЭКГ (исследование работы сердца)
Seychas my vypolnim EKG (issledovanie raboty serdtsa)

PL Wykonamy teraz zapis EKG (badanie funkcji serca)

AR نقوم الآن بفحص تخطيط القلب (لتقييم فعاليات القلب)
Naqoom al-aan bi-fahs takhteet al-qalb (li-taqyeem fa""aliyaat al-qalb)

PT Agora vamos registar um ECG (avaliação da função cardíaca)

FK Kounye la nou pral anrejistre yon ECG (evalyasyon fonksyon kè a)

EL Τώρα θα καταγράψουμε ηλεκτροκαρδιογράφημα (αξιολόγηση της καρδιακής λειτουργίας)
tOra the katagrApsume elektrokardeeogrAfeema (axeeolOgeesee tees kardeeakees leeturgEEas)

HI अब हम ईसीजी रिकॉर्ड करेंगे (हृदय क्रियाविधि का आकलन)
ab ham ECG record karenge (hridya kriyavidhi ka aaklan)

We will now perform a bronchoscopy, gastroscopy / colonoscopy

Haremos ahora una broncoscopia, gastroscopia / colonoscopia

我们现在给你做支气管镜，胃镜 / 结肠镜
wǒ mén xiàn zài gěi nǐ zuò zhī qì guǎn jìng, wèi jìng / jiē cháng jìng

Nous allons maintenant réaliser une bronchoscopie / une gastroscopie / une colonoscopie

Wir machen eine Bronchoskopie / Gastroskopie / Koloskopie

Bây giờ chúng tôi sẽ soi phế quản, soi bao tử, soi kết tràng

Le faremo ora una broncoscopia / gastroscopia / colonoscopia

이제 기관지 내시경 검사 / 위 내시경 검사 / 결장 내시경 검사를 하겠습니다
I-je gi-gwan-ji nae-si-gyeong geom-sa / wi nae-si-gyeong geom-sa / gyeol-jang nae-si-gyeong geom-sa-reul ha-get-seum-ni-da

Сейчас мы выполним бронхоскопию, гастроскопию / колоноскопию
Seychas my vypolnim bronkhoskopiyu, gastroskopiyu / kolonoskopiyu

Przeprowadzimy teraz bronchoskopię / gastroskopię / kolonoskopię

نقوم الآن بفحص منظار شعبات الرئة \ منظار المعدة \ منظار الأمعاء
Naqoom al-aan bi-fahs: mindhaar shu"baat ar-ri'ah / mindhaar al-mi"adah / mindhaar al-am"aa'

Agora vamos realizar uma broncoscopia / gastroscopia / colonoscopia

Kounye la nou pral fè yon bwonkoskopi / gastwoskopi / kolonoskopi

Τώρα θα κάνουμε βρογχοσκόπηση, γαστροσκόπηση / κολονοσκόπηση
tOra the kAnume vroghoskOpeesee, gastroskOpeesee / kolonoskOpeesee

अब हम आपकी ब्रॉन्कोस्कॉपी, गेस्ट्रोस्कॉपी / कॉलोनोस्कॉपी करेंगे....
ab ham aapki bronchoscopy, gastroscopy / colonoscopy karenge

Examination of the lung / stomach / intestine with a tube

ES Examen del pulmón / estómago / intestino con un tubo

ZH 检查肺部 / 胃 / 肠道
jiǎn chá fèi bù / wèi / cháng dào

FR Nous allons maintenant réaliser l'examen du poumon / de l'estomac / de l'intestin à l'aide d'un tube

DE Untersuchung der Lunge / des Magens / Darms mit einem Schlauch

VI Khám phổi / bao tử / ruột bằng một chiếc ống

IT Esame dei polmoni / dello stomaco / dell'intestino con una sonda

KO 폐 / 위 / 장 튜브 검사
pye / wi / jang tyu-beu geom-sa

RU Обследование легких / желудка / кишки с помощью зонда
Obsledovanie legkikh / zheludka / kishki s pomoshch'yu zonda

PL Badanie płuc / żołądka / jelit używając rurki

AR نقوم الآن بفحص الرئة \ المعدة \ الأمعاء بإستعمال أنبوبة
Naqoom al-aan bi-fahs ar-ri'ah / al-mi"adah / al-am"aa' bi-isti"maal anboubah

PT Exame do pulmão / estômago / intestino com um tubo

FK Egzamin poumon / vant / intestine ak yon tib

EL Εξέταση του πνεύμονα / στομαχιού / εντέρων με ένα σωληνάριο
exEtasee tu pnEvmona / stomaheeU / edEron me Ena soleenAreeo

HI ट्यूब के साथ फेफड़ों / पेट / आंत्र संबंधी जांच
tube ke saath phephRon / pet / aantr sambandhi jaanch

24 Diagnosis

This is a mild / severe disease

S Se trata de una enfermedad leve / grave

H 这是一个小病 / 严重疾病
zhè shì yī gè xiǎo bìng / yán zhòng jí bìng

R Ceci est une maladie anodine / sévère

E Es handelt sich um eine leichte / schwere Erkrankung

VI Đây là căn bệnh nhẹ / nghiêm trọng

Questa è una malattia non grave / grave

O 이것은 가벼운 / 심각한 질병입니다
I-geo-seun ga-byeo-un / sim-gak-han jil-byeong-im-ni-da

U Это легкая / тяжёлая болезнь
Eto legkaya / tyazhyolaya bolezn'

L Jest to łagodna / poważna choroba

R هذا مرض خفيف \ شديد
Haadhaa maradh khafeef / shadeed

T Esta doença é ligeira / aguda

K Sa a se yon maladi ki pa grav / grav

L Αυτή είναι νόσος ήπιας / σοβαρής μορφής
aftEE EEne nOsos EEpeeas / sovarEEs morfEEs

HI यह एक सौम्य/उग्र रोग है
yeh ek saumya / ugra rog hai

The following disease was identified ... (alphabetically)

ES Se encontró la siguiente enfermedad ... (en orden alfabético)

ZH 以下疾病被诊断出来了
yǐ xià jí bìng bèi zhěn duàn chū lái le

FR La maladie suivante a été identifiée (par ordre alphabétique)

DE Es handelt sich um folgende Erkrankung ... (alphabetisch)

VI Đã phát hiện thấy có căn bệnh sau đây ... (theo thứ tự bảng chữ cái)

IT È stata diagnosticata la seguente malattia ... (in ordine alfabetico)

KO 다음의 질병이 확인되었습니다 ... (알파벳 순서로)
Da-eum-ui jil-byeong-i hwa-gin-doe-eot-seum-ni-da ... (al-pa-bet sun-seo-ro)

RU Была обнаружена следующая болезнь ... (в алфавитном порядке)
Byla obnaruzhena sleduyushchaya bolezn' ... (v alfavitnom poryadke)

PL Rozpoznano, że choroba jest następująca ... (alfabetycznie)

AR تم تحديد المرض التالي ... (بالترتيب الأبجدي)
Tamma tahdeed al-maraddh at-taalee ... (bit-tarteeb al-abjadee)

PT A doença que se segue foi identificada ... (alfabeticamente)

FK Yo te jwen maladi swivan an ... (alfabetik)

EL Αναγνωρίστηκε η ακόλουθη νόσος ... (αλφαβητικά)
anagnorEEsteeke ee akOluthee nOsos ... (alfaveeteekA)

HI निम्न रोग की पहचान हुई है ...(वर्णमाला के क्रम से)
nimn rog ki pehchaan huii hai ... (varNmaala ke kram se)

abscess / alcohol intoxication / allergy / asthma / luxation

S absceso / intoxicación alcohólica / alergia / asma / luxación

H 溃疡 / 酒精中毒 / 过敏 / 哮喘 / 脱臼
Kui yang / jiu jing zhong du / guo min / xiao chuan / tuo jiu

R abcès / intoxication alcoolique / allergie / asthme / luxation

E Abszess / Alkoholvergiftung / Allergie / Asthma / Ausrenkung

I áp-xe / nhiễm độc rượu / dị ứng / bệnh suyễn / trật khớp

T ascesso / intossicazione da alcol / allergia / asma / lussazione

O 고름 / 알콜 중독 / 알레르기 / 천식 / 탈구
go-reum / al-kol jung-dok / al-le-reu-gi / cheon-sik / tal-gu

U абсцесс / алкогольная интоксикация / аллергия / астма / вывих
abstsess / alkogol'naya intoksikatsiya / allergiya / astma / vyvikh

L ropień / odurzenie alkoholowe / alergia / astma / zwichnięcie

R تدمل \ التسمم بالكحول \ حساسية \ ضيق النفس (اسمة) \ خلع
Tadammul / at-tasammum bil-kuhoul / hassaasiyah / ddhayq an-nafas (asmah) / khala'

T abcesso / intoxicação alcoólica / alergia / asma / luxação

K absè / anpwazonman tafya / aleji / opresyon / dejewentaj

L απόστημα / μέθη / αλλεργία / άσθμα / εξάρθρημα
apOsteema / mEthee / alergEEa / Asthma / exArthreema

I व्रण / शराब से उत्पन्न मादकता / एलर्जी / दमा / किसी अंग का विस्थापन
vraN / sharaab se utpanna maadakta / allergy / damaa / kisi ang ka visthaapan

bacterial disease / herniated disc / bladder inflammation

ES infección bacteriana / hernia discal / inflamación de la vejiga

ZH 细菌疾病 / 椎间盘突出症 / 膀胱炎
Xi jun ji bing / zhui jian pan tu chu zheng / pang guang yan

FR maladie bactérienne / hernie discale / inflammation de la vessie

DE Bakterielle Erkrankung / Bandscheibenvorfall / Blasenentzündung

VI bệnh do vi khuẩn / trật đĩa đệm / viêm bàng quang

IT malattia batterica / ernia del disco / infiammazione della vescica

KO 박테리아성 질병 / 디스크 이탈 / 방광 염증
bak-te-ri-a-seong jil-byeong / di-seu-keu i-tal / bang-gwang yeom-jeung

RU бактериальное заболевание / грыжа межпозвоночного диска / воспаление мочевого пузыря
bakterial'noe zabolevanie / gryzha mezhpozvonochnogo diska / vospalenie mochevogo puzyrya

PL choroba bakteryjna / przepuklina krążka międzykręgowego / zapalenie pęcherz

AR مرض جرثومي \ قرص مفتق فى العمود الفقري \ إلتهاب المثانة
Maradh jarthoumi / qars mufattaq fil-amoud al-faqari / iltihaab al-mathanah

PT Doença bacteriana / disco herniado / inflamação da bexiga

FK enfeksyon mikwòb / èni diskal / enflamasyon vesi

EL βακτηριακή νόσος / δισκοκήλη / φλεγμονή ουροδόχου κύστης
vakteereeakEE nOsos / deeskokEElee / flegmonEE urodOhu kEEstees

HI बैक्टिरीयल रोग / डिस्क में हर्निया / मूत्राशय में सूजन......
bacterial rog / disc mein hernia / mootrashay mein soojan

appendicitis / anemia / bruise / blood disease

apendicitis / anemia / equimosis / enfermedad de la sangre

盲肠炎 / 贫血 / 擦伤 / 血液疾病
Mang chang yan / pin xue / ca shang / xue ye ji bing

appendicite / anémie / contusion / maladie du sang

Blinddarmentzündung / Blutarmut / Bluterguss / Bluterkrankung

viêm ruột thừa / thiếu máu / bầm tím / bệnh liên quan tới máu

appendicite / anemia / contusione / malattia del sangue

맹장염 / 빈혈 / 멍 / 혈액 질병
maeng-jang-yeom / bin-hyeol / meong / hyeo-raek jil-byeong

аппендицит / анемия / кровоизлияние / болезнь крови
appenditsit / anemiya / krovoizliyanie / bolezn' krovi

zapalenie wyrostka robaczkowego / anemia / choroba krwi

التهاب الزائدة \ فقر الدم \ كدمة \ مرض الدم
Iltihaab az-zaa'idah / faqr ad-damm / kadmah / maradh ad-damm

apendicite / anemia / contusão / doença do sangue

apendisit / anemi / ven anfle / maladi nan san

σκωληκοειδίτιδα / αναιμία / μώλωπας / αιματολογική νόσος
skoleekoeedEEteeda / anemEEa / mOlopas / ematologeekEE nOsos

एपेन्डिसाइटिस / रक्ताभाव / खरोंच / रक्त रोग.....
appendicitis / raktaabhaav / kharonch / rakta rog

blood clot / coagulation defect / hypertension

ES embolia / trombosis / defecto de la coagulación / hipertensión

ZH 血凝块 / 凝血缺陷 / 高血压
Xue ning kuai / ning xue que xian / gao xue ya

FR caillot de sang / défaut de la coagulation / hypertension

DE Blutgerinnsel / Blutgerinnungsstörung / Bluthochdruck

VI máu đóng cục / máu khó đông / cao huyết áp

IT grumo di sangue / difetto di coagulazione / ipertensione

KO 응혈 / 응고 결함 / 고혈압
eung-hyeol / eung-go gyeol-ham / go-hyeo-rap

RU сгусток крови / нарушение коагуляции / гипертензия
sgustok krovi / narushenie koagulyatsii / gipertenziya

PL skrzep krwi / zaburzenie krzepnięcia krwi / nadciśnienie

AR جلطة دم \ مشكلة في التخثر \ إرتفاع ضغط الدم
Jultah damm / mushkilah at-takhaththur / irtifaa' ddhaght ad-damm

PT coágulo sanguíneo / defeito da coagulação / hipertensão

FK boul san / defòmasyon koagilasyon / ipetansyon

EL θρόμβος αίματος / ανωμαλία πήξης αίματος / υπέρταση
thrOmvos Ematos / anomalEEa pEExees Ematos / eepErtasee

HI रक्त का थक्का / स्कन्दन की कमी / हाइपरटेन्शन.....
rakta ka thakka / skandan ki kami / hypertension.

intestinal obstruction / dementia / depression / diabetes

ES obstrucción intestinal / demencia / depresión / diabetes

ZH 肠梗阻 / 失智症 / 抑郁症 / 糖尿病
Chang geng zu / shi zhi zheng / yi yu zheng / tang niao bing

FR obstruction intestinale / démence / dépression / diabète

DE Darmverschluss / Demenzerkrankung / Depression / Diabetes

VI tắc ruột / mất trí / trầm cảm / tiểu đường

IT occlusione intestinale / demenza / depressione / diabete

KO 장폐색 / 치매 / 우울증 / 당뇨병
jang-pye-saek / chi-mae / u-ul-jeung / dang-nyo-byeong

RU непроходимость кишечника / деменция / депрессия / диабет
neprokhodimost' kishechnika / dementsiya / depressiya / diabet

PL obstrukcja jelita / otępienie / depresja / cukrzyca

AR إنسداد أمعائي \ جنون \ إكتئاب \ مرض السكر
Insidaad am'aa'ie / junoon / ikti'aab / maraddh as-sukkar

PT obstrução intestinal / demência / depressão / diabetes

FK obstriksyon nan intestine / foli / depresyon.sik

EL εντερική απόφραξη / άνοια / κατάθλιψη / διαβήτης
entereekEE apOfraxee / Aneea / katAthleepsee / deeavEEtees

HI आंत में अवरोध / मनोभ्रंश / डिप्रेशन / मधुमेह....
aant mein avrodh / manobhransh / depression / madhumeh.

diarrhea / inflammation / common cold / biliary colic

ES diarrea / inflamación / resfrío común / cólico biliar

ZH 腹泻 / 急性炎症 / 伤风感冒 / 胆瘘
Fu xie / ji xing yan zheng / shang feng gan mao / dan lou

FR diarrhée / inflammation / rhume banal / colique biliaire

DE Durchfallerkrankung / Entzündung / Erkältung / Gallenkolik

VI tiêu chảy / sưng viêm / cảm lạnh thông thường / đau bụng do túi mật

IT diarrea / infiammazione / raffreddore comune / colica biliare

KO 설사 / 염증 / 일반 감기 / 담즙 산통
seol-sa / yeom-jeung / il-ban gam-gi / dam-jeup san-tong

RU понос / воспаление / простуда / печёночная колика
ponos / vospalenie / prostuda / pechyonochnaya kolika

PL biegunka / zapalenie / przeziębienie / kolka żółciowa

AR إسهال \ إلتهاب \ زكام عادي \ مغص صفراوي
ls-haal / iltihaab / zukkaam 'aadee / maghs safrawi

PT diarreia / inflamação / constipação / cólica biliar

FK dyare / enflamasyon / la grip / kolik bilyè

EL διάρροια / φλεγμονή / κοινό κρυολόγημα / κολικός των χοληφόρων
deeAreea / flegmonEE / keenO kreeolOgeema / koleekOs ton holeefOron

HI अतिसार / सूजन / सामान्य जुखाम / पित्ताश्मरी के दबाव से उत्पन्न दर्द.
atisaar / soojan / samanya jukham / pittashamri ke dabaav se utpanna dard.

vascular disease / joint disease / ulcer / skin disease

ES enfermedad vascular / artropatía / úlcera / dermatosis

ZH 血管病 / 关节病 / 溃疡 / 皮肤病
Xue guan bing / guan jie bing / kui yang / pi fu bing

FR Maladie vasculaire / maladie articulaire / ulcère / maladie de la peau

DE Gefäßkrankheit / Gelenkserkrankung / Geschwür / Hautkrankheit

VI bệnh huyết mạch / bệnh khớp / lở loét / bệnh về da

IT malattia vascolare / malattia delle articolazioni / malattia della pelle

KO 혈관 질병 / 관절 질병 / 궤양 / 피부 질병
hyeol-gwan jil-byeong / gwan-jeol jil-byeong / gwe-yang / pi-bu jil-byeong

RU болезнь сосудов / болезнь суставов / язва / кожная болезнь
bolezn' sosudov / bolezn' sustavov / yazva / kozhnaya bolezn'

PL choroba naczyniowa / choroba stawów / wrzód / choroba skórna

AR مرض وعائي \ مرض المفاصل \ قرحة \ مرض البشرة
Maradh wi'aa'ie / maraddh al-mafaasil / qurhah / maradh al-bashrah

PT doença vascular / doença das articulações / úlcera / doença da pele

FK enfeksyon vaskilè / enfeksyon jweinti / enfeksyon nan po

EL αγγειοπάθεια / πάθηση αρθρώσεων / έλκος / δερματική νόσος
aggeeopAthea / pAtheesee arthrOseon / Elkos / dermateekEE nOsos

HI वाहिनियों का रोग /जोड़ो का रोग /अल्सर /चर्म रोग..
vahinion ka rog / jodon ka rog / ulcer / cherma rog

cardiac infarction / cardiac insufficiency / cardiac arrhythmias

ES infarto del miocardio / insuficiencia cardiaca / arritmias cardiacas

ZH 心肌梗塞 / 心功能不全 / 心律失常
Xin ji geng se / xin gong neng bu quan / xin lv shi chang

FR infarctus du myocarde / insuffisance cardiaque / arythmies cardiaques

DE Herzinfarkt / Herzinsuffizienz / Herzrhythmusstörungen

VI nhồi máu cơ tim / thiếu năng tim / chứng loạn nhịp tim

IT infarto cardiaco / insufficienza cardiaca / aritmia cardiaca

KO 심근 경색 / 심부전증 / 심장성 부정맥
sim-geun gyeong-saek / sim-bu-jeon-jeung / sim-jang-seong bu-jeong-maek

RU инфаркт миокарда / сердечная недостаточность / аритмия сердца
infarkt miokarda / serdechnaya nedostatochnost' / aritmiya serdtsa

PL zawał serca / niewydolność serca / arytmie serca

AR نوبة قلبية \ ضعف قلبي \ إضطراب قلبي
Noubah qalbiyah / ddha'f qalbee / idhtiraab qalbee

PT enfarte cardíaco / insuficiência cardíaca / arritmias cardíacas

FK kriz kadyak / ensifyans kadyak / arytmi kadyak

EL έμφραγμα / καρδιακή ανεπάρκεια / καρδιακές αρρυθμίες
Emfragma / kardeeakEE anepArkeea / kardeeakEs areethmEEes

HI ह्रदय में रोधगलन / ह्रदय के कार्य में कमी / दिल की असाधारण धड़कन....
hriday mein rodhgalan / hriday ke karya mein kami / dil ki asadharan dhadkan

meningitis / immune disease / infection / bone fracture

ES meningitis / trastorno inmunitario / infección / fractura ósea

ZH 脑膜炎 / 免疫疾病 / 感染 / 骨折
Nao mo yan / mian yi ji bing / gu zhe

FR méningite / maladie immunitaire / infection / fracture

DE Hirnhautentzündung / Immunkrankheit / Infektion / Knochenbruch

VI viêm màng não / bệnh liên quan tới hệ miễn dịch / nhiễm trùng / gãy xương

IT meningite / malattia del sistema immunitario / infezione / frattura ossea

KO 뇌막염 / 면역 질병 / 감염 / 뼈 골절
noe-mag-yeom / myeon-yeok jil-byeong / gam-yeom / ppyeo-gol-jeol

RU менингит / иммунная болезнь / инфекция / перелом кости
meningit / immunnaya bolezn' / infektsiya / perelom kosti

PL zapalenie opon mózgowych / choroba immunologiczna / zakażenie / złamanie kości

AR إلتهاب السحايا \ مرض الجهاز المناعى \ إلتهاب \ كسر عظام
Iltihaab as-sahaayaa / maradh al-jihaaz al-manaa'ee / iltihaab / kasr 'idhaam

PT meningite / doença auto-imune / infecção / fractura óssea

FK mennenjit / enfeksyon nan system iminitè / zo kase, frakti

EL μηνιγγίτιδα / ασθένεια του ανοσοποιητικού / λοίμωξη / κατάγματα οστού
meeneegEEteeda / asthEneea tu anosopee-eeteekU / lEEmoxee / katAgmata ostU

HI मेनिनजाइटिस / प्रतिरोधक प्रणाली रोग / संक्रमण / हड्डी का फ्रेक्चर......
meningitis / pratirodhak praNali rog / sankramaN / haddi ka fracture

seizure / cancer / hepatitis / pulmonary embolism

ES crisis convulsiva / cáncer / hepatitis / embolia pulmonar

ZH 癫痫 / 癌症 / 肝炎 / 肺栓塞
Dian xian / ai zheng / gan yan / fei shuan se

FR attaque / cancer / hépatite / embolie pulmonaire

DE Krampfanfall / Krebserkrankung / Leberentzündung / Lungenembolie

VI tai biến mạch máu não / ung thư / bệnh viêm gan / tắc mạch phổi

IT convulsioni / cancro / epatite / embolia polmonare

KO 간질 발작 / 암 / 간염 / 폐 색전증
gan-jil / am / gan-yeom / pye saek-jeon-jeung

RU судороги / рак / гепатит / эмболия лёгких
sudorogi / rak / gepatit / emboliya lyogkikh

PL drgawki / rak / zapalenie wątroby / zator tętnicy płucnej

AR صرعة \ سرطان \ إلتهاب الكبد \ جلطة رئوية
Sar'ah / sirataan / iltihaab al-kabad / jultah ri'awiyah

PT crises / cancro / hepatite / embolismo pulmonar

FK kriz / kansè / hepatit / anabolism pulmonè

EL επιληπτική κρίση / καρκίνος / ηπατίτιδα / πνευμονική εμβολή
epeeleepteekEE krEEsee / karkEEnos / eepatEEteeda / pnevmoneekEE emvolEE

HI दौरा / कैंसर / हिपेटाइटिस / फेफड़ों की ६ मणीओ में अवरो ६ ६.....
daura / cancer / hepatitis / fefdon ki dhamnion mein avrodh

pneumonia / gastrointestinal inflammation / stomach ulcer

S
neumonía / inflamación gastrointestinal / úlcera gástrica

H
肺炎 / 肠胃炎 / 胃溃疡
Fei yan / chang wei yan / wei kui yang

R
pneumonie / inflammation gastro-intestinale / ulcère gastique

E
Lungenentzündung / Magen-Darm-Entzündung / Magengeschwür

VI
viêm phổi / viêm bao tử / loét bao tử

T
polmonite / infiammazione gastrointestinale / ulcera allo stomaco

O
폐렴 / 위장 염증 / 위 궤양
pye-ryeom / wi-jang yeom-jeung / wi gwe-yang

U
пневмония / воспаление желудочно-кишечного тракта / язва желудка
pnevmoniya / vospalenie zheludochno-kishechnogo trakta / yazva zheludka

L
zapalenie płuc / zapalenie żołądkowo-jelitowe / wrzód żołądka

R
إلتهاب الرئة \ إلتهاب المعدة والأمعاء \ قرحة فى المعدة
Iltihaab ar-ri'ah / iltihaab al-ma'idah wal-am'aa / qurhah al-ma'idah

T
pneumonia / inflamação gastrointestinal / úlcera do estômago

K
nemoni / enflamasyon gastwointestinal / ilsè nan vant

L
πνευμονία / γαστρεντερική φλεγμονή / έλκος στομάχου
pnevmonEEa / gastredereekEE flegmonEE / Elkos stomAhu

II
न्यूमोनिया / आन्त्रशोथ में सूजन / पेट में अल्सर....
pneumonia / aantrashoth mein soojan / pet mein ulcer

malaria / nerve: trapped / neurologic disease / renal disease

ES malaria / nervio: atrapado / enfermedad neurológica / enfermedad renal

ZH 疟疾 / 神经:被困 / 神经系统疾病 / 肾脏疾病
Nue ji / shen jing: bei kun / shen jing xi tong ji bing / shen zang ji bing

FR malaria / nerf coincé / maladie neurologique / maladie rénale

DE Malaria / Nerv: eingeklemmt / Nervenerkrankung / Nierenerkrankung

VI bệnh sốt rét / dây thần kinh: bị chèn / bệnh về thần kinh / bệnh thận

IT malaria / nervo compresso / malattia neurologica / malattia renale

KO 말라리아 / 신경: 폐색 / 신경 질병 / 신장 질병
mal-la-ri-a / sin-gyeong: pye-saek / sin-gyeong jil-byeong / sin-jang jil-byeong

RU малярия / ущемление нерва / неврологическое заболевание / болезнь почек
malyariya / ushchemlenie nerva / nevrologicheskoe zabolevanie / bolezn' pochek

PL malaria / nerw: uwięziony / choroba neurologiczna / choroba nerek

AR مرض الملاريا \ عصب مقروص \ مرض عصبي \ مرض كلوي
Maradh al-malaariyaa / asab maqroos / maraddh asabi / maradh kilawi

PT malária / nervo comprimido / doença neurológica / doença renal

FK malaria / nè; atrape / enfeksyon nuwolojik / maladi (enfeksyon) nan ren

EL ελονοσία / νεύρο: παγιδευμένο / νευροπάθεια / νεφροπάθεια
elonosEEa / nEvro: pageedevmEno / nevropAtheea / nefropAtheea

HI मलेरिया / तन्त्रिकाः फंसी हुई / स्नायुरोग / गुर्दे का रोग....
malaria / tantrika: phansi hui / snayurog / gurde ka rog

renal colic / parasitic disease / fungal infection

cólico renal / parasitosis / infección micótica

肾绞痛 / 寄生虫病 / 真菌感染
Shen jiao tong / ji sheng chong bing / zhen jun gan ran

colique rénale / maladie parasitaire / infection par les champignons

Nierenkolik / Parasitäre Erkrankung / Pilzinfektion

đau bụng do thận / bệnh nấm ký sinh / nhiễm nấm

colica renale / malattia da parassita / infezione fungina

신성 산통 / 기생충 질병 / 진균(곰팡이) 감염
sin-seong san-tong / gi-saeng-chung jil-byeong / jin-gyun(gom-pang-i) gam-yeom

почечная колика / паразитоз / грибковая инфекция
pochechnaya kolika / parazitoz / gribkovaya infektsiya

kolka nerkowa / choroba pasożytnicza / zakażenie grzybicze

مغص كلوي \ مرض تطفلي \ إلتهاب فطري او عفني
Maghs kilawi / maraddh tataffuli / iltihaab futri au 'afani

cólica renal / doença parasitária / infecção micótica

kolik ren / enfeksyon parazit / enfeksyon fongis

κολικός νεφρού / παρασιτική ασθένεια / μυκητιασική λοίμωξη
koleekOS nefrU / paraseeteekEE asthEneea / meekeeteeaseekEE IEEmoxee

गुर्दे में दर्द / परजीवीय रोग / फंगल रोग...
gurde mein dard / parjiviya rog / fungal rog

psychiatric or mental disorder / rheumatic disease

ES trastorno psiquiátrico o mental / enfermedad reumática

ZH 精神病或神经错乱 / 风湿性疾病
Jing shen bing huo shen jing cuo luan / feng shi xing ji bing

FR trouble psychiatrique ou mental / maladie rhumatismale

DE Psychiatrische oder Psychische Erkrankung / Rheuma

VI bệnh tâm thần hay rối loạn tâm thần / bệnh thấp khớp

IT disturbo psichiatrico o mentale / malattia reumatica

KO 정신 장애 / 류마티스성 질병
jeong-sin jang-ae / ryu-ma-ti-seu-seong jil-byeong

RU психическое расстройство / ревматизм
psikhicheskoe rasstroystvo / revmatizm

PL schorzenie psychiatryczne lub umysłowe / choroba reumatyczna

AR إضطراب نفساني او عقلي \ مرض رثوي
Iddhtiraab nafsaani aw 'aqli / maradh ri'awi

PT perturbação psiquiátrica ou doença mental / doença reumática

FK maladi sikyatrik oswa mantal / maladi rumatism

EL ψυχιατρική ή διανοητική διαταραχή / ρευματοπάθεια
pseeheeatreekEE ee deeanoeeteekEE deeatarahEE / revmatopAthea

HI मनोवैज्ञानिक या मानसिक रोग / आमवात रोग...
manovaigyanik ya mansik rog / aamvaat rog

thyroid disease / stroke / metabolic disease

enfermedad tiroidea / apoplejía / enfermedad metabólica

甲状腺疾病 / 中风 / 代谢性疾病
Jia zhuang xian ji bing / zhong feng / dai xie xing ji bing

maladie de la glande thyroïde / apoplexie / maladie métabolique

Schilddrüsenerkrankung / Schlaganfall / Stoffwechselstörung

bệnh tuyến giáp / đột quỵ / bệnh về chuyển hóa

disturbo della tiroide / ictus / malattia del metabolismo

갑상선 질병 / 뇌졸증 / 신진대사 질병
gap-sang-seon jil-byeong / noe-jol-jeung / sin-jin-dae-sa jil-byeong

болезнь щитовидной железы / инсульт / нарушение обмена веществ
bolezn' shchitovidnoy zhelezy / insul't / narushenie obmena veshchestv

choroba tarczycy / udar / choroba metaboliczna

مرض فى الغدة الدرقية \ ضربة \ مرض أيضى
Maradh fil-ghuddah ad-darqiyah / ddharbah / maradh aydhi

doença da tireóide / acidente vascular / doença metabólica

maladi tiwoyid / estwok / maladi metabolic

ασθένεια του θυροειδούς / εγκεφαλικό επεισόδιο / ασθένεια του μεταβολισμού
asthEneia tu theeroeedUs / egefaleekO epeesOdeeo / asthEneea tu metavoleesmU

थायरोइड / हमला / चयापचयी रोग......
Thyroid / humla / chayapachyi rog

Thrombosis / tuberculosis / overdose / overweight / hypoglycemia

ES Trombosis / tuberculosis / sobredosis / sobrepeso / hipoglucemia

ZH 血栓 / 结核 / 服药过量 / 超重 / 低血糖
Xue shuan / jie he / fu yao guo liang / di xue tang

FR Thrombose / tuberculose / surdosage / excès de poids / hypoglycémie

DE Thrombose / Tuberkulose / Überdosis / Übergewicht / Unterzucker

VI Chứng huyết khối / bệnh lao / sử dụng quá liều / mập phì / hạ đường huyết

IT Trombosi / tubercolosi / overdose / sovrappeso / ipoglicemia

KO 혈전증 / 결핵 / 마약 과용 / 체중과다 / 저혈당
hyeol-jeon-jeung / gyeol-haek / ma-yak gwa-yong / che-jung-gwa-da / jeo-hyeol-dang

RU Тромбоз / туберкулёз / передозировка / избыточная масса тела / гипогликемия
Tromboz / tuberkulyoz / peredozirovka / izbytochnaya massa tela / gipoglikemiya

PL Zakrzepica / gruźlica / przedawkowanie / nadwaga / hipoglikemia

AR تجلط \ مرض السل \ جرعة زائدة \ زيادة الوزن \ نقص سكر الدم
Tajallut / maradh as-sull / jur'ah zaa'idah / ziyadah al-wazn / naqs sukkar ad-damm

PT trombose / tuberculose / overdose / excesso de peso / hipoglicemia

FK Boul san / tibekilòz / twòb gwo dòz / gra / hipoglysemi

EL θρόμβωση / φυματίωση / υπερβολική δόση / υπερβολικό βάρος / υπογλυκαιμία
thrOmvosee / feematEEosee / eepervoleekEE dOsee / eepervoleekO vAros / eepogleekemEEa

HI थ्रोम्बोसिस / तपैदिक / अतिखुराक / मोटापा / रक्त में ग्लूकोज़ की कमी...
Thrombosis / tapaidik / atikhurak / motapa / rakta mein glucose ki kami

suppuration / intoxication / injury / luxation / sprain

S   supuración / intoxicación / lesión / luxación / esguince

H   化脓 / 中毒 / 伤害 / 脱臼 / 扭伤
Hua nong / zhong du / shang hai / tuo jiu / niu shang

R
E   suppuration / intoxication / blessure / luxation / foulure

  Vereiterung / Vergiftung / Verletzung / Verrenkung / Verstauchung

I
T   nhiễm trùng vết thương / nhiễm độc / chấn thương / trật khớp / bong gân

  suppurazione / intossicazione / lesione / lussazione / slogatura

O   화농 / 중독 / 상해 / 탈구 / 염좌
hwa-nong / jung-dok / sang-hae / ta-lgu / yeom-jwa

U   нагноение / интоксикация / травма / вывих / растяжение
nagnoenie / intoksikatsiya / travma / vyvikh / rastyazhenie

L   ropienie / odurzenie / uszkodzenie / złamanie / skręcenie

R   تقيح \ تسمم \ جرح \ خلع \ لي المفصل
Taqayyuh / tasammum / jarh / khala' / lay al-mifsal

T   Supuração / intoxicação / lesão / luxação / entorce

K   bay pi / anpwazonman / andomaje / dejwentaj / foule, antòs

L   πυόρροια / δηλητηρίαση / τραυματισμός / εξάρθρημα / διάστρεμμα
peeOreea / deeleeteerEEasee / travmateesmOs / exArtheema / deeAstrema

HI   पस बनना / मादकता / चोट / किसी अंग का विस्थापन / मोच......
pus banna / maadakta / kisi ang ka visthapan / moch

viral disease / strain / duodenal ulcer

ES enfermedad viral / tensión / úlcera duodenal

ZH 滤过性毒菌病 / 扭伤 / 十二指肠溃疡
Lv guo xing du jun bing / niu shang / shi er zhi chang kui yang

FR maladie virale / claquage / ulcère duodénal

DE Viruskrankheit / Zerrung / Zwölffingerdarmgeschwür

VI bệnh do vi-rút / chứng căng cơ / loét tá tràng

IT malattia virale / stiramento / ulcera duodenale

KO 바이러스성 질병 / 과다운동 / 십이지장 궤양
ba-i-reo-seu-seong jil-byeong / gwa-da-un-dong / sib-i-ji-jang gwe-yang

RU вирусная болезнь / растяжение связок / язва двенадцатиперстной кишки
virusnaya bolezn' / rastyazhenie svyazok / yazva dvenadtsatiperstnoy kishki

PL choroba wirusowa / uszkodzenie powysiłkowe / wrzód dwunastnicy

AR مرض فيروسي \ شد، لي \ قرحة إثنا عشرية
Maraddh fierousi / shidd, lay / qurhah ithnaa'ashariyah

PT doença viral / distensão / úlcera duodenal

FK enfeksyon viral / foule / ilsè nan ti trip

EL ιική νόσος / διάστρεμμα / έλκος δωδεκαδακτύλου
ee-eekEE nOsos / deeAstrema / Elkos dodekadaktEElu

HI विषाणु रोग / तनाव / ग्रहणी अल्सर
vishaNu rog / tanaav / grahNi ulcer

You have a tumor

S Tiene un tumor

H 你有一个肿瘤
nǐ yǒu yī gè zhǒng liú

R Vous avez une tumeur

E Sie haben einen Tumor

I Quý vị có khối u

T Lei è affetto da tumore

O 종양이 있으십니다
Jong-yang-i i-seu-sim-ni-da

U У вас опухоль
U vas opukhol'

L Ma Pan(i) nowotwór

R عندك تورم
'indak / 'indik tawarrum

T Tem um tumor

K Ou gen yon timè

L Έχετε όγκο
Ehete Ogo

I आपको फुलाव है
aapko phulav hai

You have a genital disease / breast disease

ES   Tiene una enfermedad genital / enfermedad de la mama

ZH   你有一个生殖性疾病 / 乳房疾病
     nǐ yǒu yī gè shēng zhí xìng jí bìng / rǔ fáng jí bìng

FR   Vous avez une maladie génitale / une maladie du sein

DE   Sie haben eine Erkrankung der Geschlechtsorgane / Brust

VI   Quý vị có bệnh ở vùng sinh dục / bệnh ở vú

IT   Lei è affetto da una malattia genitale / al seno

KO   생식기 질병 / 유방 질병이 있으십니다
     Saeng-sik-gi jil-byeong / yu-bang jil-byeong-i i-seu-sim-ni-da

RU   У вас заболевание половых органов / заболевание молочной железы
     U vas zabolevanie polovykh organov / zabolevanie molochnoy zhelezy

PL   Ma Pan(i) chorobę narządów płciowych / chorobę piersi

AR   عندك مرض تناسلي \ مرض الثدي
     'indak / 'indik maraddh tanaasuli / maraddh ath-thadiy

PT   Tem uma doença genital / doença da mama

FK   Ou gen yon maladi afè prive nou / maladi tete

EL   Έχετε νόσο γεννητικών οργάνων / νόσο μαστού
     Ehete nOso geneeteekOn orgAnon / nOso mastU

HI   आपको जननांग रोग / स्तन रोग है
     aapko jannang rog / stan rog hai

You have had a premature birth / miscarriage

ES   Tuvo un parto prematuro / aborto

ZH   你曾经早产过一次 / 流产过一次
nǐ céng jīng zǎo chǎn guò yī cì / liú chǎn guò yī cì

FR   Avez-vous eu une naissance prématurée / une fausse couche

DE   Sie haben eine Frühgeburt / Fehlgeburt

VI   Quý vị đẻ non / bị sảy thai

IT   Lei ha avuto un parto prematuro / aborto spontaneo

KO   조기 분만 / 유산을 하셨습니다
Jo-gi bun-man / yu-sa-neul ha-syeot-seum-ni-da

RU   У вас были преждевременные роды / выкидыш
U vas byli prezhdevremennye rody / vykidysh

PL   Miała Pani przedwczesny poród / poronienie

AR   اصيبت بولادة قبل الأوان \ إسقاط
Usibti bi-wilaadah qabl al-awaan \ isqaat

PT   Teve um parto prematuro / aborto natural

FK   Ou te genyen yon akouchman premature / foskouch

EL   Είχατε πρόωρο τοκετό / αποβολή
EEhate prOoro toketO / apovolEE

HI   आपको कालपूर्व शिशु / गर्भपात हुआ है
aapko kaalpurva shishu / garbhapaat hua hai

You are pregnant

ES	Está embarazada
ZH	你怀孕了 nǐ huái yùn le
FR	Vous êtes enceinte
DE	Sie sind schwanger
VI	Quý vị đang mang thai
IT	Lei è incinta
KO	임신하셨습니다 Im-sin-ha-syeot-seum-ni-da
RU	Вы беременны Vy beremenny
PL	Jest Pani w ciąży
AR	انت حامل Inti haamil
PT	Está grávida
FK	Ou ansent
EL	Είστε έγκυος EEste Egeeos
HI	आप गर्भवती हैं aap gharbhavati hain

You are (not yet) in the initial phase of delivering your baby

ES   Ya (todavía no) está en la fase inicial del parto

ZH   你是在（还没在）产程的初始阶段
nǐ shì zài (hái méi zài) chǎn chéng de chū shǐ jiē duàn

FR   Vous (n') êtes (pas encore) à la phase initiale de l'accouchement de votre bébé

DE   Die Geburt beginnt (noch nicht)

VI   Quý vị đang (vẫn chưa) ở giai đoạn bắt đầu trở dạ

IT   Lei è (non è ancora) nella fase iniziale del parto

KO   분만 초기 단계입니다 (단계가 아직 아닙니다)
Bun-man cho-gi dan-gye-im-ni-da (dan-gye-ga a-jik a-nim-ni-da)

RU   У вас (ещё не) начались роды
U vas (eshchyo ne) nachalis' rody

PL   (Jeszcze nie) jest Pani w początkowej fazie porodu

AR   انت (ما زال لست) فى مرحلة الولادة الأولى
Inti (maa zaal lastee) fi marhalah al-wiladah al-oolaa

PT   Está (ainda não está) na fase inicial do parto do seu bebé

FK   Ou nan (poko nan) staj inisyal pou akouche pitit ou.

EL   (Δεν) είστε (ακόμη) στην αρχική φάση τοκετού
(den) EEste (akOmee) steen arheekEE fAsee toketU

HI   आप अभी बच्चे को जन्म देने की शुरुआती अवस्था में हैं (नही हैं)
aap abhi bachche ko janma dene ki shuruaati avastha mein hain (nahi hain)

He / she has a childhood disease

ES Él / ella tiene una enfermedad de la niñez

ZH 他 / 她 得了儿童高发病
tā / tā dé le ér tóng gāo fā bìng

FR Il (elle) a une maladie d'enfance

DE Er / Sie hat eine Kinderkrankheit

VI Bé mắc một căn bệnh thường gặp ở trẻ nhỏ

IT Lui / lei è affetto / a da malattia infantile

KO 그가 유년기 질병이 있습니다
Geu-ga yu-nyeon-gi jil-byeong-i it-seum-ni-da

RU У него / нее детская болезнь
U nego / neyo detskaya bolezn'

PL On / ona ma chorobę wieku dziecięcego

AR عنده \ عندها مرض طفلي
'indoh / 'indhaa (to a female) maraddh tifli

PT Ele / ela tem uma doença infantil

FK Li gen yon maladi ke timoun genyen

EL Αυτός / Αυτή έχει παιδική ασθένεια
aftOs / aftEE Ehee pedeekEE asthEneea

HI उसे बचपन से उत्पन्न रोग है ......
usey bachpan se utpanna rog hai

diphtheria / pertussis / polio / measles

S difteria / tos ferina / poliomielitis / sarampión

H 白喉 / 百日咳 / 脊髓灰质炎 / 麻疹
bái hóu / bǎi rì ké / jǐ suí huī zhì yán / má zhěn

R diphtérie / coqueluche / poliomyélite / rougeole

E Diphtherie / Keuchhusten / Kinderlähmung / Masern

I bệnh bạch hầu / ho gà / bệnh bại liệt / bệnh sởi

T difterite / pertosse / polio / morbillo

O 디프테리아 / 백일해 / 소아마비 / 홍역
di-peu-te-ria / bae-gil-hae / so-a-ma-bi / hong-yeok

U дифтерия / коклюш / полиомиелит / корь
difteriya / koklyush / poliomielit / kor'

L błonicę / koklusz / paraliż dziecięcy / odrę

R خناق \ سعال ديكي \ شلل الأطفال \ الحصبة
Khanaaq / su'aal deekiy / shalal al-atfaal / al-hassbah

T difetria / tosse convulsa / poliomielite / sarampo

K difteri / koklich / polyo / lawoujòl

L διφθερίτιδα / κοκκύτης / πολιομυελίτιδα / ιλαρά
deeftherEEteeda / kokEEtees / poleeoomee-elEEteeda / eelarA

H डिफ्थीरिया / काली खाँसी / पोलियो / खसरा.
diphtheria / kaali khaansi / polio / khasraa

mumps / German measles / chickenpox

ES parotiditis / rubéola / varicela

ZH 流形性腮腺炎 / 风疹 / 水豆
liú xíng xing sāi xiàn yán / fēng zhěn / shuǐ dòu

FR oreillons / rubéole / varicelle

DE Mumps / Röteln / Windpocken

VI bệnh quai bị / bệnh ban đào / bệnh đậu mùa

IT parotite / rosolia / varicella

KO 볼거리 / 풍진 / 수두
bol-geo-ri / pung-jin / su-du

RU свинка / краснуха / ветряная оспа
svinka / krasnukha / vetryanaya ospa

PL świnkę / różyczkę / ospę

AR النكاف \ الحصبة الألمانية \ جدري الماء
An-nakaaf / al-hassbah al-almaaniyah / judaree al-maa'

PT papeira / rubéola / varíola

FK malmouton / lawoujòl alman / varisel

EL μαγουλάδες / ερυθρά / ανεμοβλογιά
magulAdes / ereethrA / anemovlogeeA

HI कनपेड़ / जर्मन खसरा / छोटी चेचक
kanped / German khasraa / chhoti chechak

25 Treatment, Instruction

You will need the following treatment

S Va a necesitar el siguiente tratamiento

H 你需要以下治疗
nǐ xū yào yǐ xià zhì liáo

R Vous avez besoin du traitement suivant

E Sie werden folgende Behandlung brauchen

I Quý vị sẽ cần biện pháp điều trị sau đây

T Lei ha bisogno del seguente trattamento

O 다음의 치료를 받으셔야 합니다
da-eum-ui chi-ryo-reul ba-deu-syeo-ya ham-ni-da

U Вы нуждаетесь в следующем лечении
Vy nuzhdaetes' v sleduyushchem lechenii

L Będzie Panu(i) potrzebować następującego leczenia

AR سوف تكون \ تكونين بحاجة إلى العلاج التالي
Saufa takoon [male] / takooneen [female] bi-haajah ilaa al-"ilaaj at-taali

T Precisará do tratamento seguinte

K W ap bezwen tretman swivan an

EL Θα χρειαστείτε την ακόλουθη θεραπεία
tha hreeastEEte teen akOluthee therapEEa

HI आपको निम्नलिखित इलाज की जरूरत होगी ...
Aapko nimnlikhit ilaaj ki jaroorat hogi

an injection / an infusion / tablets / ointment / medicinal drops / suppositories

ES una inyección / solución intravenosa / pastillas / pomada / gotas medicinales / supositorios

ZH 打针 / 打点滴 / 片剂 / 膏剂 / 滴剂 / 浑悬剂
dǎ zhēn / dǎ diǎn dī / piàn jì / gāo jì / dī jì / hùn xuán jì

FR une injection / une tisane / des comprimés / un onguent (pommade) / des gouttes / des suppositoires

DE eine Spritze / eine Infusion / Tabletten / Salbe / Tropfen / Zäpfchen

VI tiêm thuốc / truyền thuốc / uống thuốc viên / thoa thuốc mỡ / nhỏ thuốc / thuốc đạn

IT un'iniezione / un'infusione / compresse / pomata / gocce medicinali / supposte

KO 주사 / 링겔 / 정제 / 연고 / 물약 / 좌약
ju-sa / ring-gel / jeong-je / yeon-go / mur-yak / jwa-yak

RU укол / инфузия / таблетки / мазь / лечебные капли / свечи
ukol / infuziya / tabletki / maz' / lechebnye kapli / svechi

PL zastrzyku / wywaru / tabletek / maści / kropli / czopków

AR حقنة \ تزريق \ حبات \ مرهم \ القطرات الدوائية \ التحميلات
Huqnah / tazreeq / habbaat / marham / al-qutraat ad-dawaa'iyah / at-tahmilaat

PT Uma injecção / uma infusão / comprimidos / pomada / drageias medicinais / supositórios

FK yon piki / yon enfuzyon / grenn / pomade / gout medikal / sipozitwa

EL μια ένεση / μια έκχυση / δισκία / αλοιφή / φαρμακευτικές σταγόνες / υπόθετα
mEEa Enesee / mEEa Ekheesee / deeskEEa / aleefEE / farmakefteekEs stagOnes / eepOtheta

HI इंजेक्शन / काढ़ा / गोलियां / मरहम / औष ६ ीय बूंदें / बत्ती
Injecton / kadha / goliyan / marham / ausdhiya bundein / batti

a wound suture / a plaster bandage / a bandage

sutura de la herida / vendaje de yeso / vendaje

伤口缝合 / 打石膏 / 打绷带
shāng kǒu féng hé / dǎ shí gāo / dǎ bēng dài

une suture de plaie / une bande plâtrée / un bandage

eine Wundnaht / einen Gipsverband / einen Verband

khâu vết thương / bó bột / băng bó vết thương

una sutura della ferita / un'ingessatura / una fasciatura

상처 봉합 / 깁스 붕대 / 붕대
sang-cheo bong-hap / gip-seu bung-dae / bung-dae

ушивание раны / гипсовая повязка / повязка
ushivanie rany / gipsovaya povyazka / povyazka

szwu / plastra / bandażu

خيط جرح \ ضماد جبسي \ ضماد
Khayt jarhh / dhammad jibsi / dhammaad

Uma sutura da ferida / uma ligadura de gesso / uma ligadura

koud yon blesi / yon plat / yon bandaj elastik

ράμματα τραύματος / ένα έμπλαστρο / έναν επίδεσμο
rAmata trAvmatos / Ena Eblastro / Enan epEEdesmo

घाव का टांका / प्लास्टर पट्टी / पट्टी
Ghaav ka tanka / plastar patti / patti

massage / physical therapy / ergotherapy

ES	masaje / fisioterapia / ergoterapia
ZH	按摩 / 物理治疗 / ergo治疗 àn mó / wù lǐ zhì liáo / ergo zhì liáo
FR	Un massage / de la physiothérapie / de l'ergothérapie
DE	Massage / Krankengymnastik / Ergotherapie
VI	xoa bóp / vật lý trị liệu / trị liệu bằng phương pháp vận động
IT	massaggio / fisioterapia / erogoterapia
KO	마사지 / 물리치료 / 인간공학 치료 ma-sa-ji / mul-li-chi-ryo / in-gan-gong-hak chi-ryo
RU	массаж / физиотерапия / трудотерапия massazh / fizioterapiya / trudoterapiya
PL	masażu / fizjoterapii / ergoterapii
AR	التدليك \ العلاج الجسماني \ العلاج الوظائفي At-tadleek / al-"ilaaj al-jismaani / al-"ilaaj al-wadhaa'ifi
PT	Massagem / terapia física / ergoterapia
FK	masaj / terapi fizik / ergoterapi
EL	μαλάξεις / φυσικοθεραπεία / εργοθεραπεία malAxees / feeseekotherapEEa / ergotherapEEa
HI	मालिश / शारीरिक इलाज / पेशी का इलाज maalish / sharirik ilaaj / peshi ka ilaaj

surgery / chemotherapy / radiation therapy

cirugía / quimioterapia / radioterapia

手术 / 化疗 / 放疗
shǒu shù / huà liáo / fàng liáo

de chirurgie / de chimiothérapie / de radiothérapie

eine Operation / eine Chemotherapie / Strahlentherapie

giải phẫu / hóa học trị liệu / phóng xạ trị liệu

chirurgia / chemoterapia / radioterapia

수술 / 화학요법 / 방사능 치료
su-sul / hwa-hag-yo-beop / bang-sa-neung chi-ryo

операция / химиотерапия / лучевая терапия
operatsiya / khimioterapiya / luchevaya terapiya

operacji / chemoterapii / radioterapii

عملية جراحية \ العلاج الكيماوي \ العلاج الشعاعي
"Amaliyah jaraahiyah / al-"ilaaj al-kimaawi / al-"ilaaj ash-shu"aa"i

Cirurgia / quimioterapia / terapia a radiação

operasyon / kimoterapi / terapi radiasyon

χειρουργείο / χημειοθεραπεία / ραδιοθεραπεία
heerurgEEo / heemeeotherapEEa / radeeotherapEEa

सर्जरी / रसायन उपचार / विकिरण उपचार
Surgery / rasayan upchar / vikiran upchar

Do you agree with this?

ES ¿Está usted de acuerdo?

ZH 你同意这样做吗？
nǐ tóng yì zhè yàng zuò ma?

FR Etes-vous d'accord avec cela?

DE Sind Sie damit einverstanden?

VI Quý vị có đồng ý với điều này không?

IT È d'accordo con questo?

KO 여기에 동의하십니까?
yeo-gi-e dong-ui-ha-sim-ni-kka?

RU Вы согласны с этим?
Vy soglasny s etim?

PL Czy Pan(i) się z tym zgadza?

AR هل توافق \ توافقين على هذا؟
Hal tuwaafiq / tuwaafiqeen "alaa hadhaa?

PT Concorda com isto?

FK Eske ou dako a sa?

EL Συμφωνείτε με αυτό;
seemfonEEte me aftO?

HI क्या आप इससे सहमत हैं?
Kya aap isse sahmat hain?

The medication must be taken as follows ...

ES El medicamento debe tomarse como sigue ...

ZH 该药品用法如下 ...
gāi yào pǐn yòng fǎ rú xià ...

FR Ce médicament doit être pris comme suit ...

DE Das Medikament muss folgendermaßen genommen werden ...

VI Cần phải dùng thuốc như sau ...

IT Il farmaco va assunto in questo modo ... .

KO 약을 다음과 같이 복용하셔야 합니다 ...
ya-geul da-eum-gwa ga-chi bo-gyong-ha-syeo-ya ham-ni-da ...

RU Лекарство следует принимать следующим образом ...
Lekarstvo sleduet prinimat' sleduyushchim obrazom ...

PL Lek ten należy przyjmować w następujący sposób ...

AR يجب أخذ الدواء كما يلى ...
Yajib akhdh ad-dawaa' kamaa yalee ...

PT O medicamento tem que ser tomado da seguinte maneira ...

FK Fòk ou pran medikaman an nan fason swivan an ...

EL Τα φάρμακα πρέπει να λαμβάνονται ως εξής ...
ta fArmaka prEpee na lamvAnonte os exEEs ...

HI यह दवा निम्न रूप से ली जानी जरूरी है ...
Yeh dawaa nimn roop se lee jani jaroori hai ...

one teaspoon / tablespoon / hourly / ... times daily / every ... days

ES	una cucharadita / una cucharada / cada hora / ... veces al día / cada ... días
ZH	一茶匙 / 汤匙 / 每小时 / ... 次每天 / 一次每 ... 天 yī chá shí / tāng shí / měi xiǎo shí / ... cì měi tiān / yī cì měi ... tiān
FR	une cuillère à thé / une cuillère à soupe / par heure / ... fois par jour / tous les ... jours
DE	einen Teelöffel / Esslöffel / stündlich / ... mal täglich / alle ... Tage
VI	một thìa cà phê / một muỗng canh / hàng giờ / ... lần mỗi ngày / ... ngày một lần
IT	un cucchiaino / cucchiaio / all'ora / ... volte al giorno / ogni ... giorni
KO	한 티스푼 / 테이블 스푼 / 매 시간 / 하루에 ... 번 / ... 일 마다 han ti-seu-pun / te-i-beul seu-pun / mae si-gan / ha-ru-e ... beon / ... il ma-da
RU	одна чайная ложка / столовая ложка / каждый час / ... раз в день / каждые ... дня(дней) odna chaynaya lozhka / stolovaya lozhka / kazhdyi chas / ... raz v den' / kazhdye ... dnya(dney)
PL	jedną łyżeczkę / łyżkę stołową / co godzinę ... razy dziennie / co ... dni
AR	ملعقة كبيرة واحدة \ ملعقة صغيرة واحدة \ بالساعة \ ... مرة باليوم \ كل ... يوم Mil"aqah kabiirah wahidah / mil"aqah saghiirah wahidah / bis-saa"ah / ... marrah bil-youm / kull ... youm
PT	Uma colher de chá / uma colher de sopa / de hora a hora / ... vezes por dia / todos os ... dias
FK	yon ti kwiye / gwo kwiye / chak inhè tan / ... fwa pa jou / chak ... jou
EL	ένα κουταλάκι του γλυκού / κουταλάκι της σούπας / κάθε ώρα / ... φορές ημερησίως / κάθε ... ημέρες Ena kutalAkee tu gleekU / kutalAkee tees sUpas / kAthe Ora / ... forEs eemereesEEos / kAthe ... eemEres
HI	एक छोटा चम्मच / बड़ा चम्मच / घंटावार / रोज ... बार / प्रत्येक ... दिन Ek chhota chammach / baRa chammach / ghantavaar / roj ... bar / Pratyek ... din

Please apply ointment thinly / liberally

Por favor aplique una capa delgada / generosa de pomada

请薄薄地 / 适量地涂上药膏
qǐng báo báo de / shì liàng de tú shàng yào gāo

S'il vous plaît, appliquez cet onguent en couche mince / généreusement

Die Salbe bitte dünn / großzügig auftragen

Vui lòng thoa một lớp thuốc mỡ mỏng / tùy ý

Applichi un sottile strato di pomata / applicare abbondantemente la pomata

연고를 얇게 / 많이 바르십시오
yeon-go-reul yal-ge / ma-ni ba-reu-sip-si-o

Пожалуйста, наносите мазь тонким / толстым слоем
Pozhaluysta, nanosite maz' tonkim / tolstym sloem

Maść należy nakładać cienką / grubą warstwą

الرجاء المسح بالمرهم خفيفاً \ بكمية محترمة
Ar-rajaa' al-mas'h bil-marham khafifan / bi-kamiyyah muhtaramah

Aplicar, por favor, pouca / muita pomada

Tanpri aplike pomade la lejerman / anpil

Παρακαλώ να απλώνετε την αλοιφή σε αραιή / γενναιόδωρη ποσότητα
parakalO na aplOnete teen aleefEE se areEE / geneOdoree posOteeta

कृपया थोड़ा / अधिक मरहम लगाएं
Kripya thoda / adhik marham lagayein

Please take this medication for the following period ...

ES Por favor tome este medicamento durante el periodo siguiente ...

ZH 请在以下时间用药 ...
qǐng zài yǐ xià shí jiān yòng yào ...

FR S'il vous plaît, prenez ce médicament pendant la période suivante ...

DE Das Medikament bitte über folgenden Zeitraum nehmen ...

VI Vui lòng dùng loại thuốc này trong khoảng thời gian như sau ...

IT Assuma questo farmaco per il seguente periodo ...

KO 다음 기간 동안 이 약을 복용하십시오 ...
da-eum gi-gan dong-an i ya-geul bo-gyong-ha-sip-sio ...

RU Пожалуйста, принимайте это лекарство в течение следующего срока ...
Pozhaluysta, prinimayte eto lekarstvo v techenie sleduyushchego sroka ...

PL Lekarstwo należy przyjmować przez następujący okres czasu ...

AR الرجاء اخذ هذا الدواء للفترة التالية ...
Ar-rajaa' akhdh hadha ad-dawaa' lil-fatrah at-taaliyah ...

PT Queira tomar este medicamento durante o período seguinte ...

FK Tanpri pran medikaman sa pandan peryòd swivan an ...

EL Παρακαλώ να πάρετε αυτό το φάρμακο για την ακόλουθη χρονική περίοδο ...
parakalO na pErnete aftO to fArmako geeA teen akOluthee hroneekEE perEEodo ...

HI कृपया यह दवा निम्नलिखित अवधि तक लें ...
Kripya yeh dawaa nimanlikhit awadhi tak lein ...

... days / ... weeks / ... years / in the morning / at noon / in the evening ...

ES ... días / ... semanas / ... años / en la mañana / al mediodía / en la tarde / hasta que se acabe el medicamento

ZH ... 天 / ... 周 / ... 年 / 在早上 / 中午 / 晚饭后 ...
... tiān / zhōu / nián / zài zǎo shàng / zhōng wǔ / wǎn fàn hòu

FR ... Jours / ... semaines / ... années / le matin / à midi / le soir ...

DE ... Tage / ... Wochen / ... Jahre / morgens / mittags / abends ...

VI ... ngày / ... tuần / ... năm / vào buổi sáng / vào buổi trưa / vào buổi tối ...

IT ... giorni / ... settimane / ... anni / al mattino / a mezzogiorno / alla sera ...

KO ... 일 동안 / ... 주 동안 / ... 년 동안 / 아침에 / 정오에 / 저녁에 ...
... il dongan / ... ju dong-an / ... nyeon dong-an / a-chi-me / jeong-o-e / jeo-nyeo-ge ...

RU ... дня(дней) / ... недели(недель) / ... года(лет) / утром / днём / вечером ...
... dnya(dney) / ... nedeli(nedel') / ... goda(let) / utrom / dnyom / vecherom ...

PL ... dni / ... tygodni / ... lat / rano / w południe / wieczorem ...

AR ... يوماً \ ... اسبوعاً \ ... سنة \ بالصباح \ بالظهر \ بالمساء ...
... youman / ... usbou"an / ... sanah / bis-sabaah / bidh-dhuhr / bil-masaa' ...

PT ... dias / ... semanas / ... anos / de manhã / ao meio-dia / de noite ...

HK ... jou / ... semen / ... ane / nan matin / a midi / nan aswe ...

EL ... ημέρες / ... εβδομάδες / ... έτη / το πρωί / το απόγευμα / το βράδυ ...
... eemEres / ... evdomAdes / ... Etee / to proEE / to apOgevma / to vrAdee ...

HI ... दिन/ ... हफ्ते/ ... वर्ष/ सुबह में / दोपहर में / शाम में ...
... din / ... haphate ... varsha / subah mein / dopahar mein / shaam mein ...

until the medication is used up

ES hasta que el medicamento se acabe

ZH 直到药用完
zhí dào yào yòng wán

FR jusqu'à ce que le médicament soit épuisé

DE bis die Packung aufgebraucht ist

VI cho tới khi dùng hết thuốc

IT fino a quando il farmaco è finito

KO 약이 떨어질 때까지
ya-gi tteo-reo-jil ttae-kka-ji

RU пока лекарство не закончится
poka lekarstvo ne zakonchitsya

PL aż do zużycia

AR حتى يُستهلك الدواء كله
Hattaa yustahlak ad-dawaa' kulloh

PT até ter consumido todo o medicamento

FK jis lè medikaman an fini.

EL έως ότου τελειώσετε το φάρμακο
Eos Otu teleeOsete to fArmako

HI जब तक दवा समाप्त नहीं हो जाती
Jab tak dawaa samaapt nahi ho jati

Please take this medication by ...

Por favor, para tomar este medicamento ...

用这个药时请 ...
yòng zhè gè yào shí qǐng ...

S'il vous plaît, prenez ce médicament en ...

Das Medikament bitte ...

Vui lòng dùng loại thuốc này bằng cách ...

Assuma questo farmaco ...

이 약을 ...
I ya-geul ...

Принимать это лекарство следует так ...
Prinimat' eto lekarstvo sleduet tak ...

Lekarstwo należy przyjmować w następujący sposób ...

الرجاء اخذ هذا الدواء من خلال ...
Ar-rajaa' akhdh hadha ad-dawaa' mil khilaal ...

Queira tomar este medicamento ...

Tanpri pran medikaman sa an ...

Παρακαλώ να παίρνετε αυτό το φάρμακο ...
parakalO na pErnete aftO to fArmako ...

कृपया यह दवा इस प्रकार लें ...
Kripya yeh dawaa is prakaar lein ...

swallowing it (with water) / dissolving it in water / chewing it

ES páseselo (con agua) / disuélvalo en agua / mastíquelo

ZH 吞下（用水）／用水溶化／嚼碎
tūn xià (yòng shuǐ) / yòng shuǐ róng huà / jiáo shuì

FR en l'avalant (avec de l'eau) / en le dissolvant dans de l'eau / en le mâchant

DE (mit Wasser) schlucken / in Wasser auflösen / zerkauen

VI nuốt (cùng với nước) / hòa tan trong nước / nhai

IT inghiottendolo (con acqua) / sciogliendolo in acqua / masticandolo

KO 삼키십시오(물과 함께) / 물에 타 드십시오 / 씹어 드십시오
sam-ki-sip-si-o(mul-gwa ham-kke) / mu-re ta deu-sip-sio / ssi-beo deu-sip-sio

RU запивать его (водой) / растворять его в воде / жевать его
zapivat' ego (vodoy) / rastvoryat' ego v vode / zhevat' ego

PL połykać (z wodą) / rozpuszczać w wodzie / żuć

AR البلع (بالماء) \ تحليله في الماء / مضغه
Al-bala" (bil-maa') / tahleeloh fil-maa / madhghoh

PT engolindo-o (com água) / dissolvendo-o em água / mastigando-o

FK vale l (ak dlo) / fon li nan dlo / mache l

EL καταπίνοντας το (με νερό) / διαλύοντας το σε νερό / μασώντας το
katapEEnodas to (me nerO) / deealEEodas to se nerO / masOdas to

HI इसे (पानी के साथ) निगलना／इसे पानी में घोलकर／इसे चबाकर ...
Ise (paani ke saath) nigalnaa / ise paani mein gholkar / ise chabaakar---

dissolving it in the mouth / gargling / inhalation / vaginal (anal) insertion

disuélvalo en la boca / haga gárgaras / inhálelo / introdúzcalo en la vagina (el ano)

口中含化 / 漱口 / 吸入 / 放入阴道 / 肛门
kǒu zhōng hán huà / shù kǒu / xī rù / fàng rù yīn dào / gāng mén

en le laissant fondre dans la bouche / en gargarisant / en inhalation / en insertion vaginale (anale)

im Mund auflösen / gurgeln / inhalieren / vaginal (anal) einführen

ngậm tan trong miệng / súc miệng / hít / đưa vào âm đạo (hậu môn)

sciogliendolo in bocca / facendo gargarismi / inalazioni / mediante inserimento vaginale (anale)

입 안에서 녹여서 드십시오 / 가글 하십시오 / 흡입하십시오 / 질내에 (항문에) 삽입하십시오
ip-a-ne-seo no-gyeo-seo deu-sip-si-o / ga-geul ha-sip-sio / heu-bi-pa-sip-si-o / jil-lae-e (hang-mu-ne) sa-bi-pa-sip-sio

сосать его во рту / полоскать рот / делать ингаляции / вводить во влагалище (прямую кишку)
sosat' ego vo rtu/poloskat' rot/delat' ingalyatsii/vvodit' vo vlagalishche (pryamuyu kishku)

rozpuszczając je w ustach / płucząc nim gardło / wdychając je / wprowadzając je pochwowo (analnie)

تحليله في الفم \ بالغرغرة \ بالإستنشاق \ إدخاله في الفرج (او الدبر)
Tahleeloh fil-famm \ bil-ghargharah \ bil-istinshaaq \ idkhaaloh fil-farj (aw ad-dubur)

dissolvendo-o na boca / gargarejando / por inalação / inserção vaginal (anal)

fon li nan bouch ou / gargarize / respire / mete l nan vajin (anal)

διαλύοντας το στο στόμα / με γαργάρες / με εισπνοές / με κολπική (πρωκτική) εισαγωγή
deealEEodas to sto stoma / me gargАres / me eespnoEs / me kolpeekEE (prokteekEE) eesagogEE

इसे मुंहमेंघोलकर / गरारेकर / भाप / योनिक(गुदीय)निवेशन
Ise muh mein gholkar / garare kar / bhaap / yonik (gudeeya) niveshan

You / he / she must remain hospitalized for ... days

ES Usted / él / ella debe hospitalizarse durante ... días

ZH 你 / 他 / 她 需要住院治疗 ... 天
nǐ (tā / tā) xū yào zhù yuàn zhì liáo ... tiān

FR Vous / il / elle doit rester hospitalisé(e) ... jours

DE Sie müssen / er / sie muss ... Tage im Krankenhaus bleiben

VI Quý vị / anh ta / cô ta phải nằm viện trong ... ngày

IT Lei / lui / lei deve rimanere in ospedale per ... giorni

KO 당신 / 그 / 그녀는 ... 일 동안 입원하셔야 합니다
dang-sin / geu / geu-nyeo-neun ... il dong-an i-bwon-ha-syeo-ya ham-ni-da

RU Вас / его / её следует оставить в больнице ещё на ... дня(дней)
Vas / ego / eyo sleduet ostavit' v bol'nitse eshchyo na ... dnya(dney)

PL Musi Pan(i) / on / ona pozostać w szpitalu na ... dni

AR عليك \ عليه \ عليها البقاء في المستشفى لـ ... يوم
"Alayk / "Alayh / "Alayha al-baqaa' fil-mustashfaa li ... youm

PT Você / ele / ela tem que ficar hospitalizado(a) durante ... dias

FK Fòk ou / li rete nan lopital pou ... jou

EL Εσείς / Αυτός / Αυτή πρέπει να νοσηλευτείτε / νοσηλευτεί για ... ημέρες.
esEEs / aftOs / aftEE prEpee na noseeleftEEte / noseeleftEE geeA ... eemEres.

HI आपको / उसे ... दिनों के लिए अस्पताल में रहना जरूरी है
Aapko / use ... dinon ke liye aspataal mein rahana jaroori hai

Please inhale the oxygen

Por favor inhale el oxigeno

请吸氧气
qǐng xī yǎng qì

S'il vous plaît, inhalez l'oxygène

Atmen Sie / atme den Sauerstoff ein

Vui lòng hít thở khí ôxy

Inali l'ossigeno

산소를 흡입하십시오
san-so-reul heu-bi-pa-sip-si-o

Пожалуйста, дышите кислородом
Pozhaluysta, dyshite kislorodom

Proszę wdychać ten tlen

الرجاء إستنشاق الأكسجين
Ar-rajaa' istinshaaq al-oxygen

Aspire o oxigénio, por favor

Tanpri respire oksigen lan

Παρακαλώ εισπνεύσετε το οξυγόνο
parakalO eespnEfsete to oxeegOno

कृपया सांस के साथ ऑक्सीजन खींचे
Kripya sans ke sath oxygen kheechei

This medication will cause vomiting

ES — Este medicamento le va a causar vómito

ZH — 这个药会导致呕吐
zhè gè yào huì dǎo zhì ǒu tù.

FR — Ce médicament peut entraîner des vomissements

DE — Dieses Medikament führt zum Erbrechen

VI — Thuốc này sẽ gây ói mửa

IT — Questo farmaco provocherà vomito

KO — 이 약은 구토를 일으킵니다
I ya-geun gu-to-reul i-reu-kim-ni-da

RU — Это лекарство вызывает рвоту
Eto lekarstvo vyzyvaet rvotu

PL — Ten lek spowoduje wymioty

AR — هذا الدواء يسبب القيء
Hadha ad-dawaa' yusabbib al-qay'

PT — Este medicamento provocará vómitos

FK — Medikaman sa a pral koze vomisman

EL — Το φάρμακο αυτό θα προκαλέσει εμετό
to fArmako aft0 tha prokalEsee emet0

HI — इस दवा के कारण उल्टी होगी
Is dawaa ke karaN ulti hogi

I must insert this tube into your / his / her stomach

S Necesito introducir este tubo en el estómago

H 我必须将这个管子放进你的／他的／她的胃里
wǒ bì xū jiāng zhè gè guǎn zǐ fàng jìn nǐ de / tā de / tā de wèi lǐ.

R Je dois introduire ce tube dans votre estomac

E Ich muss diesen Schlauch in Ihren / seinen / ihren Magen einführen

VI Tôi phải đưa chiếc ống này vào trong bao tử của quý vị / anh ta / cô ta

T Devo inserire questo tubicino nel suo stomaco

O 제가 당신의 / 그의 / 그녀의 배에 이 튜브를 삽입해야 합니다
je-ga dang-si-nui / geu-ui / geu-nyeo-ui bae-e i tyu-beu-reul sa-bi-pae-ya ham-ni-da

U Я должен ввести этот зонд в ваш / его / её желудок
Ya dolzhen vvesti etot zond v vash / ego / eyo zheludok

PL Muszę wprowadzić tę rurkę do Pana(i) / jego / jej żołądka

AR يجب على إدخال هذه الأنبوبة فى معدتك \ معدته \ معدتها
Yajib "alayyi idkhaal hadhihi al-anboubah fi ma"idatak / ma"idatoh / ma"idathaa

PT Devo introduzir este tubo no seu estômago / no estômago dele / dela

K Fòk mwen mete tib sa a nan vant ou / li

EL Πρέπει να εισάγω αυτό το σωληνάκι στο στομάχι σας / του / της
prEpee na eesAgo aftO to soleenAkee sto stomAhee sas / tu / tees

HI मुझे यह ट्यूब आपके / उसके पेट में डालना जरूरी है
Mujhe yeh tube aapke / uske pet mei daalna jaroori hai

Please relax / please swallow

ES	Por favor relájese / por favor trague
ZH	请放松 / 请吞咽 qǐng fàng sōng / qǐng tūn yàn
FR	S'il vous plaît, détendez-vous / s'il vous plaît, avalez
DE	Entspannen (Sie sich) / Schlucken (Sie)
VI	Vui lòng thả lỏng / vui lòng nuốt
IT	Si rilassi / deglutisca
KO	편하게 있으십시오 / 삼키십시오 pyeon-ha-ge i-seu-sip-si-o / sam-ki-sip-si-o
RU	Пожалуйста, расслабьтесь / пожалуйста, глотайте Pozhaluysta, rasslab'tes' / pozhaluysta, glotayte
PL	Proszę się rozluźnić / proszę przełknąć
AR	الرجاء التريح \ الرجاء الإبتلاع Ar-rajaa' at-tarayyuh / ar-rajaa' al-ibtilaa"
PT	Descontraia-se, por favor / engula, por favor
FK	Tanpri rilaks / tanpri vale
EL	Παρακαλώ χαλαρώσετε / Παρακαλώ καταπιείτε parakalO halarOsete / parakalO katapeeEEte
HI	कृपया आराम करें / कृपया निगलें Kripya aaraam karein / kripya niglein

We must bring the fever down

ES   Tenemos que bajar la fiebre

ZH   我们必须控制高烧
wǒ mén bì xū kòng zhì gāo shāo

FR   Nous devons faire baisser la fièvre

DE   Wir müssen das Fieber senken

VI   Chúng tôi phải làm hạ sốt

IT   Dobbiamo abbassare la febbre

KO   열을 내려야 합니다
yeo-reul nae-ryeo-ya ham-ni-da

RU   Нам надо понизить температуру
Nam nado ponizit' temperaturu

PL   Musimy obniżyć gorączkę

AR   علينا تخفيف الحمى
"Alaynaa takhfeef al-hummaa

PT   Temos que fazer baixar a febre

FK   Fòk nou bese lafyèv la

EL   Πρέπει να κατεβάσουμε τον πυρετό
prEpee na katevAsume ton peeretO

HI   हमें बुखार कम करना होगा
Hamein bukhaar kam karna hoga

I will try to extract it

ES Voy a tratar de sacarlo

ZH 我要试着取出来它
wǒ yào shì zhe qǔ chū lái tā

FR Je vais essayer de l'extraire

DE Ich werde versuchen, es herauszuholen

VI Tôi sẽ cố gắng rút / lấy nó ra

IT Proverò ad estrarlo

KO 그것을 빼내려고 시도하겠습니다
geu-geo-seul ppae-nae-ryeo-go si-do-ha-get-seum-ni-da

RU Я постараюсь вытащить это
Ya postarayus' vytashchit' eto

PL Spróbujemy dokonać ekstrakcji

AR سوف احاول خلعه
Saufa uhaawil khal"oh

PT Vou tentar extraí-lo

FK Mwen pral eseye retire l

EL Θα προσπαθήσω να το εξάγω
tha prospathEEso na to exAgo

HI मैं इसे निकालने का प्रयास करूंगा
Mein ise nikalne ka prayaas karoonga

Put no strain / only minimal strain on your leg / arm

No haga esfuerzo / evite hacer esfuerzo con la pierna / el brazo

你的腿 / 胳膊不能用力 / 仅能用一点点力
nǐ de tuǐ / gē bó bù néng yòng lì / jǐn néng yòng yī diǎn diǎn lì

Ne faites pas d'effort / seulement un minimum d'effort avec votre jambe / votre bras

Sie dürfen das Bein / den Arm nicht / nur wenig belasten

Không ép / chỉ ép nhẹ lên chân / cánh tay của quý vị

Non metta nessuna tensione / solo una tensione minima nella gamba / braccio

팔 / 다리에 힘을 주지 마십시오 / 최소의 힘만 주십시오
pal / da-ri-e hi-meul ju-ji ma-sip-si-o / choe-so-ui him-man ju-sip-si-o

Никаких нагрузок / только минимальные нагрузки на вашу ногу / руку
Nikakikh nagruzok / tol'ko minimal'nye nagruzki na vashu nogu / ruku

Proszę całkowicie nie obciążać / ograniczyć do minimum obciążanie nogi / ręki

لا تحمل \ تحملين رجلك \ ذراعك بالضغط \ حمل \ حملي رجلك \ ذراعك بضغط خفيف فقط
La tuhammil / tuhammileen rijlak / dhiraa"ak bidh-dhaght / hammil / hammilee rijlak / dhiraa"ak bi-dhaght khafeef faqat

Não exerça pressão / só um pouco de pressão sobre a perna / o braço

Pa mete presyon / selmen yon ti presyon sou janm / bra w

Μη βάζετε πίεση / να βάζετε ελάχιστη πίεση στο κάτω άκρο / άνω άκρο σας
mee vAzete pEEesee / na vAzete elAheestee pEEesee sto kAto Akro / Ano Akro sas

अपनी टांग / भुजा पर जोर न दें / न्यूनतम जोर दें
apni tang / bhuja par Jor na dein / nyuntam jor dein

You must use crutches

ES	Deberá usar muletas
ZH	你必须用拐 nǐ bì xū yòng guǎi
FR	Vous devez utiliser des béquilles
DE	Sie müssen Krücken benutzen
VI	Quý vị phải dùng nạng
IT	Deve usare le stampelle
KO	목발을 사용하셔야 합니다 mok-ba-reul sa-yong-ha-syeo-ya ham-ni-da
RU	Вы должны использовать костыли Vy dolzhny ispol'zovat' kostyli
PL	Musi Pan(i) używać kul
AR	يجب أن تستعمل العكازات Yajib an tasta"mil / tasta"mileen al-"ukkaazaat
PT	Tem que usar muletas
FK	Fòk ou sevi ak bekil
EL	Πρέπει να χρησιμοποιήσετε πατερίτσες prEpee na hreeseemopeeEEsete paterEEtses
HI	आपको बैसाखी प्रयोग करनी जरूरी है Aapko baisakhi prayog karni jaroori hai

You must go to the dentist

ES Debe ir al dentista

ZH 你需要看牙科医生
nǐ xū yào kàn yá kē yī shēng

FR Vous devez aller chez le dentiste

DE Sie müssen zum Zahnarzt gehen

VI Quý vị phải đi khám nha sĩ

IT Deve andare dal dentista

KO 치과 의사한테 가셔야 합니다
chi-gwa ui-sa-han-te ga-syeo-ya ham-ni-da

RU Вы должны обратиться к стоматологу
Vy dolzhny obratit'sya k stomatologu

PL Musi Pan(i) pójść do dentysty

AR عليك بزيارة طبيب الأسنان
"Alayk bi-ziyaarah tabib al-asnaan

PT Tem que ir ao dentista

FK Fòk ou al kay dantis

EL Πρέπει να πάτε στον οδοντίατρο
prEpee na pAte ston ododEEatro

HI आपको दंतचिकित्सक के पास जाना जरूरी है
Aapko dantchikitsak ke paas jana jaroori hai

Please avoid the following food products

ES Por favor evite los alimentos siguientes

ZH 请不要吃以下食品
qǐng bù yào chī yǐ xià shí pǐn

FR S'il vous plaît, évitez les aliments suivants

DE Vermeiden Sie folgende Nahrungsmittel

VI Vui lòng kiêng dùng các loại thực phẩm sau đây

IT Eviti i seguenti alimenti

KO 다음의 식품을 삼가십시오
da-eu-mui sik-pu-meul sam-ga-sip-si-o

RU Пожалуйста, воздержитесь от следующих продуктов питания
Pozhaluysta, vozderzhites' ot sleduyushchikh produktov pitaniya

PL Proszę unikać następujących produktów żywnościowych

AR الرجاء الإبتعاد عن المنتوجات الغذائية التالية
Ar-rajaa' al-ibti"aad "an al-mantoujaat al-ghadhaa'iyah at-taaliyah

PT Evite, por favor, os seguintes produtos alimentares

FK Tanpri evite pwodwi manje swivan yo

EL Παρακαλώ να αποφεύγετε τα ακόλουθα τρόφιμα
parakalO na apofEvgete ta akOlutha trOfeema

HI कृपया निम्नलिखित भोजन उत्पादों से बचें
Kripya nimnlikhit bhojan utpadon se bachein

Milk products / fried foods / fatty foods / hot foods

S Leche y derivados / alimentos fritos / alimentos grasosos / alimentos irritantes

H 奶制品 / 油炸食品 / 高脂肪食品 / 烫的食品
nǎi zhì pǐn / yóu zhá shí pǐn / gāo zhī fáng shí pǐn / tàng de shí pǐn

R Des produits laitiers / des aliments frits / de la nourriture grasse / des aliments trop épicés

E Milchprodukte / Gebratenes / Fettiges / Scharfes

I Các loại thực phẩm làm từ sữa / đồ thực phẩm chiên / thức ăn có nhiều chất béo / đồ ăn nóng

T Latticini / fritto / grassi / cibi piccanti

O 유제품 / 튀긴 식품 / 고지방 식품 / 매운 식품
yu-je-pum / twi-gin sik-pum / go-ji-bang sik-pum / mae-un sik-pum

U Молочные продукты / жареная пища / жирная пища / горячая пища
Molochnye produkty / zharenaya pishcha / zhirnaya pishcha / goryachaya pishcha

L Nabiału / potraw smażonych / potraw tłustych / potraw ostro przyprawionych

R متنوجات حليبية \ مأكولات مقلية \ مأكولات حارة
Mantoujaat halibiyah / ma'koulaat maqliyah / ma'koulaat haarrah

T Produtos lácteos / fritos / comidas gordas / comidas picantes

K Pwodwi lèt / manje ki fri / manje ki gen gres / manje cho

L Γαλακτοκομικά προϊόντα / τηγανητά φαγητά / λιπαρά φαγητά / ζεστά φαγητά
galaktokomeekA proeeOda / teeganeetA fageetA / leeparA fageetA / zestA fageetA

I दुग्ध उत्पाद / तला भोजन / वसायुक्त भोजन / गर्म भोजन
Dugdha utpaad / tala bhojan / vasaayukt bhojan / garam bhojan

Please call me / us if the fever does not go down / goes up

ES Por favor llámeme / llámenos si la fiebre no baja / si la fiebre sube

ZH 请联系我 / 我们，如果你高烧不退 / 上升
qǐng lián xì wǒ / wǒ mén, rǔ gāo nǐ gāo shāo bù tuì / shàng shēng

FR S'il vous plaît, appelez-moi / nous, si la fièvre ne descend pas / si elle monte

DE Bitte rufen Sie mich / uns, wenn das Fieber nicht sinkt / steigt

VI Vui lòng gọi cho tôi / chúng tôi nếu không hạ sốt / sốt cao hơn

IT Mi / ci telefoni se la febbre non si abbassa / si alza

KO 열이 내리지 / 올라가지 않으면 저 / 우리한테 전화하십시오
yeo-ri nae-ri-ji / ol-la-ga-ji a-neu-myeon jeo / u-ri-han-te jeon-hwa-ha-sip-si-o

RU Пожалуйста, позвоните мне / нам, если температура не спадет / поднимется
Pozhaluysta, pozvonite mne / nam, esli temperatura ne spadet / podnimetsya

PL Proszę do mnie / nas zadzwonić, jeśli gorączka nie spadnie / podwyższy się

AR الرجاء الإتصال بي \ بنا إذا لم يخف الحمى \ إذا زاد الحمى
Ar-rajaa' al-ittisaal bi / binaa idha lam yakhuff al-hummaa / idhaa zaad al-hummaa

PT Queira telefonar-me / -nos, se a febre não descer / subir

FK Tanpri rele m / nou si lafyèv la pa bese / monte

EL Παρακαλώ να μου / μας τηλεφωνήσετε εάν ο πυρετός δεν κατέβει / ανέβει
parakalO na mu / mas teelefonEEsete eAn o peeretOs den katEvee / anEvee

HI यदि बुखार कम न हो / बढ़े, कृपया मुझे / हमें call करें
yadi bukhaar kam na ho / badhe, kripya mujhe / hamein call karein

Please call me / us if your child refuses to drink

Por favor llámeme / llámenos si el niño no quiere beber

请联系我 / 我们，如果你的孩子拒绝饮水
qǐng lián xì wǒ / wǒ mén, rǔ gǔo nǐ de hái zǐ jù jué yǐn shuǐ

S'il vous plaît, appelez-moi (nous), si votre enfant refuse de boire

Bitte rufen Sie mich / uns, wenn Ihr Kind nicht trinken will

Vui lòng gọi cho tôi / chúng tôi nếu con quý vị không chịu uống

Mi / ci telefoni se il bambino rifiuta di bere

아이가 안 마시려고 하면 저 / 우리한테 전화하십시오
a-i-ga an ma-si-ryeo-go ha-myeon jeo / u-ri-han-te jeon-hwa-ha-sip-si-o

Пожалуйста, позвоните мне / нам, если ваш ребенок откажется пить
Pozhaluysta, pozvonite mne / nam, esli vash rebenok otkazhetsya pit'

Proszę do mnie / nas zadzwonić, jeśli dziecko odmówi przyjmowania napoju

الرجاء الاتصال بي \ بنا إذا رفض طفلك الشرب
Ar-rajaa' al-ittisaal bi / binaa idha rafadh tiflak ash-sharb

Queira telefonar-me / -nos, se o(a) seu(sua) filho(a) se recusar a beber

Tanpri rele m / nou si pitit ou a refize bouwe

Παρακαλώ να μου / μας τηλεφωνήσετε εάν το παιδί σας αρνηθεί να πιει
parakalO na mu / mas teeleefonEEsete eAn to pedEE sas arneetheE na peeEE

यदि आपका बच्चा पीने से मना करता है, कृपया मुझे / हमें कॉल करें
Yadi aapka bachcha peene se manaa karta hai, kripya mujhe / hamein call karein

Please call me / us if your child continues to vomit

ES Por favor llámeme / llámenos si el niño sigue vomitando

ZH 请联系我 / 我们，如果你的孩子继续呕吐
qǐng lián xì wǒ / wǒ mén, rǔ gǔo nǐ de hái zǐ jì xù ǒu tù

FR S'il vous plaît, appelez-moi (nous), si votre enfant continue de vomir

DE Bitte rufen Sie mich / uns, wenn Ihr Kind immer noch erbricht

VI Vui lòng gọi cho tôi / chúng tôi nếu con quý vị vẫn ói mửa

IT Mi / ci telefoni se il bambino continua a vomitare

KO 아이가 구토를 계속하면 저 / 우리한테 전화하십시오
a-i-ga gu-to-reul gye-sok-ha-myeon jeo / u-ri-han-te jeon-hwa-ha-sip-sio

RU Пожалуйста, позвоните мне / нам, если у вашего ребёнка будет
продолжаться рвота
Pozhaluysta, pozvonite mne / nam, esli u vashego rebyonka budet prodolzhat'sya rvota

PL Proszę do mnie / nas zadzwonić, jeśli dziecko będzie nadal wymiotować

AR الرجاء الإتصال بي \ بنا إذا استمر طفلك يتقيأ
Ar-rajaa' al-ittisaal bi / binaa idha stamarr tiflak yataqayya'

PT Queira telefonar-me / -nos, se o seu filho continuar a vomitar

FK Tanpri rele m / nou si pitit ou a kontinye vomi

EL Παρακαλώ να μου / μας τηλεφωνήσετε εάν το παιδί σας συνεχίσει να κάνει εμετό
parakalO na mu / mas teelefonEEsete eAn to pedEE sas seenehEEsee na kAnee emetO

HI यदि आपका बच्चा लगातार उल्टी करता है, कृपया मुझे / हमें कॉल करें
Yadi aapka bachcha lagaataar ulti kartaa hai, kripya mujhe / hamein call karein

Please call me / us if the diarrhea worsens ...

ES Por favor llámeme / llámenos si la diarrea empeora ...

ZH 请联系我 / 我们，如果腹泻加重 ...
qǐng lián xì wǒ / wǒ mén, rǔ gǔo fù xiè jiā zhòng

FR S'il vous plaît, appelez-moi (nous), si la diarrhée s'aggrave ...

DE Bitte rufen Sie mich / uns, wenn der Durchfall sich verschlimmert ...

VI Vui lòng gọi cho tôi / chúng tôi nếu tiêu chảy ngày càng nặng hơn ...

IT Mi / ci telefoni se la diarrea peggiora ...

KO 설사가 악화되면 저 / 우리한테 전화하십시오 ...
seol-sa-ga ak-hwa-doe-myeon jeo / u-ri-han-te jeon-hwa-ha-sip-si-o ...

RU Пожалуйста, позвоните мне / нам, если понос усилится ...
Pozhaluysta, pozvonite mne / nam, esli ponos usilitsya ...

PL Proszę do mnie / nas zadzwonić, jeśli biegunka pogorszy się ...

AR الرجاء الإتصال بي \ بنا إذا اشتد الإسهال ...
Ar-rajaa' al-ittisaal bi / binaa idha shtadd al-is'haal ...

PT Queira telefonar-me / -nos, se a diarreia piorar ...

FK Tanpri rele m / nou si dyare a vin pli mal ...

EL Παρακαλώ να μου / μας τηλεφωνήσετε εάν η διάρροια χειροτερέψει ...
parakalO na mu / mas teelefonEEsete eAn ee deeAreea heeroterEpsee ...

HI यदि अतिसार अधिक बिगड़ जाता है, कृपया मुझे / हमें कॉल करें
Yadi atisaar adhik bigad jata hai, kripya mujhe / hamein call karein

... your child does not urinate within the next 8 hours

ES ... su niño no orina en las 8 horas siguientes

ZH ... 你的孩子八个小时内不小便
... nǐ de hái zǐ bā gè xiǎo shí nèi bù xiǎo biàn

FR S'il vous plaît, appelez-moi (nous), si votre enfant n'urine pas au cours des 8 prochaines heures

DE ... Ihr Kind in den nächsten 8 h nicht uriniert

VI ... con quý vị không đi tiểu trong 8 giờ tới

IT ... se il bambino non urina nelle prossime 8 ore

KO 앞으로 8시간 이내에 아이가 소변을 보지 않으면 ...
a-peu-ro 8-si-gan i-nae-e a-i-ga so-byeo-neul bo-ji a-neu-myeon ...

RU ... ваш ребёнок не помочится в течение следующих 8 часов
... vash rebenok ne pomochitsya v techenie sleduyushchikh 8 chasov

PL ... jeśli dzicko nie odda moczu w ciągu następnych ośmiu godzin

AR ... إذا لم يتبول طفلك في أثناء ٨ ساعات قادمة
... idhaa lam yatabawwil tiflak fi athnaa' 8 saa"aat qaadimah

PT ... o(a) seu(sua) filho(a) não urinar dentro das próximas 8 horas

FK ... pitit ou a pa pipi nan pwochen 8 hè tan yo

EL ... το παιδί σας δεν ουρήσει εντός των επόμενων οκτώ ωρών
... to pedEE sas den urEEsee edOs ton epOmenon oktO orOn

HI ... आपका बच्चा अगले 8 घंटों में मूत्र नहीं करता
... Aapka bachcha agle 8 ghanton mein mootra nahin kartaa

... your child continues to have breathing problems

... su niño sigue teniendo dificultad para respirar

... 你的孩子继续有呼吸困难
... nǐ de hái zǐ jì xù yǒu hū xī kùn nán

Si votre enfant continue à avoir des problèmes respiratoires ...

... Ihr Kind weiterhin Probleme beim Atmen hat

... con quý vị vẫn có các vấn đề về hô hấp

... se il bambino continua a d avere problemi respiratori

아이가 계속 호흡곤란을 느끼면 ...
a-i-ga gye-sok ho-heup-gol-la-neul neu-kki-myeon ...

... у вашего ребёнка продолжатся проблемы с дыханием
... u vashego rebyonka prodolzhatsya problemy s dykhaniem

... jeśli dziecko będzie w dalszym ciągu miało trudności z oddychaniem

... إذا إستمر طفلك أن يعاني من مشاكل التنفس
... idhaa stamarr tiflak an yu"aani min mashaakil at-tanaffus

... o(a) seu(sua) filho(a) continuar a ter problemas respiratórios

... pitit ou a kontinye gen pwoblem respirasyon

... το παιδί σας συνεχίσει να έχει αναπνευστικά προβλήματα
... to pedEE sas seenehEEsee na Ehee anapnefsteekA provlEEmata

... आपके बच्चे को सांस लेने में लगातार परेशानी
... Aapke bachche ki sans lene mein lagaataar pareshani

Please give your child ...

ES Por favor déle a su niño ...

ZH 请给你的孩子 ...
qǐng gěi nǐ de hái zǐ ...

FR S'il vous plaît, donnez à votre enfant ...

DE Geben Sie Ihrem Kind ...

VI Vui lòng cho con quý vị ...

IT Dia al bambino ...

KO 아이한테 다음을 주십시오 ...
a-i-han-te da-eu-meul ju-sip-si-o ...

RU Пожалуйста, дайте вашему ребёнку ...
Pozhaluysta, dayte vashemu rebyonku ...

PL Proszę dziecku podawać ...

AR ... الرجاء إعطاء طفلك
Ar-rajaa' i"taa' tiflak ...

PT Por favor, dê ao(à) seu(sua) filho(a) ...

FK Tanpri bay pitit ou ...

EL Παρακαλώ να δώσετε στο παιδί σας ...
parakalO na dOsete sto pedEE sas ...

HI कृपया अपने बच्चे को दें ...
Kripya apne bachche ko dein ...

non-carbonated water/tee/electrolytes/apple juice with water/large amounts of liquid

ES agua no gaseosa/té/electrólitos / jugo o zumo de manzana con agua / mucho líquido

ZH 不含糖的水 / 茶 / 含电解质饮料 / 苹果汁加水 / 大量液体
bù hán táng de shuǐ / chá / hán diàn jiě zhì yǐn liào / píng guǒ zhī jiā shuǐ / dà liàng yè tǐ

FR de l'eau non gazeuse / du thé / des électrolytes / du jus de pomme dilué avec de l'eau / de grandes quantités de liquides

DE stilles Wasser / Tee / Elektrolyte / Apfelsaft mit Wasser / viel Flüssigkeit

VI uống nước không có ga / trà / chất điện giải / nước táo cùng với nước / thật nhiều chất lỏng

IT acqua non gassata / tè / elettroliti / succo di mela con acqua / grandi quantità di liquidi

KO 탄산가스가 포화되지 않은 물 / 차 / 전해액 / 물로 희석시킨 사과 주스 / 다량의 액체
tan-san-ga-seu-ga po-hwa-doe-ji a-neun mul / cha / jeon-hae-aek / mul-lo hui-seok-si-kin sa-gwa ju-seu / da-ryang-ui aek-che

RU негазированную воду / чай / солевой раствор / разведенный водой яблочный сок / обильное питьё
negazirovannuyu vodu / chai / solevoy rastvor / razvedennyi vodoy yablochnyi sok / obil'noe pit'yo

PL niegazowaną wodę / herbatę / elektrolity / sok jabłkowy / dużo płynów

AR ماء غير مكرين \ الشاي \ سوائل الیكترولایت \ عصیر تفاح مع الماء \ كمیات كبیرة من السوائل
Maa' ghayr mukarban / ash-shaay / sawaa'il electrolyte / "aseer tuffaah ma" al-maa' / kammiyaat kabiirah min as-sawaa'il

PT água sem gás/chá/electrólitos/sumo de maçã com água/grandes quantidades de líquido

FK dlo non karbonize / te / elektwolyt / ji pom ak dlo / anpil likid

EL νερό χωρίς ανθρακικό / τσάι / ηλεκτρολύτες / χυμό μήλου με νερό / μεγάλες ποσότητες υγρών
nerO horEEs anthrakeekO / tsAee / eelektrolEEtes / heemO mEElu me nerO / megAles posOteetes eegrOn

HI गैर-कार्बोनेटिड पानी / चाय / इलेक्ट्रोलाइट / पानी के साथ सेब का जूस / अधिक मात्रा में तरल
Gair-carbonated paani / chai / electrolytes / paani ke saath seb ka joos / adhik maatra mein taral

Bananas / apple sauce / cereals with cream / cooked rice / soy-based foods

ES Plátanos/puré de manzana / cereal con crema / arroz hervido / alimentos de soya (soja)

ZH 香蕉／苹果酱／麦片加奶／米饭／豆制品
xiāng jiāo / píng guǒ jiàng / mài piàn jiā nǎi / mǐ fàn / dòu zhì pǐn

FR Des bananes / de la compote de pomme / des céréales avec de la crème / du riz cuit / des aliments à base de soja

DE Bananen / Apfelmus / Getreide mit Sahne / gekochten Reis / Sojakost

VI Chuối / nước sốt táo / ngũ cốc sấy khô với kem / cơm / các loại đồ ăn làm bằng đậu nành

IT Banane / mele cotte / cereali con crema / riso cotto / alimenti a base di soia

KO 바나나 / 사과 소스 / 크림과 먹는 씨리얼 / 밥 / 간장콩으로 만든 음식
ba-na-na / sa-gwa so-seu / keu-rim-gwa meong-neun ssi-ri-eol / bap / gan-jang-kong-eu-ro man-deun eum-sik

RU Бананы / яблочное пюре / хлопья со сливками / приготовленный рис / соевые продукты
Banany / yablochnoe pyure / khlop'ya so slivkami / prigotovlennyi ris / soevye produkty

PL Banany / tarte jabłko / płatki zbożowe ze śmietaną / ugotowany ryż / potrawy na bazie soi

AR الموز \ صلصة التفاح \ الحبوب مع الكريم \ الرز المطبوخ \ مأكولات تحتوي على مادة السوي
Al-mooz / salsah at-tuffaah / al-huboub ma" al-krem / ar-ruzz al-matboukh / ma'koulaat tahtawi "ala maadah al-soy

PT Banana/compota de maçã/cereais com leite gordo/arroz cozido/alimentos à base de soja

FK Fig / sos pom / sereyal ak krem / diri ki kwit / manje a baz soja

EL Μπανάνες / λιωμένο μήλο / δημητριακά με κρέμα / μαγειρεμένο ρύζι / φαγητά από σόγια
banAnes / leeomEno mEElo / deemeetreeakA me krEma / mageeremEno rEEzee / fageetA apO sOgeea

HI केला / सेब की सॉस / क्रीम के साथ अन्न / पके हुए चावल / सोया आ ६ ारित भोजन
kela / seb ki sauce / creem ke saath anna / pake hue chaawal / soya aadhaarit bhojan

Do not allow your child to leave the house / to stay in bed

ES No permita que el niño salga de la casa / se quede en cama

CH 不要让你的孩子离开房间 / 呆在床上
bù yào ràng nǐ de hái zǐ lí kāi fáng jiān / dāi zài chuǎng shàng

FR Ne pemettez pas à votre enfant de quitter la maison / de rester au lit

DE Lassen Sie Ihr Kind nicht rausgehen / im Bett bleiben

VI Không cho con quý vị ra khỏi nhà / nằm trên giường

IT Non lasci che il bambino esca da casa / rimanga a letto

KO 아이가 집 밖으로 나가도록 / 침대에 누워 있도록 하지 마십시오
a-i-ga jip ba-kkeu-ro na-ga-do-rok / chim-dae-e nu-wo it-do-rok ha-ji ma-sip-si-o

RU Не позволяйте ребёнку уходить из дома / оставаться в постели
Ne pozvolyaite rebyonku ukhodit' iz doma / ostavat'sya v posteli

PL Proszę nie pozwolić by dziecko wychodziło z domu / leażało w łóżku

AR لا تسمح \ تسمحي لطفلك ترك البيت \ البقاء فى السرير
Laa tasmah / tasmahii li-tiflak tark al-bayt / al-baqaa' fis-sareer

PT Não deixe o(a) seu(sua) filho(a) sair de casa / ficar na cama

K Pa kite pitit soti deyo kay la / pou li rete nan kaban li

EL Μην αφήσετε το παιδί σας να βγει από το σπίτι / να μείνει στο κρεβάτι
meen afEEsete to pedEE sas na bgee apO to spEEtee / na mEEnee sto krevAtee

HI अपने बच्चे को घर न छोड़ने दें / बिस्तर में रहने दें
Apne bachche ko ghar na chhodne dein / bistar mein rahne dein

There is no helpful medication available

ES No existen medicamentos útiles

ZH 目前没有效药
mù qián méi yǒu yǒu xiào yào

FR Il n'y a aucun médicament disponible

DE Es gibt keine Medikamente, um zu helfen

VI Hiện không có loại thuốc nào có tác dụng

IT Non esiste un farmaco efficace disponibile

KO 도움이 될 약이 현재 없습니다
do-u-mi doel ya-gi hyeon-jae eop-seum-ni-da

RU Действенного лекарства нет
Deystvennogo lekarstva net

PL Nie ma skutecznego lekarstwa

AR لا يوجد دواء مساعد
Laa youjad dawaa' musaa"id

PT Não existe nenhum medicamento disponível para o tratamento

FK Pa gen okenn medikaman ki ka ede kounye la a

EL Δεν υπάρχει διαθέσιμο φάρμακο που θα βοηθούσε
den eepArhee deeathEseemo fArmako pu tha voeethUse

HI यहां कोई मददगार दवा उपलब्ध नहीं है
Yahaan koi madadgaar dawaa uplabdha nahin hain

We must wait until it heals by itself

Debemos esperar a que se cure solo

我们只有等它自己康复
wǒ mén zhǐ yǒu děng tā zì jǐ kāng fù

Nous devons attendre qu'il (elle) guérisse de lui-même (d'elle-même)

Wir müssen warten, bis es von selbst abheilt

Chúng ta phải chờ nó tự lành

Bisogna aspettare fino a quando guarisce da solo

저절로 낫기를 기다려야 합니다
jeo-jeol-lo nat-gi-reul gi-da-ryeo-ya ham-ni-da

Нам надо ждать, когда всё пройдёт само собой
Nam nado zhdat', kogda vsyo proydyot samo soboy

Musimy poczekać aż samo się wyleczy

يجب أن ننتظر حتى يُشفى بنفسه
Yajib an nantadhir hattaa yushfaa bi-nafsih

Temos que esperar até que se cure por si só

Fòk nou tan ke li geri pou kont li

Πρέπει να περιμένουμε να θεραπευτεί από μόνο του
prEpee na pereemEnume na therapeftEE apO mOno tu

हमें इसके स्वयं ठीक होने तक इंतजार करना होगा
Hamein iske swayam theek hone tak intjaar karna hoga

Arabic

Important note: Certain grammatical changes occur in Arabic depending on whether one is addressing a male or a female. You may notice that some of the transliterated words have the ending "-ak," which indicates "your." For example, "rijlak" means "your leg," where "your" is assumed to refer to a male. When addressing a female, please change/adjust the ending to "-ik," or "-ikee," or in the case of Iraqi, Bedouin, Saudi and Gulf patients, to "-itch." The proper pronunciation of this possessive suffix differs sometimes considerably from dialect to dialect, and thus all the pronunciation options have not been directly included in the text. These pronunciation and dialect differences, incidentally, are not typically indicated in the written form of the Arabic language.

Letter/Symbol	Pronunciation
"	The quotation mark is used to indicate the sound of the letter "ayn" in Arabic, which has no real equivalent in any Western language. It is basically the sound of a slight constriction of the throat, such as with the "u" in "uh" or "ugh." Do not over-emphasize the constricted sound, as this will make pronouncing the rest of the word excessively difficult.
Q	Spoken like a "k" but farther back in the throat. Note that in some Arabic dialects, especially those of Saudi Arabia and the Gulf, it sounds like the letter "g" in "go."
Dh	Like the "th" in "this" or "them" but NOT in "think" or "thing."
Th	Like the "th" in "thing."
Gh	Roughly like the French r.
Vowels	Pronounce the vowels as steadily as possible, with as little "gliding" or shifting as found in English.

Chinese

There are eight dialects in China, and though they have nearly the same grammar and word pool, the pronunciation is quite different. It is good to keep in mind that the Chinese language has several different tones. The first tone is a steady high sound, e.g. mā (as in mother). The second sound rises from mid-level tone to high, e.g. má (as in hemp). The third tone has a mid-low to low descent that rises again to the middle level, e.g. mǎ (as in horse). The fourth is a high-falling short tone, e.g. mà (as in scold). There is also a "light tone", a short, unstressed, "neutral" tone that is used for all unstressed syllables.

Symbol	Eglish Equivalent	Mandarin Example
ai	wide	lái
an	ant	yǎn
ao	loud	lǎo
a	large	pà
b	bob	bīng
c	cats	céng
ch	chat	chī
d	dig	dùn
e	fur	nè
ei	reid	wěi
en	an	bèn
f	fan	féng
g	good	gè
h	hit	hǎn
i	see	lí
ie	yeh	jiē
iu	you	liú
j	junk	jí
k	kit	kě
l	like	láng
m	mat	míng
n	note	niú

ou	bowl	kóu
o	ward	wó
p	pop	péi
q	cheat	qí
r	rat	rè
s	sit	sǎ
sh	ship	shí
t	tip	tū
u	look	lú
ui	way	cuī
uo	ward	guò
w	wait	wáng
x	sheath	xíng
y	york	yū
z	kids	zǐ
zh	judge	zhāng
ang	aunt	kàng
eng	lung	lěng
ing	wing	níng
ong	long	hong

Creole

Nasal Sounds are pronounced partially through the nose, but without the pronunciation of the letter "n". There are really no exact equivalents in the English language but may be close to some sounds.

Letters	Pronunciation	Examples
ch	as in shown	chache (to show)
e	as in day	ede (to help)
è	as in leg	mèsi (thank you)
g	always "hard" sound, i.e. "go"	gen (to have)
i	as in bee	isit (here)
j	avoid "d" in front of words starting with this letter	jou (day)
o	as in toe	zo (bone)
ò	as in paw	zòrey (ear)
ou	as in food	ou (you)
r	rolled, pronounced at the back of the throat	respire (to breath)
s	always pronounced as the letter "s" and never as a "z"	prese (in a hurry)
y	as in yes	pye (foot), zòrèy (ear)
Nasal Sounds		
an	somewhat like **aim**	dan (teeth), nan (in, into)
en	as in Chopin	pen (bread)
on	somewhat like **don't**	non (no/name)

French

People usually encounter difficulties when trying to pronounce French words because many sounds are not found in the English language. This is particularly true for the nasal sounds. Here, we try to illustrate the correct French pronunciation as closely as possible. Consonants that are not listed are very similar in pronunciation to their English counterparts.

Letter	Pronunciation	Example
Vowels		
[a]	like a in father	madame, la salle, là
[e]	similar to a in take, but closed	café, manger, regardez
[E]	like the second a in marmalade	lait, il met, il est, merci
[i]	short, like ee in meet	il, l'amie, lycée
[O]	open o like in more	la porte, Paul, alors
[o]	closed o like in go	mot, allô, aussi, eau
[ø]	sound like in her without the r	un peu, deux
[œ]	like [ø] but more open	neuf, sœur
[@]	sound between [œ] and [ø], like indefinite article "a" in English	le, melon
[u]	like oo in spoon	ou, où, bonjour
[y]	same vowel as [i], but rounded	tu, rue, salut
[~E]	nasal [E]	enfin, faim, plein, bien, un
[~O]	nasal [o]	bon, montre, il tombe
[ā]	nasal [a]	dans, je prends
Half consonants		
[j]	pronounced as y	famille, travail, pied, yeux
[w]	fleeting [u]-sound, no syllable, belongs to following vocal	oui, voilà
[H]	fleeting [y]-sound, no syllable, belongs to following vocal	cuisine, je suis, huit
Consonants		
[s]	hard s like in sit	sœur, Pascal, c'est ça
[z]	pronounced as z	maison, chaise
[S]	pronounced like sh in she	chaise, je cherche
[Z]	like s in vision	je, bonjour
[J]	like soft n in onion	cognac, il gagne

Greek

The accent is placed on the syllable with the capitalized vowel.
For example, in pOnos (πόνος = pain) the first syllable is emphasised.

Letter		Pronunciation
A	α	„a" short as in car
AY	αυ	„af" as craft
B	β	„v" as verb
ΜΠ	μπ	„b" as back
ΝΤ	ντ	„d" as dort
Γ	γ, γε, γι	„g" as gamma
Δ	δ	„ds"
E	ε	„e" short as in bet
EE	εε	„ee"long as in sleep
EY	ευ	„ef" or „if"
Z	ζ	„ts"
H	η	„i" as ideal
Θ	θ	as „th" in englisch
I	ι	„i" as with
EI, OI, YI	ει, οι, υι	„i" as with
K	κ	„k" as kappa
Λ	λ	„l" as lambda
M	μ	„m" as mouth
N	ν	„n" as no
Ξ	ξ	„x" as maximal
O	ο	long „o" as in home
OY	ου	long „u" as flute
Π	π	„p" as passion
P	ρ	„r" as red
Σ	σ, ς	„s" as sun
T	τ	„t" as tongue
Y	υ	„i" as with
Φ	φ	„pfi"
X	χ	„ch"
Ψ	ψ	„psi"
Ω	ω	„o" as omega

Italian

Italian spelling is largely phonetic, in other words, letters have the same pronunciation irrespective of the word and context in which they appear. Some exceptions to this simple rule are listed in the table below. Most Italian polysyllabic words are usually stressed on the penultimate syllable – ristorante, venire, giornale – while others are stressed on the last syllable. When the latter is the case, the last vowel is accented, for example, the grave accent (`) on the ending vowel "i" or "e" in martedì or perciò, or the acute accent (´) on the ending "e" in perché. The circumflex accent (ˆ) suggests the contraction of two letters "i".

Letter	Pronunciation	Example
a	like "a" in afternoon	accento
c, cc	before consonants and vowels a, o, u, regular, like "c" at beginning of words class or cloud	classe, banco
	before vowels e, i like in "cello, chilly"	accento, dieci
ch, cch	like the letter "k"	che, pacchi
ci, cci	before a, o, u like in "chilly"	ciao!
e	like "e" in content	che
g, gg	before consonants and before a, o, u, regular, like in "grand" before e, i like in "gentle"	grande gente
gh	like in "gills"	ghiaccio
gi, ggi	like in "gin"	mangiare
gl	like in "million"	figlio
gn	like in "cognac"	bagno
h	always silent, never spoken	ho
i	like "i" in "ski"	si
o	like "o" in "low"	nove
qu	like in "Kuala Lumpur"	acqua
r	like in „real", strong, trilled	mare
s	soft, like in "sole" or "house"	sole, sera
	between two vowels hard like in "freezer"	rosa
sc	before consonants and a, o, u like in "flask" before e, i like "sh" in "shut"	scrivere, scusi pesce, uscita
sci	before a, o, u like "sh" in "shut", ("i" is silent)	lasciare, sciopero
sp	like in "crisp"	sport
st	like in "list"	Stato
u	like "u" in true	uno
Double consonants are distinguishable:		bel-lo
Each single vowel is distinguishable in vowel combinations:		E-uropa

Korean

The Romanization of the Korean language has last been updated by the Korean Department of Culture and Tourism in the year 2000.

There is a space between each word and each syllable of a word is identified by hyphens (-). Each syllable is to be pronounced as a single sound.

Letter	Pronunciation
Consonants	
ch	china
g	good
j	joy
jj	judge
kk	kitchen
pp	Paul
s	similar to "sh" sound in English
ss	sun
tt	ten
Vowels	
a	ah
ae	bad
e	bed
eo	but
eu	peut (French)
i	beet (sometimes long, sometimes short)
o	short
oe	Sir
y	yes
u	spoon (sometimes long, sometimes short)
w	won

Polish

The Polish language consists of many sibilants and combinations of them, often within one word, and it distinguishes between hard, hardened and soft consonants. Particularities of pronunciation are given in the table below. Letters not given are pronounced like in English.

Letter	Pronunciation	Example
ą	before f, w, s, ś, sz, rz, z, ż, ź and ch like a nasal "o"; before b and p like "om"; before g and k like "Congo" or "monk"; otherwise "on"	wąż
c	like "ts" in "cats", also like German "z" in "Zeit", before i like ć	cukier
ć	sound between "c" and "cz", like "cheap"	ćma
e	like e in "spelling"	plecy
ę	before f, w, s, ś, sz, rz, z, ż, ź and ch like a nasal "e", before b and p like "em", before g and k like "length"; otherwise "en", at the end of a word generally pronounced "e"	język
g	always hard like in "gold"	nogach
h	like a hard "ch"	humor
i	like "ee" in "eel"	zanim
j	like "y" in "yes"	jakies
ł	like English "w"	łódź
n	before i „ń"	nowela
ń	like soft n in "onion"	koń
o	like o in "on", not like in "alone"	koń
ó	like "oo" in "spoon"	sól
s	before i like „ś"	bas
ś	sound between "s" and „sz", like in "she"	śnić
u	like "oo" in "spoon"	zupa
w	like English "v"	waga
y	like i in "sit"	syn
z	before i like „ź"	zupa
ż	a hard „zh" like in „garage"	żurnal
ź	sound between "z" and „ż", pronounced like soft „zh"	gruźlica
Polish letter combinations		
au	like "ow"	
ch	like a hard "ch"	dach
cz	like „tsh" in "putsch"	Czech
sz	a hard „sh"	szal
rz	a hard „zh" like in „garage"	rzecz
rz	after p, t, k and ch a soft „sh"	przerwa

Portuguese

The following pronunciation guidelines are applicable to European Portuguese. Letters not listed are pronounced like in English. Words that end in the vowels a, e, o or the consonants s, m are usually stressed on the penultimate vowel. Words that end in i, u or in consonants are stressed on the last syllable. If there is an exception to this rule, accents are placed (acute á or circumflex â). Syllables with tilde (ã) are always stressed if no other syllable has an acute or a circumflex.

Letter(s)	Pronunciation	Example
Vowels		
A	like "a" in afternoon	talha
a, á	open a	alto, árvore
e, ê	like "e" in "cafe"	medo, você
-e	as final sound like "i" in "ski" but short, almost swallowed	leite, vale
e, é	open "e" like in "content"	resto
i	like "i" in "ski"	ninho
Ô	closed "o" like in "Olga"	avô
-o	as final sound like u from "true" but shorter	santo
o, ó	in word interior or as final sound accentuated, open "o" like in "loft"	morte nó
u	like "u" in "true"	Portugal
Diphthong with:		
o or u	Sound between "u" and "w"	ao, mau
l	like English "y"	nacional
Nasal vowels		
am, an, ã	nasal "a"	campo
em, en	nasal "e"	lembrar
un, um	nasal "u"	um, untar
im, in	nasal "i"	limbo
õ, om, on	nasal "o" similar to "o" in French "on"	limões
Consonants		
ca, co, cu	like English "c"	casa

ça, ce, ci, ço, çu	soft, sharp "s" like in "grass"	cedo, maçã
ch	soft "sh" like in "shut"	cheque
ga, go	like English "g" in "goal"	gato
ge, gi	like "j" in "journal"	gelo
gua	"g" with deep "u"	água
gue, gui	like "go", the "u" is silent	guia
h	always silent, never spoken	harpa
j	like "j" in "journal"	jogo
-l	deep "l"	Portugal
lh	like "lj"	alho, filho
nh	like "ny" in "canyon"	ninho
qua, quo	sound like "k" with a deep "u"	quanto
que, qui	like the letter "k"	aquel, aqui
r, -r	similar to "r" in "interest", stronger than English "r"	coro, caro mar
rr	very strong "r", always trilled	carro
s, ss	as initial sound or in word interior like "grass"	sapo, assado
-s	as final sound like "bush"	galinhas
vowel-s-vowel	like "s" in "weasel"	raso
v	like "v" in "veil"	vento
x	like "sh" in "shut", but softer	caixa, texto
x	in word interior soft, sharp "s" like in "grass"	próximo
z, exa, exe, exi, exo, exu	like "s" in "weasel"	exame, natureza

Russian

This pronunciation guide is intended to help pronounce Russian words written by Latin letters. The suggested system for romanization of Russian is relatively intuitive for anglophones to pronounce. Although it is not a true phonetic key, it helps to suggest the necessary sounds by using the sounds of well known words so they can be then applied to pronounce the Russian words.

Letters	Transliteration keys	Examples
А а	a	a as in father
Б б	b	b as in but
В в	v	v as in van
Г г	g	g as in get
Д д	d	d as in dress
Е е	e	ye as in yesterday
Ё ё	yo	yo as in yonder
Ж ж	zh	zh as in measure or g as in beige
З з	z	z as in zoo
И и	i	ee as in meet
Й й	y	y as in toy or as in yoga
К к	k	k as in class
Л л	l	l as in love
М м	m	m as in mother
Н н	n	n as in name
О о	o	o as in bottle
П п	p	p as in paper
Р р	r	r as in error
С с	s	s as in smile
Т т	t	t as in ten
У у	u	u as in cool
Ф ф	f	f as in farm
Х х	kh	h as in loch
Ц ц	ts	ts as in its or as in tsunami
Ч ч	Ch	ch as in chess
Ш ш	sh	sh as in fish or ship
Щ щ	shch	shch as in fresh chicken or as in Spanish sherry
Ъ ъ	" (quote marks)	the "hard sign", has no sound of its own, used to separate a consonant from a following sound
Ы ы	y	i as in bill (with the tongue tip a little bit further back)
Ь ь	' (apostrophe)	the "soft sign", makes the preceding consonant soft like the first n in onion
Э э	e	e as in bet
Ю ю	yu	yu as in Yugoslavia
Я я	ya	ya as in yard

Spanish

The Spanish alphabet has 30 letters. Words ending with a vowel, n or s are stressed on the next to the last syllable, e.g. ayudar (to help)
The last syllable is stressed in words ending with consonants other than n or s, e.g. calor
Any word that follows a different stress pattern must have an accent on the vowel of the stressed syllable, e.g. corazón (heart).

Letter	Name	Pronunciation
A	a	like 'a' in afternoon
B	be	softer than English 'b'
C	ce	like 'k' in 'key' before a, o, u or consonants, before e, i like 'th' in 'then' is the pronunciation in Spain; c like 's' in 'say' in Latin America
CH	che/ce hache	like 'ch' in chest
D	de	softer than English 'd'
E	e	like 'e' in contents
F	efe	same as 'f' in English
G	ge	mostly like 'g' in 'guess' like h before e, i, but ...gui..., ...gue... is spoken as 'g' in 'guess'
H	hache	silent
I	i	like 'i' in 'ski'
J	jota	similar to the 'h' in 'hospital'
K	ka	like 'k' in 'key'
L	ele	like 'l' in 'lemon'
LL	elle/doble ele	like 'y' in 'yellow'
M	eme	same as in English
N	ene	same as in English
Ñ	eñe	like 'ny' in 'canyon'
O	o	like 'o' in 'low'
P	pe	same as in English
Q	cu	like 'k'
R	ere	similar to 'r' in 'interest', stronger than English 'r'
RR	erre	strong spanish 'r', always trilled
S	ese	like 'ss' in 'stress'i
T	te	between English 't' and 'd'
U	u	like 'u' in 'true'
V	ve/uve	like English 'b'
W	uve doble	similar to 'w' in 'word'
X	equis	like 's', 'ks'
Y	i griega	like 'y' in 'yes'
Z	zeta	like 's'; before e and i like the English 'th' in Spain like 's' in Latin America

Spanish

The Spanish alphabet has 28 letters, words ending with a vowel and ones are stressed on the last or the last syllable, pronounced as...

the last syllable is stressed on words ending with consonants other than s, r... vowel, a word which follows a different stress pattern may have an accent on the vowel of the stressed syllable pronounced here.

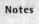

Notes

A concise clinical reference guide for medical interns and residents

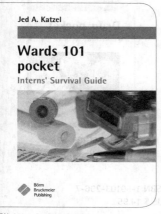

Jed A. Katzel

Wards 101 pocket
Interns' Survival Guide

Börm
Bruckmeier
Publishing

ISBN 978-1-59103-336-6
US $ 19.95

- Basics like important scales & scores, H&P, wrtiting notes & orders

- The latest management and therapeutic recommendations for conditions in over 15 specialities

- More than 200 figures and tables for quick access to all important information

- Including neurology, ID, psychiatry, geriatrics, pediatrics and many more

- Extra-information: normal values, medical formulas, common abbreviations, statistics

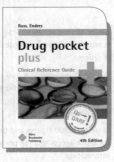
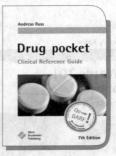
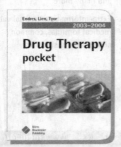

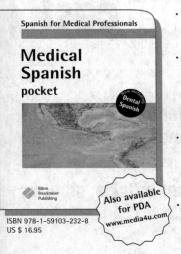

Börm Bruckmeier Publishing
PO Box 388
Ashland, OH 44805

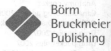

Börm
Bruckmeier
Publishing

Phone: 888-322-6657
Fax: 419-281-6883

Name		E-mail		
Address				
City		State		Zip

Subtotal

Sales Tax, add only for: CA 8%; OH 6.25% | + **Sales Tax**

Shipping & Handling for US address: | + **S&H**
UPS Standard: 10% of subtotal with a minimum of $5.00
UPS 2nd Day Air: 20% of subtotal with a minimum of $8.00

= **Total**

Credit Card: ❑ Visa ❑ Mastercard ❑ Amex ❑ Discover
Card Number

Exp. Date   Signature

For foreign orders, quantity rebate, optional shipping and payment please inquire:
service@media4u.com

Books and Pocketcards also available at ...   www.media4u.com

Börm Bruckmeier Products

	COPIES		PRICE/COPIES		PRICE
Anatomy pocket		x	US $ 16.95	=	
Canadian Drug pocket 2008		x	US $ 14.95	=	
Differential Diagnosis pocket		x	US $ 14.95	=	
Drug pocket 2007		x	US $ 12.95	=	
Drug pocket plus 2007		x	US $ 19.95	=	
Drug Therapy pocket 2006–2007		x	US $ 16.95	=	
ECG pocket		x	US $ 16.95	=	
ECG Cases pocket		x	US $ 16.95	=	
EMS pocket		x	US $ 14.95	=	
Homeopathy pocket		x	US $ 14.95	=	
Medical Abbreviations pocket		x	US $ 16.95	=	
Medical Classifications pocket		x	US $ 16.95	=	
Medical Spanish pocket		x	US $ 16.95	=	
Medical Spanish Dictionary pocket		x	US $ 16.95	=	
Medical Spanish pocket plus		x	US $ 22.95	=	
Medical Translator pocket		x	US $ 19.95	=	
Normal Values pocket		x	US $ 12.95	=	
Respiratory pocket		x	US $ 16.95	=	
Wards 101 pocket		x	US $ 19,95	=	
Alcohol Withdrawal pocketcard		x	US $ 3.95	=	
Antibiotics pocketcard 2007		x	US $ 3.95	=	
Antifungals pocketcard		x	US $ 3.95	=	
ECG pocketcard		x	US $ 3.95	=	
ECG Evaluation pocketcard		x	US $ 3.95	=	
ECG Ruler pocketcard		x	US $ 3.95	=	
ECG pocketcard Set (3)		x	US $ 9.95	=	
Echocardiography pocketcard Set (2)		x	US $ 6.95	=	
Epilepsy pocketcard Set (2)		x	US $ 6.95	=	
Geriatrics pocketcard Set (3)		x	US $ 9.95	=	
History & Physical Exam pocketcard		x	US $ 3.95	=	
Medical Abbreviations pocketcard Set (2)		x	US $ 6.95	=	
Medical Spanish pocketcard		x	US $ 3.95	=	
Medical Spanish pocketcard Set (2)		x	US $ 6.95	=	
Neurology pocketcard Set (2)		x	US $ 6.95	=	
Normal Values pocketcard		x	US $ 3.95	=	
Pediatrics pocketcard Set (3)		x	US $ 9.95	=	
Periodic Table pocketcard		x	US $ 3.95	=	
Psychiatry pocketcard Set (2)		x	US $ 6.95	=	
Vision pocketcard		x	US $ 3.95	=	

pockets

pocketcards